Global New Drug Development

Global New Drug Development

An Introduction

Jan A. Rosier
University College Dublin, Ireland

Mark A. Martens
Consultant in Pre-clinical Development and Toxicology, Belgium

Josse R. Thomas
University of Leuven, Belgium

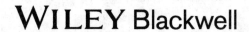

WILEY Blackwell

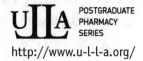

POSTGRADUATE PHARMACY SERIES

http://www.u-l-l-a.org/

Library of Congress Cataloging-in-Publication Data

Rosier, Jan A., author.
  Global new drug development : an introduction / Jan A. Rosier, Mark A. Martens, and Josse R. Thomas.
      p. ; cm.
  Includes bibliographical references and index.
  ISBN 978-1-118-41488-0 (cloth)
  I. Martens, Mark A., author. II. Thomas, Josse R., author. III. Title.
  [DNLM: 1. Drug Discovery. 2. Drug Industry–organization & administration. QV 745]
  RS420
  615.1′9–dc23

                                                                      2014013906

A catalogue record for this book is available from the British Library.

Contents

Series Foreword

ULLA postgraduate Pharmacy Series

The ULLA Pharmacy Series is an innovative series of introductory text books for postgraduate students and researchers in the pharmaceutical sciences.

This series is produced by the ULLA Consortium (European University Consortium for Pharmaceutical Sciences). The Consortium is a European academic collaboration in research and teaching of the pharmaceutical sciences that is constantly growing and expanding. The Consortium was founded in 1992 and consists of pharmacy departments from leading universities throughout Europe including:

- Faculty of Pharmacy, Uppsala University, Sweden
- School of Pharmacy, University College London, UK
- Leiden/Amsterdam Center for Drug Research, University of Leiden and Vrije Universiteit Amsterdam, The Netherlands
- Drug Research Academy, Faculty of Health and Medical Sciences, University of Copenhagen, Denmark
- Faculty of Pharmacy, Paris-Sud University, France
- Department of Pharmacy, University of Parma, Italy
- Faculty of Pharmaceutical Sciences, University of Leuven (KU Leuven), Belgium
- Faculty of Pharmacy, University of Helsinki, Finland

The editorial board for the ULLA series consists of several academics from these European Institutions who are all experts in their individual field of pharmaceutical science.

Previous titles include:

Pharmaceutical Toxicology
Paediatric Drug Handling
Molecular Biopharmaceutics

International Research in Healthcare
Facilitating Learning in Healthcare
Biomedical and Pharmaceutical Polymers
Inhalation Drug Delivery

The titles in this ground breaking series are primarily aimed at PhD students and will also have global appeal to postgraduate students undertaking masters or diploma courses, undergraduates for specific courses, and practising pharmaceutical scientists.

Further information can be found at www.ullapharmsci.org.

Preface

This book is written for students in pharmacy, veterinary and human medicine, chemistry and life sciences who have chosen to study drug development, and for any reader who would like to gain a better insight into drug development. The complete life cycle of a new drug is described in this book, with an emphasis on drug development. It should be regarded as an introduction and is intended to help students and interested readers on their way to exploration and self-tuition.

The objective of this book is neither to serve as a comprehensive textbook that describes detailed drug development methods and processes nor to offer comparative overviews of regulatory guidelines. Other books have been published that address specific aspects of drug development and discuss legislation and guidelines issued by national and international authorities in greater detail. For example, *in vitro* and *in vivo* laboratory techniques that are used during the discovery and development of new drugs are described in great detail in a number of textbooks, but their integration, relevance and interdependency into the larger context of drug development is lacking. It is the intention of this book to fill the gap between detailed descriptions of isolated drug development processes, techniques and approaches and general overviews of pharmaceutical R&D that provide no insight into the interactions between all the activities that constitute a full new drug development process.

On reading this book the reader will have gained a better understanding of the multidisciplinary character of drug development, the interaction between the different scientific disciplines involved and the terms and concepts used. He/she will have gained more confidence in accessing relevant internet websites and databases for specific guidance offered by regulatory agencies and drug development organisations. If the interested reader wants to delve deeper into specific aspects of drug development, references are given to specialised books, publications of the peer-reviewed literature and regulatory guidelines.

Although drug development is a structured process, it allows for the adaptation of the several steps to be taken due to the specific needs of the therapeutic area, the nature of the drug and its route of administration. Since the concept of the book is an introduction to drug development we chose to limit the scope to the development of small molecules with a preference for the oral route of administration. The development of large molecule drugs (e.g. monoclonal antibodies, oligonucleotides) and vaccines – also referred to as biologic(al)s or biopharmaceuticals – are not discussed because the strategies followed in their development are different from those applied in the 'traditional' approach of small molecules. The development of biologicals requires a separate book.

An introduction to drug development necessarily includes an introduction to the legislation and regulatory guidelines that govern these processes. However, it is not the ambition of this book to offer a detailed description of all relevant guidelines nor does it quote texts from these guidelines. It has been written from the viewpoint of a drug development team and the individuals who are involved in and committed to the development of a drug and takes the reader through the consecutive steps, while referring to relevant guidelines when needed. For practical reasons preference is given to guidelines issued by the International Conference on Harmonisation (ICH), the European Medicines Agency (EMA) and the US Food and Drug Administration (US FDA).

Regulatory authorities from around the world use different terms to describe processes and phases in drug development. For example, the European Union (EU) guidelines refer to a 'pre-authorisation phase' to discuss the processes that take place before the drug is granted a marketing authorisation. The US FDA uses the term 'pre-approval phase' to denote the same stage of development. In this book preference is given to the terminology used by the regulatory authorities of the region in the world where the regulatory process applies. For example, the term IND (Investigational New Drug) Application is used for a clinical trial authorisation in the USA, whereas the term Clinical Trial Application (CTA) is used for the same process in the EU. When processes are discussed that are applicable to both regions in the world preference is given to the terminology generally used by drug development teams. In very specific cases, the differences in terminology are clearly explained to avoid confusion.

Jan A. Rosier
Mark A. Martens
Josse R. Thomas

Acknowledgements

We would like to thank Arthur Van Aerschot, professor in medicinal chemistry and head of the Department of Pharmaceutical and Pharmacological Sciences at the University of Leuven (KU Leuven) who invited us to write a book on drug development as part of the ULLA series of textbooks in pharmaceutical sciences.

We are also indebted to the experts in drug research and development, regulatory sciences and pharmaceutical business who were so kind as to review parts of the book that belong to their field of expertise and offered their comments:

Bart De Spiegeleer, expert in drug quality and registration, professor at the Faculty of Pharmaceutical Sciences of Ghent University (UGent); Luc Janssens, senior director worldwide CMC regulatory affairs at Janssen R&D, Belgium; Kenny Simmen, vice-president infectious diseases discovery at Janssen R&D, Belgium; Gerben Van 't Klooster, vice-president drug development at Galapagos, Belgium; Araz Raoof, vice-president and global functional head discovery sciences at Janssen R&D, Belgium; Jan De Hoon, clinical pharmacologist, professor at the Faculty of Medicine of the University of Leuven (KU Leuven) and head of the Center for Clinical Pharmacology of the university hospitals of Leuven (UZ Leuven), Belgium; Katelijne De Nys, radiation oncologist, professor at the Faculty of Medicine of the University of Leuven (KU Leuven), head of the Clinical Trial Center of the university hospitals of Leuven (UZ Leuven) and president of the committee for reimbursement of drugs (CTG-CRM) at the National Institute for Insurance of Disease and Invalidity (RIZIV-INAMI), Belgium; Lieven Annemans, health economist, professor at the Faculty of Medicine and Health Sciences of Ghent University (UGent) and at the Faculty of Pharmacy of the Vrije Universiteit Brussel (VUB), Belgium; and Marijke Van Zieleghem, group product manager, marketing department, Servier Benelux, Belgium.

We are grateful to the reviewers who were appointed by Wiley as experts in the field of drug development for the help they provided to us in the early phases of the writing of this book: Michael Coleman, professor of toxicology at Aston University, Birmingham, UK and Louis Lazo Radulovic, adjunct professor of toxicology at the University of Michigan, USA.

We would also like to thank the students in pharmaceutical sciences of the University of Leuven (KU Leuven) who read certain parts of the book and provided feedback on the content and the clarity of the texts: Sophie Bogaert, Anne Calsius, Christel Claes, Barbara Mertens, Chloé Scheldeman and Eveline Wijckmans.

The authors wish to thank the staff of Wiley Publishers, particularly Fiona Seymour, senior project editor, who steered us through this project with great patience.

The understanding and support of our families, sometimes taken for granted, was key to the successful completion of this book. Therefore we would like to dedicate this book to our spouses, children and grandchildren.

Jan A. Rosier
Mark A. Martens
Josse R. Thomas

Abbreviations

ACE	Angiotensin-Converting Enzyme
ADME	Absorption, Distribution, Metabolism and Excretion
ADR	Adverse Drug Reaction
AE	Adverse Event
AF	Assessment factor
AIDS	Acquired Immuno-Deficiency Syndrome
ALARP	As Low As Reasonably Practicable
AMS	Accelerator Mass Spectrometry
APD	Action Potential Duration
API	Active Pharmaceutical Ingredient
ARR/RD	Absolute Risk Reduction or Risk Difference
ASMF	Active Substance Master File
AUC	Area Under the Curve (plasma concentration versus time curve of a drug)
BCOP	Bovine Corneal Opacity and Permeation (assay)
BCS	Biopharmaceutics Classification System
BIA	Budget Impact Analysis
CABG	Coronary Artery Bypass Graft (surgery)
CAM	ChorioAllantoic Membrane
CAPA	Corrective And Preventive Actions
CBA	Cost-Benefit Analysis
CDER	Center for Drug Evaluation and Research (FDA)
CEA	Cost-Effectiveness Analysis
CEP	Certificate of the European Pharmacopoeia
CER	Comparative Efficacy/Effectiveness Research
CHMP	Committee for Medicinal Products for Human use (EMA)
CI	Confidence Interval
Cl_{tot}	Total Body Clearance
CMA	Cost-Minimization Analysis
C_{max}	Maximum Plasma Concentration

CMC	Chemistry, Manufacturing, and Controls
CNS	Central Nervous System
CoG	Cost of Goods
CRA/CSM	Clinical Research Associate or Clinical Study Monitor
CRF	Case Report Form
CRO	Contract Research Organisation
CRP	C-Reactive Protein
CT	(X-ray) Computed Tomography
CTA	Clinical Trial Application or Clinical Trial Authorisation or Clinical Trial Agreement
CTD	Common Technical Document
CUA	Cost-Utility Analysis
CV	Cardiovascular
DMC/DSMB	Data Monitoring Committee or Data and Safety Monitoring Board
DMF	Drug Master File
EA	Environmental Assessment (USA)
EAD	Early After Depolarisation
EBM	Evidence-Based Medicine
EC	European Commission
EC_{50}	Concentration at which an Effect is observed in 50% of the tested population
ECG	Electrocardiogram
EEA	European Economic Area (European Union plus Norway, Iceland and Liechtenstein), sometimes described as the 'European Community' or 'Europe' or the 'European region'
EMA	European Medicines Agency
EoPh2	End of Phase 2
EP	Endpoint
EPAR	European Public Assessment Report
ERA	Environmental Risk Assessment (EU)
ETT	Exercise Tolerance Test
EU	European Union, currently 28 Member States
EudraCT	European Clinical Trials Database
EWG	Expert Working Group (ICH)
FAS	Full Analysis Set
FDA	Food and Drug Administration (USA)
FDC	Fixed-Dose Combination
FIH	First In Human clinical trial, also known as First in Man (FIM)
GCP	Good Clinical Practice(s)

GLP	Good Laboratory Practice(s)
GMP	Good Manufacturing Practice(s)
GVP	Good Phamacovigilance Practices
GxP	Generic abbreviation to describe GMP, GLP and GCP
HED	Human Equivalent Dose
HEK	Human Embryonic Kidney (cells)
hERG	Human-ether-à-go-go-gene, coding for the human potassium channel
HET-CAM	Hen's Egg Test on the ChorioAllantoic Membrane
HIV	Human Immunodeficiency Virus
HPLC	High-Performance (Pressure) Liquid Chromatography
HTA	Health Technology Assessment
IB	Investigator's Brochure
IC_{50}	Concentration at which 50% Inhibition is observed
ICER	Incremental Cost-Effectiveness Ratio
ICF	Informed Consent Form
ICH	International Conference on Harmonisation (of technical requirements for registration of pharmaceuticals for human use)
IEC/IRB	Independent Ethics Committee (EU and other countries), Institutional Review Board (USA)
IL-4	Interleukin-4, cytokine that targets B-cells, T-cells, macrophages and mast cells
IMP	Investigational Medicinal Product
IMPD	Investigational Medicinal Product Dossier
IND	Investigational New Drug
IR	Infrared (spectroscopy)
ISO	International Organisation for Standardization
ITT	Intention To Treat (analysis)
IWG	Implementation Working Group (ICH)
K_{oc}	Soil Adsorption Coefficient (corrected for Organic Carbon content)
LC-MS/MS	(High-Pressure) Liquid Chromatography coupled to tandem Mass Spectrometry
LC_{50}	Concentration at which Lethality is observed in 50% of the tested population
LLNA	Local Lymph Node Assay (skin sensitisation test in the mouse)
Log P_{ow}	Logarithm of the Partition coefficient octanol/water (also referred to as log K_{ow})
LSC	Liquid Scintillation Counting
MA	Marketing Authorisation

MAA	MA Application
MABEL	Minimal Anticipated Biological Effects Level
MACE	Major Adverse Cardiac/Cardiovascular Events
MAD	Multiple Ascending Dose
MAH	MA Holder
MALDI-MS	Matrix-Assisted Laser Desorption/Ionisation Mass Spectrometry
MEEC	Maximum Expected Environmental Concentration (USA)
MRSD	Maximum Recommended Safe starting Dose
MRI	Magnetic Resonance Imaging
MS	Mass Spectrometry
MS/MS	Tandem Mass Spectrometry
MTD	Maximum Tolerated Dose
NADPH	Nicotinamide Adenine Dinucleotide Phosphate (reduced)
NCE	NormoChromatic Erythrocytes
NDA	New Drug Application
NMR	Nuclear Magnetic Resonance
NNH	Number Needed to Harm
NNT	Number Needed to Treat
NOAEL	No-Observed-Adverse-Effect Level
NOEC	No-Observed-Effect-Concentration
NPV	Net Present Value
OECD	Organisation for Economic Co-operation and Development
OPM	Operating Manual
P-gp	P-glycoprotein (transporter protein)
PAI	Pre-Approval Inspection
PAMPA	Parallel Artificial Membrane Permeation/Permeability Assay
PASS	Post-Authorisation Safety Study
PBPK	Physiologically Based PharmacoKinetic (modelling)
PBRER	Periodic Benefit-Risk Evaluation Report
PCE	PolyChromatic Erythrocytes
PCI	Percutaneous Coronary Intervention
PDCO	Paediatric Committee (EMA)
PEC	Predicted Environmental Concentration (EU)
PET	Positron Emission Tomography
PFC	Plaque Forming Cell (assay)
PI	Prescribing Information (Equivalent in the USA and other countries of the SmPC in Europe)
PIP	Paediatric Investigation Plan
pKa	Acid/Base Constant
PK/PD	Pharmacokinetics/Pharmacodynamics (relationship)
PMS	Post-Marketing Surveillance
PNEC	Predicted No-Effect Concentration (EU)

PP	Per-Protocol (analysis)
PRAC	Pharmacovigilance Risk Assessment Committee (EMA)
PSUR	Periodic Safety Update Report
PV	PharmacoVigilance
QA	Quality Assurance
QALY	Quality-Adjusted Life-Year
QbD	Quality by Design
QC	Quality Control
QMS	Quality Management System
QRM	Quality Risk Management
QT (interval)	Time between the start of the Q wave and the end of the T wave on the ECG
QTc	QT interval corrected for heart rate
RCT	Randomised Controlled Trial
REA	Relative Effectiveness Assessment
REMS	Risk Evaluation and Mitigation Strategies
RH	Relative Humidity
RLG	Radioluminography
RMP	Risk Management Plan
ROS	Reactive Oxygen Species
RR	Relative Risk
OR	Odds Ratio
HR	Hazard Ratio
S9	Supernatant of induced liver homogenate centrifuged at 9000g
S9-mix	S9 fraction with NADPH generating system
SAD	Single Ascending Dose
SEDDS	Self-Emulsifying Drug Delivery Systems
SIMS	Secondary Ion Mass Spectrometry
SmPC	Summary of Product Characteristics (EU)
SOP	Standard Operating Procedure
SPECT	Single-Photon Emission Computed Tomography
SWOT	Strengths, Weaknesses, Opportunities and Threats (analysis)
$t\frac{1}{2}$	(Plasma) elimination half-life
T_3	Triiodothyronine
T_4	Thyroxine
TdP	Torsade(s) de Pointes
TFT	TriFluoroThymidine
t_{max}	Time at which the maximum (plasma) concentration is reached
TNF	Tumour Necrosis Factor
TQT	Thorough QT (study)
TSH	Thyroid Stimulating Hormone

TTC	Threshold of Toxicological Concern
UDP-GT	Uridine diphospho-glucuronyl transferase
UDS	Unscheduled DNA Synthesis
USP	US Pharmacopoeia
UV	UltraViolet (spectroscopy)
V_d	Volume of Distribution
WBA	Whole Body Autoradiography

Introduction

The objective of this book is to introduce students and interested individuals to the principles of the development of small drug molecules, and to an overview of all the steps and processes that are required to bring a new drug from discovery to the marketplace. To allow the reader to become gradually more familiar with drug development the structure of the book is organised in the following 8 chapters:

Chapter 1 introduces the concept of the drug life cycle and offers the reader the context in which a drug is discovered, developed, marketed and leaves the market. The drivers for the search for a new drug, the structure of the drug life cycle, the costs and risks of drug research and development (R&D), the value of a drug for patients and society and the managerial aspects of drug R&D are presented and discussed.

Chapter 2 offers an introduction to drug discovery and design and describes phenotypic- and target-based approaches as well as the different steps of drug discovery from the identification of a disease target up to the transfer of the lead drug molecule to development. This chapter has been deliberately kept short since the emphasis of this book is on drug development and there are many other textbooks that describe the approaches followed in drug discovery in greater detail.

Chapter 3 is meant to set the scene for a more detailed description of drug development in later chapters and concentrates on general aspects of drug development such as drug development organisation and teams, the scientific disciplines involved in drug development (i.e. chemical/pharmaceutical, non clinical and clinical; also referred to in this book as drug development streams) and their interactions, phases in drug development, regulatory environment, quality management, risk management and ethics.

Chapter 4 provides more detail on the methods and techniques used in drug development, because they are often referred to in the specific chapters describing early and late drug development. The sections of this chapter are organised according to the three drug development streams.

After addressing the drug life cycle in Chapter 1, drug discovery in Chapter 2, the context in which a new drug is developed in Chapter 3, and the methods and techniques in Chapter 4, the reader is assumed to have a background that is sufficient to understand the complex activities and processes associated with the detailed description of new drug development in the following chapters.

Chapter 5 describes early drug development leading to 'proof-of-concept', i.e. the first proof that the drug candidate is safe and displays a pharmacological activity in man. This chapter is divided into the two main steps of early development: pre-clinical development leading to the first clinical trial in man, and clinical development leading to the first proof of pharmacological activity in patients.

Chapter 6 addresses late drug development and is subdivided into the phase that precedes marketing authorisation, the marketing authorisation process and the phase of drug development after marketing authorisation or the post-approval phase.

Chapters 5 and 6 are organised according to the contributions made by the three drug development streams. The integration of data from chemical/ pharmaceutical, non clinical and clinical development is discussed at each critical time point in drug development where important decisions have to be made on the further course of the development programme.

Chapter 7 is dedicated to special types of drug development such as orphan drugs, paediatric drugs, geriatric drugs and fixed-dose drug combinations.

Finally, Chapter 8 briefly focusses on the most important aspects of drug commercialisation, the last phase of the drug life cycle.

Each chapter in this book has its own set of tables, figures and references.

The book closes with an Epilogue that discusses some of the challenges of the traditional approach to new drug development and summarises a number of alternatives that seem to be gaining momentum.

1
Drug Life Cycle

1.1 Introduction

A drug life cycle is a succession of activities that starts with a research project in which new drug molecules are either discovered in nature or (semi-)synthesised or designed *de novo* in medicinal chemistry laboratories and ends when the drug is removed from the market. The process of drug discovery and design is characterised by intense intellectual creativity and biological and molecular exploration, by trial and error approaches and by frequent and recurring data collection and interpretation. Its course is largely dependent on the approaches taken by individual scientists. Once a molecule with promising characteristics is identified, it is developed into a drug product during a process known as 'drug development'. The objective of drug development is to bring safe and effective drugs to the patient. Drug development is a highly structured process that is conducted in a stepwise fashion that is also referred to as a 'stage gate process' or a 'phased review process' whereby chemical, pharmaceutical, nonclinical and clinical information is gathered, critically reviewed and assessed before a new phase of development can proceed. While the discovery of a new drug molecule is characterised by a high degree of freedom, the process of drug development is highly structured. This is due to regulations imposed upon the process by health authorities such as the US Food and Drug Administration (US FDA) and the European Medicines Agency (EMA). Every step of the process is carefully timed and linked to the previous step and the next step. It is a process that is well planned and controlled. Drug development is complex and it is characterised by failures, reiterations and reassessments of scientific data and by intensive interaction among different scientific disciplines. It is not a matter of pharmacology or medicine alone but it also involves chemical engineering, process chemistry,

Global New Drug Development: An Introduction, First Edition.
Jan A. Rosier, Mark A. Martens and Josse R. Thomas.
© 2014 John Wiley & Sons, Ltd. Published 2014 by John Wiley & Sons, Ltd.

manufacturing plant management, biostatistics, drug-delivery sciences, bio-pharmacy, materials sciences, physical chemistry, medicinal chemistry, and supply management all working together in harmony with disciplines such as pharmacology, clinical research, clinical data management, bioinformatics, bio-analytical chemistry, pharmacokinetics, toxicology and other scientific disciplines in the life sciences. On top of the challenge of making these different disciplines work together, there is the continuous uncertainty as to whether the drug candidate, at the end of a drug development process of about 6-10 years, will be demonstrated to be effective and safe in the targeted patient population. This means that the development of a new drug is a process of high risk, takes many years, requires a talented group of scientists, engineers and clinicians, consumes considerable human and financial resources and requires strong management to be successful. At the end of a development project when all scientific and medical data have become available, the quality, safety and efficacy are critically reviewed by the health authorities. The new drug will only be approved when they are convinced that the drug complies with the criteria of quality, safety and efficacy, and has a positive benefit–risk balance. As a result, the drug development organisation will receive a marketing authorisation and is allowed to put the drug on the market.

The new drug may remain on the marketplace for a considerable amount of time and new research can be initiated to show that the drug can be used for other therapeutic indications, be administered via other routes of administration or combined with other drugs. A drug, however, has a limited 'lifetime' on the market and at one point in time the decision can be taken to withdraw it from the market. Such a decision may be based on the entry of new and better drugs on the marketplace or expiry of the patent life with competition from less-expensive generic drugs as a result. Alternatively, a drug may be withdrawn from the market because it has been shown to have unacceptable side effects. This process of post-approval activities is the last and major step in the process of a drug life cycle.

1.2   Drivers of the search for a new drug

Before embarking on the search for a new drug, the R&D organisation, which can be a private company or a non-for-profit organisation, has to decide whether it is worthwhile to engage in an expensive and risky drug R&D project. According to Hill & Rang [1], the following criteria are to be considered before such a decision is taken:

I.   Strategic considerations that address the question whether the R&D organisation should embark on the drug R&D project at all (should it be done?).

II.   Scientific and technical considerations that address the question whether the project is technically feasible (can it be done?).
III. Operational considerations that address the question whether the project – if feasible – can be conducted within the boundaries of the organisation. In other words, whether the organisation has the required organisational, infrastructural, human and financial resources (can we do it?).

1.2.1 Strategic criteria

By far the most important selection criterion is whether the new drug – if developed – will meet an unmet medical need. An area of unmet medical need is a therapeutic area in which there is an absence or lack of safe and effective drugs and where the introduction of a new drug can offer benefit to patients. Strategic considerations require a thorough analysis of the epidemiology of the disease, its current pharmacotherapy and projected pharmacotherapy at the time when the new drug will be available, i.e. after approx. 7 to 12 years. The gap between what is achievable and what is desirable is analysed and a decision is made whether it is worthwhile to fill this gap. It can be large (e.g. there is no good drug available nor in development at this moment) or it can be small (e.g. there is a need for a better pharmaceutical dosage form that reduces the side effects or leads to more comfort for the patient than the current drug on the market). Unmet medical need is one of the factors affecting the future market potential of a new drug, i.e. whether the project can generate return on investment (ROI), but there are many others, to name a few: predictions of disease prevalence and incidence, acute versus chronic diseases, market share of competitors, drug regulatory hurdles, drug reimbursement policy, future patent cliffs, etc. Other strategic factors are related to the company or organisation wishing to search for the new drug, e.g. the therapeutic areas and markets a company is well established in, the focus on small molecules versus biotech products, the current and future state of the drug pipeline, the willingness to play in the blockbuster league or to focus on niches, the financial health of the company, etc.

1.2.2 Scientific and technical criteria

A drug development project should be technically feasible. It is important to consider whether the drug development 'idea' can be transformed into a scientific hypothesis that can be tested in a clinical environment. For example, although the development of drugs for AIDS prevention may be worthwhile, the translation of a scientific hypothesis ('drug X will prevent the occurrence of AIDS in a specific group of individuals') into a development plan may be very challenging if not impossible to complete because of the recruitment of volunteers for the clinical trial, the time it may take to (dis)prove the hypothesis and the ethical impact of the clinical exploration. Alternatively, the availability of a technological platform for the development of a complex dosage form such as an implant, may drive the decision to proceed. The feasibility of a project can also be hampered by projected difficulties, especially during clinical development, safety evaluation or pharmaceutical formulation research. Drugs against chronic diseases may require a much larger investment in long and expensive clinical trials than drugs to treat acute diseases. On the one hand, drugs that are developed to treat 'lifestyle diseases' such as diabetes type 2 and obesity should be very safe to use and require a considerable safety investigation before market authorisation is granted. On the other hand, drugs to treat life-threatening diseases such as cancer may show side effects that non-cancer patients would and should not tolerate. Developing a new drug can be worthwhile when a competitive advantage can be expected. This is certainly true for a 'first-in-class' drug (the innovator drug in a new therapeutic class), but also for a 'fast-follower' drug (the 2nd or 3rd one in a new class, but better than the innovator) and a 'best-in-class' drug (aiming to be the best one). These are very ambitious R&D programmes that require considerable investments when compared with the investment required for 'me too' ('I can do as well') or 'me better' ('I can do somewhat better') drugs that are easier to develop. However, 'me too' or 'me better' drugs can sometimes successfully complement a well-balanced innovative drug portfolio. Another important scientific factor is the potential to protect the intellectual property of the new drug by means of a patent, giving the owner the exclusive right to commercialise the drug for a given period of time (usually 20 years from the date of filing) which can be extended under certain conditions. The period that the drug is protected by a patent once on the marketplace is short because R&D takes a considerable amount of time. This period is important for the pharmaceutical industry to allow a return on R&D investment before generic (or biosimilars in case of biotech drugs) enter the market once the patent expires.

1.2.3   Operational criteria

A key operational criterion for the choice of a drug development project is the comparison of the required resources with the available resources. This includes the availability of staff and expertise, as well as facilities, equipment, materials and capital. Not every activity in drug R&D has to take place within the drug R&D organisation, but every activity that is outsourced has to be financed. The timescale for a complete drug R&D cycle is another important factor. Some drugs can be developed in a – relatively – short period of time such as drugs to treat acute infections, or can even be 'fast tracked' when the medical need is high, while other drugs may require many years to develop such as drugs against osteoporosis. Longer development times increase the cost and reduce the time for patent protection during commercialisation. If a company finds ways to develop drugs faster than its competitors, this 'time crunching' capacity can be an important driver for the development of a new drug.

The decision to start the search for a new drug will depend on the careful consideration of all the criteria mentioned above. The overall analysis is usually performed by operational people taking into account the strengths and weaknesses of the new drug and the drug development organisation versus the opportunities and threats in the environment and the marketplace (SWOT analysis) to name the simplest approach.

1.3 Structure of a drug life cycle

The life cycle of a drug involves four consecutive phases: drug discovery and design, drug development, regulatory review and approval, and commercialisation and marketing.

Drug discovery and design consists of an exploration phase, an assay development phase, a screening phase, a hit-to-lead phase and a lead optimisation phase. There are many sources of new drug molecules: natural sources such as micro-organisms, plants or animals or libraries of drug molecules that either have failed or have been used for other therapeutic areas. These molecules can be structurally modified and be subjected to pharmacological screening tests. Drug molecules can be modified to improve their pharmacological activity and bioavailability and to reduce toxicity before they are ready for transfer to drug development. This is described in more detail in Chapter 2. A drug molecule that is selected for development is referred to in this book as a 'drug candidate'.

Drug development can be subdivided into two major phases: early development and late development. Early development has a pre-clinical and a clinical phase whereas late development has a pre-approval and a post-approval phase. During early development the drug candidate is carefully studied with the objective to prove that its properties can justify its introduction into a late development programme. An essential principle of early development is the 'Proof-of-Concept', which means that it can be proven that the molecule does what it is purported to do in a small group of patients under well-controlled conditions. The objective of the late development part of a drug development project is to confirm that the claims of the therapeutic use in a small group of patients can be justified in large clinical trials with a large number of patients suffering from the disease the molecule is intended to treat. A candidate drug that has transferred from early development to late development is referred to in this book as a 'drug under development'.

When the final results of drug development show that the drug under development is safe and effective and can be manufactured at a high level of quality, all the data are collected, integrated and submitted to the health authorities in order to obtain authorisation for marketing. The regulatory approval process takes a considerable amount of time because the authorities responsible for granting marketing authorisation need time to carefully assess the therapeutic value and the safety of the new drug.

Once market authorisation is granted on the basis of a positive benefit–risk balance, the drug can be introduced ('launched') into the market. From this point in time pharmaceutical marketing further drives the life cycle of the drug. It takes approximately 7-12 years from the identification of a drug target in the human body to the introduction of a new drug into the market. While on the market, efforts in drug development continue to refine the manufacturing process, to improve pharmaceutical formulations and to explore new routes of administration or new therapeutic indications. During the market life of a new drug its use is continuously monitored to detect side effects to improve its safe use in clinical practice. At the end of the drug life cycle the drug can be withdrawn from the market place for various reasons. It can either be because of safety reasons, expiry of patent life or because of replacement by a superior drug of the same class. An overview of the drug life cycle is given in Figure 1.1.

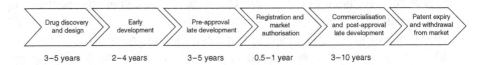

Drug discovery and design	Early development	Pre-approval late development	Registration and market authorisation	Commercialisation and post-approval late development	Patent expiry and withdrawal from market
3–5 years	2–4 years	3–5 years	0.5–1 year	3–10 years	

Figure 1.1   The drug life cycle.

1.4   Costs and risks of drug research and development

1.4.1   Cost drivers

The cost of drug R&D is considerable and is primarily driven by clinical (approx. 60% of total cost) and chemical and pharmaceutical R&D (approx. 30% of total cost). Another cost driver is the large number of studies in experimental animals required to demonstrate the nonclinical safety and efficacy of the drug. In addition, the synthesis of a new drug can be a complex undertaking that requires important investments in manufacturing plant infrastructure, equipment, chemicals and pharmaceutical drug-delivery technologies.

1.4.2 Estimates of drug development costs

It is generally accepted that the cost of a drug development project ranges from 800 million USD to approximately 1 billion USD [2, 3, 4, 5]. These figures are frequently mentioned in the literature and the lay press but have been subject to criticism because scholars observed that drug development costs are highly variable or unknown [6, 7]. For example, tax savings are not taken into account, clinical trial costs are inflated and development times are exaggerated. Alternative calculations led to drug development cost predictions ranging between 180 and 231 million USD. Still others have projected drug development costs to range between 500 million USD and more than 2 billion USD [3]. However, it is a fact that the investment required to discover and develop a new drug is substantial and involves considerable risk since it is only known at the end of late drug development whether the drug is or is not effective and safe in patients and can be put on the market.

1.5 Risks of drug R&D

There are two kinds of risk in drug R&D: therapeutic area/portfolio risk and project risk.

Therapeutic area/portfolio risk is associated with the choice of the therapeutic area in which a drug R&D organisation intends to develop new drugs. When a drug company makes the strategic decision to move into a new therapeutic area there is always the risk that no molecules can be discovered and/or designed that have a promising therapeutic activity or that even an interesting active molecule cannot be developed into a new medicinal product. Project risk is related to a given drug R&D project. This is discussed in more detail in Chapter 3.

1.5.1 Failure and success rates in drug development

The failure rate of new drug candidates to make it through the development process is called attrition. An attrition of x% means that x% of the projects has been terminated during a given phase in drug development or in drug development as a whole. High attrition means that the number of drug candidates that are introduced into the drug pipeline substantially drops during the different development phases. Zero attrition – a theoretical concept – means that all drug candidates that enter the development pipeline make it to an approved drug and are launched in the market. Attrition rates are important to management since it is an indicator of the productivity and efficiency of the drug R&D organisation. The average success rate for all therapeutic areas is approximately 11% [8]. Success rates differ according to the therapeutic area and range from 5% for oncology drugs to 20% for cardiovascular drugs. Even if a drug candidate eventually makes it through development, it is still not certain whether the application for market authorisation will be approved by the regulatory authorities. The failure rate during regulatory review by the authorities is 25%. In the case of oncology products the failure rate is as high as 30% [8]. This high failure rate may impact the potential survival of a drug company since at this stage all financial resources have been consumed and costs incurred. For small companies that have invested all their resources in a single drug, a refusal for market authorisation may result in the death of the company. The failure to bring one drug on the market can be absorbed by R&D firms with a large and diverse product portfolio but many consecutive failures may have dramatic consequences.

Although attrition is generally referred to as the failure rate for a drug development portfolio in one or more therapeutic areas, it can also be used to determine the failure rate for each phase of the drug development process. In other words, it can be determined for each transition of a drug candidate from early to late development or from marketing authorisation to approval. Approximately 60% of all the drug candidates that are tested for the first time in man (Phase 1 clinical trials) are approved for testing in exploratory pharmacology trials in patients (Phase 2 clinical trials) and approximately 20% are admitted to confirmatory pharmacology trials (Phase 3 clinical trials). Only about 10% of all drug candidates that are admitted to testing in humans make it to the marketplace. The most important reasons for attrition are efficacy, toxicity and commercial [8]. If one were able to increase the probability of technical success by decreasing attrition either for the total project or for each phase of development, productivity would increase accordingly. A detailed discussion on the possible approaches that can be used to increase R&D productivity of new drugs is beyond the scope of this book but can be found in several scholarly papers and books that address this topic [9–17].

1.5.2   Net present value

A portfolio is a collection of drug products in R&D and on the marketplace. Defining which drug development project and therapeutic areas will constitute a portfolio is a difficult task and is associated with a risk that is referred to as 'portfolio risk'. It is a strategic decision that is taken by top R&D management. For example, the decision to switch from a cardiovascular-based R&D portfolio to an ophthalmology-based R&D portfolio involves a myriad of separate decisions that involve experts from basic research, medicinal chemistry, market analysis, finance, drug development and regulatory affairs. One of the most straightforward methods to value a project is to estimate the financial benefits from it and subtract the costs to give a net value. This rather simple deduction can be sophisticated by bringing in the time-related value of money as income today is worth more than income next year and early expenditure is more costly than later expenditure. This leads to a figure called the Net Present Value (NPV) that evaluates the financial impact of a new drug R&D project and is helpful in taking strategic decisions [18]. It goes beyond the scope of this book to enter into a detailed discussion of the value of NPV but suffice it to state that projects with a negative NPV should be abandoned, while projects with a positive NPV may be considered for inclusion in the portfolio. Although the NPV calculation allows the assessment of a project on a purely financial basis, it is not, and should not be, the final answer to the question of project selection. What is required more than the financial expertise needed to perform NPV calculations is the intimate knowledge of the medical need that drives the development of a new drug. It is therefore not surprising that some drugs with a low NPV were developed and became drugs that generated considerable income for the company and benefit for the patients. The success of a new drug is therefore not always driven by financial parameters alone.

1.6   Value for patient and society

The selection of a drug development project should not only be based on NPV and shareholder return. More importantly, there should also be a return to society at large. Gradually, drug R&D companies realise that their long-term future will not only be driven by financial success but also by the realisation that they should contribute to society and provide answers to medical needs. Some major organisations have started the development of drugs for small markets with high medical need realising that the financial returns would hardly compensate the investments made. Although there are only a few of these projects it shows that the trend for contributing to society and to patients is steadily – albeit slowly – finding its place next to shareholder value contribution. Alternative approaches have been introduced such as the Health Impact Fund [17].

1.7   The end of a drug's life

Most withdrawal decisions are either driven by a substantial drop in sales or safety concerns. For example, drugs such as cisapride, grepafloxacin and terfenadine were removed from the market because of cardiovascular side effects and bromfenac and troglitazone because of hepatotoxicity. They have been on the market for only a relatively short period of time. Other drugs are removed from the market for reasons of competition because more innovative and better drugs reached the market and make the use of the original drug obsolete. Alternatively, when the end of its patent life is reached, the original drug is pushed out of the market by 'generic' drugs. Generic drugs are copies of the original drugs developed by the R&D drug industry and can be introduced in the market after it is shown that they are bioequivalent with the original drug.

1.8 Management

The development of a new drug requires a sound scientific strategy, clear planning, careful financial control, flawless execution and a correct decision-making process. Above all, it requires scientists, engineers and clinicians who are not only experts in their field, but who are also capable of understanding the other scientific disciplines sufficiently well to appreciate their impact on their own field and the fields of others involved in the project. Because of the high failure rate in new drug development they should also have a strong personal conviction about the added value of their work and the contribution they may bring to patients and society. This means that the development of a new drug is not only time consuming and expensive but also requires strong management and leadership in order to reach development milestones on time, to control budgets, to evaluate investments and to manage human resources.

In general, this process is led by a portfolio team that manages the drug portfolio of a company, while project teams manage the process of discovery and development. A portfolio team operates at the level of top management and addresses strategic questions regarding the drugs to be developed or which therapeutic area to be targeted. Once the decision is taken to start the discovery and development of a new drug in a specific therapeutic area, a project team is established that conducts the discovery project with the objective to identify a new molecule from which a new medicinal product can be developed. The drug discovery process is discussed in more detail in Chapter 2.

References

[1] Hill RG, Rang HP. (2013) Drug discovery and development. *Technology in transition*, 2nd edn, Churchill Livingstone/Elsevier, Edinburgh.
[2] Dimasi JA, Hansen RW, Grabowski HG. (2003) The price of innovation: new estimates of drug development costs, *Journal of Health Economics* **22**, 151–185.
[3] Adams CP, Van Branter V. (2006) Estimating the cost of new drug development: Is it really $802 million? *Health Affairs* **25**, 420–428.
[4] Anonymous. (2003) New estimates of drug development costs (Editorial). *Journal of Health Economics* **22**, 325–330.
[5] Anonymous. (2003) Costing drug development (Editorial). *Nature Reviews Drug Discovery* **2**, 247.
[6] Light DW, Warburton R. (2011) Demythologizing the high cost of pharmaceutical research, *Biosocieties* 1–17.

[7] Angell M. (2005) *The truth about drug companies: How they deceive us and what to do about it.* Random House, New York.

[8] Kola I, Landis J. (2004) Can the pharmaceutical industry reduce attrition rates? *Nature Reviews Drug Discovery* **4**, 711–715.

[9] Kola I. (2008) The state of innovation in drug development. *Clinical Pharmacotherapeutics & Therapy* **83**, 227–230.

[10] Booth B, Zemmil R. (2004) Prospects for productivity. *Nature Reviews Drug Discovery* **3**, 451–456.

[11] Garnier J. (2008) Rebuilding the R&D engine in big Pharma. *Harvard Business Review* **86**, 68–76.

[12] Paul SM, Mytelka DS, Dunwiddle *et al.* (2010) How to improve R&D productivity: the pharmaceutical industry's grand challenge. *Nature Reviews Drug Discovery* **9**, 203–214.

[13] Scanell JW, Blanckley A, Boldon H *et al.* (2012) Diagnosing the decline in pharmaceutical R&D efficiency. *Nature Reviews Drug Discovery* **11**, 191–200.

[14] Sams-Dodd F. (2005) Target-based drug discovery: is something wrong? *Drug Discovery Today: Targets* **10**, 139–147.

[15] Pandey M. (2003) Investment decisions in pharmaceutical R&D projects. *Drug Discovery Today* **8**, 968–971.

[16] Pritchard JF, Jurima-Romet M, Reimer MLJ *et al.* (2003) Making better drugs: decision-gates in non-clinical drug development. *Nature Reviews Drug Discovery* **2**, 542–552.

[17] Pogge T. (2010) The Health Impact Fund: Better Pharmaceutical Innovations at Much Lower Prices. In: Pogge T, Rimmer M, Rubenstein K (eds.) *Incentives for Global Health: Patent Law and Access to Essential Medicines*, Cambridge University Press, Cambridge.

[18] Goffin K and Mitchell R. (2010) *Innovation Management Strategy and Implementation using the Pentathlone Framework*, Palgrave Macmillan, New York.

2
Drug Discovery and Design

2.1   Introduction

The objective of drug discovery is to identify pharmacologically active molecules for which there are clear indications that they will reach the pharmacological target in the body in sufficient amounts such that they can exert their desired effect without producing toxicity. In drug discovery, molecules with pharmacological activity are selected from a set of existing molecules. They may be of microbiological, plant or animal origin or part of existing molecule libraries. Molecular drug design, however, creates totally new molecules that are designed to optimally fit pharmacological target macro-molecules. In this chapter some insight is offered into the drug discovery process. Drug discovery is a flexible process, as opposed to drug development, which operates in a highly regulated environment. The way in which drug discovery is conducted largely depends on the type of the drug molecules studied (e.g. small molecules, polypeptides, oligonucleotides), the under-standing of the disease biology, the screening technology applied, the route of administration and the therapeutic area. Therefore, drug discovery strategies can differ substantially among drug R&D organisations.

There are many ways to discover new drugs but the most important strate-gies that are followed are phenotypic-based or target-based approaches, and molecular drug design. A target can be a single gene, a gene product (protein) or a molecular mechanism that has been identified on the basis of genetic analysis or biological observation. In this chapter, the major drug discovery approaches are discussed first, followed by the description of the phases of a drug discovery process that is target based. The strategy explained below refers to the discovery of small molecules only and does not cover biophar-maceuticals and vaccines.

Global New Drug Development: An Introduction, First Edition.
Jan A. Rosier, Mark A. Martens and Josse R. Thomas.
© 2014 John Wiley & Sons, Ltd. Published 2014 by John Wiley & Sons, Ltd.

2.2   Approaches in drug discovery

2.2.1   Phenotypic based

The phenotypic-based approach investigates the effect of the drug molecule on disease phenotypes that are induced in cells, multicellular systems, tissues and whole organisms [1]. Phenotypic screening allows for the identification of drug molecules that modify disease phenotypes by action on one unknown target or by simultaneous action on several unknown targets. The subsequent determination of the relevant targets of drug molecules identified by phenotypic screening can be tedious, slow and sometimes even impossible. The advantage of a phenotypic approach is that drug molecules can be selected on the basis of their effect on the outcome of a disease process as a whole without being limited to one single target. This is certainly the case for the discovery of first-in-class drugs against diseases of which the biology is poorly understood. The disadvantage of the approach is that molecular design strategies that are based on singular protein targets cannot be applied to optimise the activity and reduce the toxicity of the drug molecule.

Phenotypic screening was frequently applied in the 1970s to 1990s. In the beginning of the 1980s, advances in molecular biology and protein chemistry led to the gradual replacement of the phenotypic screens by target-based screens by most drug R&D organisations. Recently, however, there is again a growing interest in phenotypic screening since this is a way of moving beyond well-defined targets from the literature to discover new therapeutic targets and new disease biology.

2.2.2   Target based

The target-based approach uses the concept of the interaction between the drug molecule and a well-defined macromolecular target [2]. When a molecule is found to bind to a well-defined target that is known to be functional in pathways that lead to disease, the identified molecule may potentially be developed into a drug to treat the disease. To be able to select a target that plays an essential role in the disease process, first the biology of the disease should be understood. This constitutes a major challenge in drug discovery. In many instances disease targets have initially been identified as a result of phenotypic screening. There are two types of targets: those that are well characterised and have been known for decades and are called "established" targets and those that have been recently discovered as a result of the Human Genome Project. A target-based approach assumes that the target is the correct site of interaction by the drug in order to exert its desired therapeutic effect. The tertiary structure of protein targets is characterised by the presence of external and internal spaces or "pockets" that are lined by amino acid residue groups (e.g., carboxyl-, amino-, hydroxyl-, aromatic-, alkyl-moieties) that can bind non-covalently small drug molecules. These bonds can be hydrogen bridges, Van der Waals forces, ion bonds or bonding based on lipophilic and aromatic affinity. As a result of this binding the normal function of the protein target is modified or inhibited, which may lead to a (favourable) biological response. Examples of such hypothesised links between target and disease are the leptin receptor in obesity [3], the low-density lipoprotein receptor in atherosclerosis [4], complement receptors in inflammation [5] and interleukin-4 in allergic diseases [6]. When a disease status can be linked to the (mal)function of such a target, the interaction of a drug molecule with this target can normalise or abolish its function with the regression or the cure of the disease as a result.

The target-based approach in drug discovery received a lot of attention because the concept could be introduced into high-throughput systems whereby the output of potentially active drug molecules could be increased substantially. However, one should realise that there still remains a very poor understanding of the biological and pharmacological impact of any given target [7]. There is an increasing concern that this approach in drug discovery has not reached the level of success that was expected. Bioactive molecules may bind strongly to a specific target *in vitro*, but at the level of the cell, tissue or the whole organism they may also impact on other biological pathways that cannot be observed in single target-based discovery programmes. A full assessment of the activity of a drug on a disease process is only possible in disease animal models (e.g. knock-out and transgenic mice) and ultimately in the clinic. Unexpected adverse effects such as secondary pharmacology (off-target) effects or toxicity may be produced and will only be detected in later phases of drug discovery or drug development [8]. Some authors argue that the general application of a target-based approach is one of the reasons why drug R&D output has declined over the past few decades [8, 9].

2.2.3 Molecular drug design

As a result of the interaction (e.g. noncovalent binding) of a drug molecule with a macromolecule that plays an essential role in the disease process, the normal function of the macromolecule can be modified or inhibited. In most instances this macromolecule is a protein (e.g. co-factor, nuclear receptor, enzyme, transporter peptide, ion gate) and it often takes several years before it can be isolated and purified and its complete 3D structure elucidated.

Molecules that have been selected by a target-based approach can be used to identify the location and nature of the molecular space they occupy in the protein by means of crystallisation of the ligand-protein complex and subsequent X-ray crystallography. The detailed knowledge of the 3D dimensions and the immediate molecular environment of the "pocket" with its binding sites allows for the modification of the molecular structure of the originally selected drug molecule by increasing the number of bonds with the target and by decreasing their distance. This is done by molecular modelling using computer graphics. Once the critical molecular characteristics of the drug molecule are known to optimally bind to the target also the limitations are known for further structural modifications of the molecule to enhance its bioavailability and to reduce its toxicity. The detailed knowledge of the binding spot in the target also allows for the design of a totally new molecular structure that optimally interacts with the target. The pharmacological activity of re-designed molecules or totally new molecules should be verified *in vitro* (e.g. enzyme-based or cell-based systems) and in experimental animal disease systems (e.g. knock-out and transgenic mice). Such new drug molecules can then be further explored for their physicochemical, pharmacokinetic, metabolic and toxicological characteristics. The role of bioinformatics is very important in molecular drug design to capture the knowledge obtained and to apply it to the design of other drug molecules

An example of a ligand-protein complex is given in Figure 2.1.

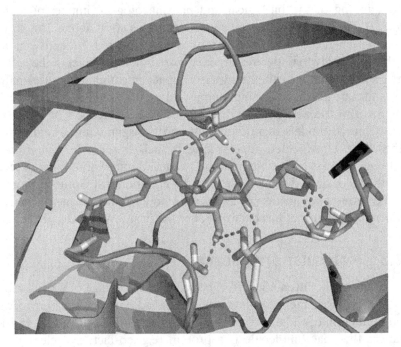

Figure 2.1   Protein-ligand interaction of darunavir in wildtype HIV protease (Source: Janssen R&D, with kind permission).

2.3   The drug discovery process

The discovery process that is described below is the target-based approach for small molecules. In general, the following phases constitute the drug discovery process: exploratory, assay development, screening, hit-to-lead, and lead optimisation [10]. This is a continuous, iterative process and ultimately leads to the selection of a drug candidate for early development. The interface

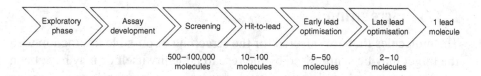

Figure 2.2   The different steps in the drug discovery process.

between drug discovery and early drug development is referred to as 'late lead optimisation'. During this phase, experts from both drug discovery and drug development interact frequently. A schematic overview of the drug discovery process is given in Figure 2.2.

2.3.1   Exploratory phase

During the exploratory phase of the drug discovery process, a review of the literature on the underlying mechanisms of the disease of interest is conducted and collaborations are initiated with academic institutions and private organisations to explore and 'validate' the molecular targets and/or endpoints that are linked to the disease process. The validation of a target is an important step in the process of target-based drug discovery. It is conducted to prove that the target is responsible for or is involved in the development of the disease. There are different ways to demonstrate this relationship and use can be made of anti-sense oligonucleotides or knock-out and transgenic animals. Sometimes animal models are used that are specific for certain disease states. For example, zebrafish have been shown to be of particular interest because of the similarity between disease-related genes in this fish species and man. This model has been used in the discovery of drugs exerting an effect on angiogenesis, inflammation or insulin regulation. The validity of a specific target as a contributing factor in a disease process increases with the number of relevant animal models in which the target modification results in phenotypic changes of the disease. The highest level of validation of a target can only be obtained from clinical research whereby the interaction with a target leads to an improvement of the disease symptoms.

2.3.2   Assay development

Once a new disease-related target is identified, a bioassay is developed to measure the change of the biological activity (e.g. enzyme activity, displacement of receptor binding) of the target in the presence of drug molecules. The assay needs to be specific for the target under study, sufficiently sensitive and reproducible and adapted for use in high-throughput automated systems. Once the assay is validated in a small-scale preliminary testing phase it can be applied at large scale for the screening of drug molecules in high-throughput systems. These high-capacity screening systems are actually robots that are capable of conducting and reading the assay at high speed for thousands of molecules.

2.3.3   Screening

The molecules that are selected for the screening of possible interaction with the target may be synthesised by the research facility itself or may have been purchased from other pharmaceutical companies or companies specialised in collections of pharmacologically active molecules. Initially, preference may be given to compounds belonging to the same therapeutic area and for which there is already some indication of safety. High-throughput screening (HTS) allows for the screening of hundreds of thousands of molecules in a relatively short period of time. When molecules are identified that show interaction with the target of a kind that they would produce a favourable therapeutic response, they are called "hits". Based on the molecular structure of the "hits" common structural characteristics may be identified that are responsible for the interaction with the target. These structural entities are called "pharmacophores" and are used for molecular modification to enhance the potency and the specificity of the interaction with the target. Medicinal chemistry plays a crucial role in optimising the structural characteristics of the selected drug molecules. This can be done by combinatorial chemistry where a vast number of molecular structures can be synthesised rapidly. The pharmacological activity of the "hits" should then be confirmed *in vitro* (e.g. in enzyme- or cell-based systems).

2.3.4   Hit-to-lead

Based on the structural and physicochemical characteristics of the molecules that have been selected from the high-throughput screening process, new molecules are synthesised with the objective to increase the interaction with the target. During this phase of optimisation, the physico-chemical, pharmacokinetic, drug metabolism and toxic properties are investigated of those molecules that have been found to show high interaction potency with the target. Physicochemical tests may, for example, include tests for aqueous and lipid solubility. At this stage of drug discovery, the selected drug molecules are subject to *in vitro* tests to assess the cytotoxicity, genotoxicity, protein binding, binding to potassium channels, microsomal metabolic stability, membrane permeability, and interaction with intestinal transporter proteins. For the detection of possible genotoxicity a simplified gene mutation assay is conducted such as the Ames screen. The binding to potassium channels *in vitro* provides some information on the possible interference of the drug molecule with the functioning of potassium channels in the cell membrane of cardiomyocytes that are essential for the re-polarisation of the heart muscle. Any blockage of this system may produce a prolongation of the QT interval of the electrocardiogram that may lead to cardiac arrhythmias. To ensure sufficient systemic exposure of the target it is important to select drug molecules that only undergo limited metabolism. This is measured by incubation with liver microsomes from various animal species and man. Membrane permeability is measured in the parallel artificial membrane permeation assay (PAMPA) where the permeation of drug molecules through an artificial membrane is assessed under different conditions. An assay that is more reliable for the *in vitro* assessment of gastro-intestinal absorption is the Caco-2 permeability assay. The advantage of this assay is that it consists of a two-compartment system separated by a human colon tumour cell culture (Caco-2 cells) which has the histological characteristics of an intestinal epithelium with microvilli and tight junctions and that expresses the transporter protein P-glycoprotein (P-gp). More details on *in vitro* absorption tests are given in Chapter 4.

If a molecule is shown to have an unfavourable property (e.g. too high plasma protein binding, mutagenic, cytotoxic), it is either discarded from the drug discovery process or further modified to eliminate the problem. This iterative process leads to a series of molecules with a high potency of inter-action with the target, acceptable bioavailability, low toxicity and metabolic stability. Less importance is attached to a low aqueous solubility or to the binding to potassium channels. Low aqueous solubility can be dealt with later in drug discovery or early drug development using appropriate drug delivery technologies. It is estimated that approximately 70% of the current drugs in R&D pipelines exhibit no or very poor aqueous solubility. Since there is only a limited relationship between binding of the drug molecule to potassium channels and the inhibition of the delayed rectifier potassium current in the ventricular muscle of the heart, more functional tests are performed later in drug discovery and drug development.

2.3.5 Lead optimisation

Lead optimisation is the last phase in drug discovery before the drug molecule is transferred to early development. In the first part of this phase, a limited number of the best possible drug candidates is selected from the lead molecules that were identified in the previous phase.

2.3.5.1 Early lead optimisation

So far, the drug molecules have been selected on the basis of *in vitro* test systems. In this phase of drug discovery more advanced *in vivo* screening systems are introduced to refine the selection process. To assess the bioavailability and the safety of lead molecules, *in vivo* pharmacokinetic and single dose toxicity assays are performed in one or more animal species using a limited number of animals. In addition to the potassium channel binding test, a more functional test i.e. the hERG patch clamp test is conducted to gain a precise idea of the possible interference of the lead molecule with the re-polarisation of the heart muscle (Section 4.3.2.1). Also, further exploration of genotoxicity is done using mammalian cells instead of bacterial systems and by expanding the number of endpoints (e.g. DNA repair, chromosome damage). If the outcome of any of these additional tests is unfavourable in view of the efficacy and/or safety profile of the lead molecule it will be eliminated from the selection process or considered for molecular re-design. In this selection process, the number of lead molecules (e.g. 10) can be reduced to a few best possible candidates for transfer to late lead optimisation.

2.3.5.2   Late lead optimisation

During late lead optimisation a drug molecule is selected to enter early development. This is done by expanding the results that have been obtained on pharmacological activity, pharmacokinetics, metabolism and toxicity. Efficacy can further be refined by using more appropriate *in vivo* animal test systems involving several experimental animal species including transgenic models. Bioavailability and toxicity can further be explored by *in vitro* screening using cultures with cells originating from organs/tissues that have been found to show toxicity in preliminary *in vivo* toxicity tests. Often advanced technologies are employed such as high-content screening where the interaction of the lead molecule with various markers of cellular toxicity is detected simultaneously. Also, a second, more appropriate, animal species can be considered to further explore toxicity (e.g., dog, monkey). The insight in microsomal metabolism can be refined by comparing *in vitro* metabolism amongst several species and the identification of the various cytochrome P450 enzymes involved in the metabolism of the selected molecules. The use of several animal species to further characterise efficacy, bioavailability and safety allows for a first attempt of allometric scaling to foresee the possible kinetic behaviour and tissue distribution or the production of toxic effects of the lead molecule in humans. Allometric scaling studies the relationship between certain pharmacokinetic or toxicological parameters in animal species of different sizes. This technique is used to predict certain characteristics of the drug candidate in man by extrapolating animal data to man based on body surface rather than on body weight and in particular on systemic exposure and pharmacokinetics. In the event of a doubtful result in the mutagenicity screen additional tests may be needed to assess the relevance of the result to man. In such cases more advanced genotoxicity testing may include *in vitro* chromosome aberration tests and *in vivo* tests with gene mutation, DNA damage, aneuploidy or chromosome damage endpoints. When some effect has been observed in the functional potassium channel (hERG) assay, additional cardiovascular safety testing may be required before making a final selection. In the case of lead molecules that are designed to be given by ocular, dermal, rectal, vaginal, respiratory or parenteral routes of administration specific local tolerance tests have to be conducted. A first screening is normally done with *in vitro* testing systems such as the bovine corneal opacity and permeability test (BCOP) and the hen chorio-allantoic membrane test (HET-CAM). Both tests are membrane based and provide the first indications of possible irritation of mucous membranes and the eye (Section 4.3.3.3). The molecules that are found to be without any effect *in vitro* can be further progressed in the discovery process. However, in the case of parenteral administration (intravenous, subcutaneous or intramuscular) additional *in vivo* tests are required to ensure safety since there exists only a poor relationship between *in vitro* outcomes and *in vivo* tolerability for parenteral applications. These types of tests (e.g., intramuscular injection in rabbits with histopathological evaluation of the site of injection) can also be conducted in this phase of drug discovery as in early development. Lead molecules, even when they exhibit a very favourable pharmacological activity, are not continued if they show parenteral intolerance unless the problem can be solved with pharmaceutical formulation technology.

The data collected thus far and those available from similar molecules are carefully assessed by a team that is composed of drug discovery and early development experts before a final selection is made. All the relevant data produced during drug discovery, their interpretation and the conclusion to proceed with drug development with the selected lead molecule are described in a document that is sometimes is referred to as the 'monograph'. This monograph serves as a basis for the early development team to build the nonclinical testing strategy necessary to progress the drug candidate to clinical testing.

References

[1] Cho YS, Kwon HJ. (2012) Identification and validation of bioactive small molecule target through phenotypic screening. *Bioorganic & Medicinal Chemistry* **20**, 1922–1928.

[2] Drew J. (2000) Drug discovery: a historical perspective. *Science* **287**, 1960–1964.

[3] Haffner SM, Mykkanen LA, Gonzalez CC *et al.* (1998) Leptin concentrations do not predict weight gain: the Mexico City Diabetes Weight Study. *International Journal of Obesity and Related Metabolic Disorders* **22**, 659–699.

[4] Hussain MM, Strickland DK, Bakillah A. (1999) The mammalian low-density lipoprotein receptor family. *Annual Review of Nutrition* **19**, 141–172.

[5] Sakiniene B, Heyman B, Tarkowski A. (1999) Interaction with complement receptor 1 (CD35) leads to amelioration of sepsis-triggered mortality but aggravation of arthritis during Staphylococcus aureus infection. *Scandinavian Journal of Immunology* **3**, 250–255.

[6] Chouchane A, Sfar I, Bousaffara R *et al.* (1999) A Repeat Polymorphism in Interleukin-4 Gene is highly Associated with Specific Clinical Phenotypes of Asthma. *International Archives of Allergy and Immunology* **120**, 50–55.

[7] Prinz F, Schlange T, Asadullah K. (2011) Believe it or not: how much can we rely on published data on potential targets? *Nature Reviews Drug Discovery* **10**, 712–713.

[8] Sams-Dodd F. (2005) Target-based drug discovery: is something wrong? *Drug Discovery Today* **10**, 139–147.

[9] Smith C. (2003) Hitting the target. *Nature* **422**, 341–347.

[10] Goodnow RA. (2006) Hit and lead identification: Integrated technology-based approaches. *Drug Discovery Today: Technologies* **3**, 367–375.

3

Drug Development: General Aspects

3.1 Introduction

Before the methods and processes of early and late drug development are discussed in Chapters 4, 5 and 6, it is necessary to become familiar with the terms and concepts that are crucial to the understanding of global new drug development. The aspects of drug development that are addressed in this chapter are the objectives of drug development, the organisations and teams, the scientific disciplines that contribute to drug development, i.e. the drug development streams and their interaction, the different phases in drug development, the regulatory environment, quality and risk management, ethics, and the global nature of drug development.

3.2 The objective of drug development

The objective of drug development is to make new drugs available to patients. To be able to do so the new drug has to comply with criteria of acceptance imposed by national and international health authorities. These criteria are drug quality, drug safety and drug efficacy and refer, respectively, to the purity and stability, the minimal toxicity and good tolerance and the capability of the drug to cure the disease or reduce its symptoms. More specifically, drug efficacy refers to the ability of a new drug to do 'more good than harm' when administered to patients in a well-defined, homogeneous target population. During the many years that it takes to develop a drug, numerous scientific data are generated, collected and reported in documents in what are called 'regulatory dossiers'. These 'regulatory dossiers' are documents that contain

Global New Drug Development: An Introduction, First Edition.
Jan A. Rosier, Mark A. Martens and Josse R. Thomas.
© 2014 John Wiley & Sons, Ltd. Published 2014 by John Wiley & Sons, Ltd.

the scientific data collected during drug development and are used to obtain approval from the national health authorities to conduct a clinical trial with humans or to market the drug, i.e. to 'register' it as a new medicine. The data needed for registration have to be produced in compliance with 'regulatory guidelines' that have been issued by regulatory authorities such as the US Food and Drug Administration (FDA) and the European Medicines Agency (EMA). For example, when a pharmaceutical scientist wants to study the stability of a new drug, he/she will need to conduct stability studies. The conditions under which these tests are performed (e.g. temperature, humidity, number of batches, sampling points) are prescribed by guidelines. These guidelines make it possible for the regulators to apply the same criteria to all drugs and to compare the results obtained during the development of different drugs. Once all the data required for the registration of a new drug have been collected, the dossier is submitted to the responsible health authorities and reviewed by scientific experts. When they are convinced that the requirements of quality, safety and efficacy are met, the drug can be approved and a marketing authorisation can be granted.

3.3   Drug development organisations and teams

The development of a new drug can be conducted by different types of drug development organisations. They can either be private companies, non-for-profit organisations or private foundations. Examples of private non-for-profit organisations are the European Organisation for the Research and Treatment of Cancer (EORTC, www. eortc.be), the Drugs for Neglected Diseases initiative (DNDi, www.dndi.org), One World Health (www.oneworldhealth.org) and the Global Alliance for Tuberculosis (TB) Drug Development (www.tballiance.org).

New drugs are developed by drug development teams supported by functional departments such as clinical operations, pharmaceutical development or toxicology. Drug development teams are often extended with academic and industrial consultants and key opinion leaders who contribute to the decision-making process. The teams may ask contract research organisations or academic research units to conduct parts of the drug development activities. For example, a team may decide to outsource the manufacturing of a new drug to a third party. It should be stressed, however, that the financial, legal and regulatory responsibility and accountability remain with the drug development organisation that is referred to as the 'sponsor' of the development of a new drug. The sponsor makes available the infrastructure (offices, laboratories, manufacturing and pilot plants) and the necessary resources (financial and human) to the drug development teams and acts as the partner with whom regulatory authorities communicate. It is not only the collaboration between the drug development organisation and its contributing partners and service providers that drives the development of a new drug, health authorities also play an important role in guiding drug development organisations during their development efforts.

Because of the multidisciplinary nature of a drug development project it is impossible for a single individual to be knowledgeable about all the contributing scientific disciplines in drug development that range from chemical engineering to clinical practice. A close collaboration among the members of a global drug development team overcomes this problem. Such a team is led by a '(global) drug development team leader' who is an experienced manager and reports to higher management. The team is composed of experts who are responsible for a specific drug development area. They represent every function that is required for the development of a drug. This representation may change during development. For example, in early development the focus is on introducing the drug candidate into man for the first time and on proving that it has a therapeutic activity in patients, whereas in late development more emphasis is laid on the commercial aspects of the drug. In general, the main functions in the team are represented by experts in:

- chemical and pharmaceutical development;
- nonclinical development;
- clinical development;
- regulatory affairs;
- finance;
- marketing;
- project management.

Each of these experts is a leader of a functional team that is in charge of the execution of the decisions taken at the level of the drug development team. Each functional team (e.g. chemical and pharmaceutical development) is composed of scientists who contribute to a specific part, (e.g. pharmaceutical development, analytical development, chemical production, chemical pilot-plant production, supply-chain management, stability investigations, packaging, and materials science). For example, the development of an appropriate dosage form such as a tablet, is led by an experienced plant manager or pharmaceutical drug delivery expert who has the required interpersonal and technical skills to do the job.

The structure of the drug development team and its relationship with the functional teams is illustrated in Figure 3.1. The composition of a team may change during development and Figure 3.2 shows a change in functional representation in the team when a drug candidate transfers from the early

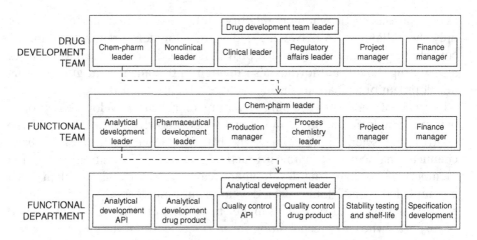

Figure 3.1 Drug development team and functional teams. API: active pharmaceutical ingredient.

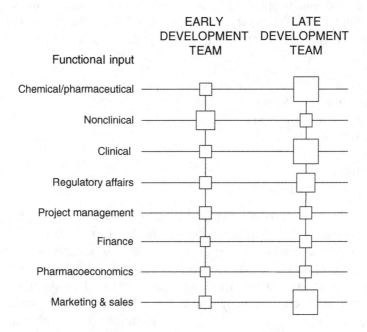

Figure 3.2 Functional input in early and late development teams.

phases of development to the later phases. The size of the squares indicates their relative contribution in the team. For example, the contribution of clinical development increases substantially upon transferring a drug candidate from early development into late development when the major clinical trials take place.

3.4   Drug development streams

The development of a new drug is a complex process. Mainly, three sets of scientific disciplines contribute to drug development: chemical and pharmaceutical development, nonclinical development and clinical development. These disciplines represent the core of the drug development team and are also referred to in this book as drug development streams. Beside the three development streams, other areas of expertise are essential in drug development such as regulatory affairs, quality management, process management, project management, clinical trial management and data management. In the end, the drug development team has to provide an answer to three pivotal questions:

- Is it possible to manufacture a high-quality active ingredient and drug product (e.g. a dosage form such as a tablet or intravenous infusion)?
- Is the drug sufficiently bioavailable and safe to be administered to healthy human volunteers and patients?
- Is the drug efficacious and safe in patients?

These questions are addressed by the chemical/pharmaceutical, nonclinical and clinical team members, respectively. Questions like "can we make the drug?", "is it safe?" and "is it efficacious?", are continuously in the minds of the team members. Examples of other questions that are addressed are the cost of production of the active ingredient and the drug product (cost of goods, CoG), pill size, pill burden, interactions with other drugs that may reduce its efficacy or increase its toxicity and the regulatory strategy that will be followed. Many drug development organisations do not conduct all these activities within their organisational boundaries but outsource them because they don't always have the expertise or human resources to conduct the myriad of studies that are required to develop a new drug. An overview of the drug development streams with their contributing functions is given in Table 3.1.

3.4.1   Chemical and pharmaceutical development

The products of chemical and pharmaceutical development are the active pharmaceutical ingredient (API) – referred to as the 'active ingredient' – and the medicinal drug product, known as the 'drug product'. The active ingredient is the pharmacologically active drug molecule, whereas the drug product is the pharmaceutical formulation that is a mixture of the active ingredient and formulating aids, i.e. excipients. The components of a pharmaceutical formulation are introduced into an appropriate dosage form such as an oral capsule. Drug products can be liquid (e.g. syrup, eye drops, nasal spray, injectable) or solid (e.g. tablet, capsule, ovule) dosage forms or can take any

Table 3.1 Drug development streams and contributing functions.

Drug development streams	Scientific discipline
Chemical and pharmaceutical development	Synthetic chemistry
	Analytical chemistry
	Stability research
	Pharmaceutical production development
	Physical chemistry
	Formulation technology and drug delivery
	Process chemistry
	Chemical engineering
	Statistics
Nonclinical development	Nonclinical pharmacology (not in the scope of this book)
	Pharmacokinetics
	Metabolism
	Toxicology
	Safety pharmacology
	Bioanalytical chemistry
	Biostatistics
Clinical development	Translational research
	Clinical medicine
	Clinical pharmacology
	Clinical toxicology
	Clinical pharmacokinetics
	Biostatistics
	Bioanalytical chemistry
	Pharmacotherapeutics
	Pharmacovigilance
	Pharmaco-epidemiology
	Pharmaco-economics

form that is deemed necessary to treat the disease (e.g. implants). In this book, the active ingredient and its formulation are referred to as the 'drug candidate' in the early phases of development and as the 'drug under development' in late development. It is referred to as a 'drug' or a 'medicine' when it is granted a marketing authorisation by the health authorities. The chemical and pharmaceutical development of a new drug focuses on the development of a production process for the active ingredient and the drug product, the development of quality specifications for both and the investigation of their stability. This is made possible through the contributions of highly integrated technical disciplines. A close collaboration between chemical development, pharmaceutical development, analytical development and manufacturing is essential to assure efficient progress during development. The scientific and technical activities that are necessary to ensure the development of a stable drug product of high quality include:

- The development and validation of a chemical production process that leads to an active ingredient of high quality. This requires expertise from synthetic, analytical and process chemistry.
- The development and validation of a pharmaceutical production process that leads to a drug product of high quality. This requires expertise from analytical chemistry, pharmaceutical production development, formulation technology and drug delivery.
- The development and validation of analytical methods for the quality control (QC) of the active ingredient and the drug product, requiring expertise from analytical chemistry, physical chemistry and quality control.
- The development of quality specifications for the active ingredient and the drug product, the investigation of the stability profile and the determination of the shelf life of the active ingredient and the drug product that requires expertise from analytical chemistry and quality control.

These development activities are also referred to as 'chemistry, manufacturing and control' or 'CMC' activities or are sometimes abbreviated as 'chem-pharm' development. Because the primary objective of chemical and pharmaceutical development is the production of a medicine of high quality, the section in the registration dossier that will be submitted for approval of a drug in the EU is referred to as the 'quality' section. In the USA, this section is known as the 'CMC' section and contains a similar data package as in the EU. The guidelines describing the chemical and pharmaceutical development and production of a new drug are discussed in the section on the regulatory environment in this chapter.

The amount of active ingredient available at the start of development is small (milligram to gram range) and is synthesised at a small scale in the medicinal chemistry laboratory. The chemical synthesis process used in discovery and early development is modified by means of process chemistry and chemical engineering techniques to gradually increase the production volume and to improve the yield and the quality of the active ingredient. Attention is also paid to the health and safety of the operators and the impact of the production process on the environment. During the development of a full-scale and cost-effective chemical and pharmaceutical production process, intellectual property (IP) issues may arise and have to be addressed. For example, if a specific chemical or pharmaceutical production process step needs to be introduced in the manufacturing of the active ingredient or the drug product, in-licensing of chemical or pharmaceutical process know-how has to be considered.

At a certain point in time during the development of the new drug, a formal transition of chemical manufacturing know-how from the chemical development department to the chemical production plant takes place. This is a crucial moment in the chemical development of a new drug and in some cases – depending on the nature of the drug and its potential commercial success – the construction of a new chemical plant is considered. This is a costly and risky enterprise since at the time of such an investment there is still no definite clinical proof that the drug is efficacious and safe. The modification of a chemical production process during scaling up may result in a change in the impurity profile of the active ingredient which may have an impact on the safety of the drug. When this change involves a new impurity or a change in the concentration of existing impurities, a risk assessment is carried out that is called "impurity qualification". Impurity qualifications may require additional toxicology testing to show that the safety of the active ingredient has remained unchanged. This is addressed in more detail in Chapter 5.

The objective of pharmaceutical development is to develop a drug product that is of high quality and assures an acceptable bioavailability of the active ingredient, sufficient to exert its therapeutic effect. Therefore, suitable formulation technologies and drug-delivery approaches are selected and introduced in the development and production processes. During the previous decades, an increasing number of poorly aqueous soluble and/or poorly permeable active ingredients have found their way into development pipelines due to the application of new drug-delivery technologies. The drug product should enable high patient compliance (e.g. acceptable pill size, limited pill burden) and acceptable pill recognition (e.g. colour, size). It should be stable for a sufficiently long time period under acceptable storage conditions and it should be manufactured using reproducible and stable processes. Analytical development plays a pivotal role in the chemical and pharmaceutical development of a new drug and is responsible for the:

- development of quality specifications for the active ingredient and the drug product;
- development and validation of analytical methods for both;
- quality control of the active ingredient and the drug product;
- assessment of the stability of the active ingredient and the drug product; and the
- proposal of retest dates/shelf lives for the active ingredient and the drug product.

Analytical development is discussed in more detail in Chapter 4.

3.4.2 Nonclinical development

Nonclinical drug development includes the sciences that address the efficacy, safety and pharmacokinetics of a drug candidate in animals and laboratory settings, as opposed to clinical drug development that studies these drug characteristics in humans (healthy volunteers or patients).

In drug development, nonclinical development is often referred to as pre-clinical development.

In this book preference is given to the term "nonclinical development" since pre-clinical development is limited to the phase of early drug development preceding the First-in-Human (FIH) clinical trial. Nonclinical development is involved in the development of a drug from late discovery to post-marketing and includes nonclinical pharmacokinetics, safety pharmacology and toxicology. In the context of this book, nonclinical pharmacology is not included in nonclinical development since the methods used and testing strategies followed are very specific to each therapeutic area and drug target and are addressed in more detail in other textbooks. Besides, the most important impact of nonclinical pharmacology on drug R&D is in the discovery phase where the drug molecules with the highest pharmacological potential have to be selected. The experience gained with nonclinical pharmacology in discovery is transferred to clinical pharmacology once the drug has been found to be safe enough to be tested in humans. Pharmacokinetics is the study of the absorption, distribution, metabolism and excretion of a drug. This is also often referred to as ADME, which is the acronym of the above-mentioned components of pharmacokinetics. The term toxicokinetics is often used when blood or plasma concentrations of the drug molecule or its metabolites are studied as a function of time in toxicology studies. Metabolism is the study of the enzymatic and non-enzymatic transformation of the drug by various organs/tissues and is an important factor in the elimination of the drug molecule from the body. In safety pharmacology the effects of the drug on vital physiological functions are studied (e.g. cardiovascular, respiratory, central nervous system functions). Toxicology refers to the study of adverse effects of drug molecules *in vitro* and in experimental animal models.

The objectives of nonclinical development in the development of a drug are:

–   selection of drug molecules in late discovery (lead optimisation phase) for release of the drug candidate to early development;
–   safety and bioavailability assessment of drug candidates for the first-in-man study;
–   safety and bioavailability assessment of drug candidates for longer-term treatment, inclusion of women of child-bearing age and children in clinical trials, combination with other drugs, introduction of new pharmaceutical formulations and routes of administration;

- assessment of the carcinogenicity potential of drugs in development;
- elucidation of mechanisms of toxic action and the assessment of their relevance to man;
- toxicology and genotoxicology qualification of drug impurities;
- safety assessment of intermediates in drug manufacturing for occupational health and safety;
- safety assessment of formulation excipients; and
- elucidation of mechanisms of toxic action in translational drug research.

The scientific and functional disciplines that contribute to the nonclinical development stream are:

- Bioanalytical chemistry that develops and validates new methods of analysis for the determination of the drug and its metabolites in body fluids and tissues. The results of this activity enable the pharmacokinetic analysis of drugs and help in the interpretation of toxicology studies.
- *In vitro* metabolism of drugs that investigates the enzymes involved in drug metabolism, differences of metabolism between species and drug–drug interactions.
- *In vivo* pharmacokinetics that investigates the kinetic behaviour of drugs and their metabolites in different animal species.
- Formulation technology to produce preparations of the drug molecule with the highest possible bioavailability for early toxicology testing.
- Toxicology in experimental animal models, comprising short- and long-term studies, genotoxicology, reproductive toxicology and long-term carcinogenicity studies.
- Safety pharmacology, comprising *in vitro* and *in vivo* cardiovascular safety studies, respiratory function studies, neurobehavioural studies and studies on gastro-intestinal function.
- Biostatistics for the interpretation of safety pharmacology and toxicity studies.
- Laboratory data management for the collection and integration of data produced in safety pharmacology and toxicology studies.
- Quality management for the application of good laboratory practices in toxicology studies and quality control of data recording and reporting.
- Nonclinical writing and document management for the reporting and integration of laboratory data for registration dossiers.

Since it is not always possible for a drug development organisation to have all these competences available, parts of nonclinical development are outsourced to contract research organisations (CRO) for large toxicology studies and/or to academic institutions when very specific mechanistic investigations have to be carried out.

3.4.3 Clinical development

The clinical development stream is considered to be the most complex part of the drug development process. It also absorbs considerable financial and human resources.

The objectives of the clinical development of a drug candidate are to:

– study its pharmacological and pharmacokinetic characteristics in healthy volunteers and patients;
– determine the dose range and dosing regimen needed to demonstrate therapeutic efficacy and safety in the targeted patient population;
– study drug-drug and drug-food interactions;
– demonstrate a positive benefit/risk ratio in patients, with a competitive advantage over existing treatment options;
– determine its optimal conditions of use in clinical practice;
– explore new indications, formulations and drug combinations.

The core activity in clinical drug development is the clinical trial, i.e. an experiment that involves human subjects, either healthy volunteers or patients, investigating the effects of the drug under study. Guideline E8 'General considerations for clinical trials', issued in 1997 by ICH (International Conference on Harmonisation, see Section 3.6.2.3), introduced the classification of clinical trials with drugs into 4 main categories according to their objectives: human pharmacology trials, therapeutic exploratory trials, therapeutic confirmatory trials and therapeutic use trials [1]. An overview of the different types of clinical trials arranged according to their objectives is given in Table 3.2.

A rational clinical drug development plan starts with human pharmacology trials and then moves to the exploratory, confirmatory, and therapeutic use trials. Therefore, human pharmacology and therapeutic exploratory studies are typically performed in early clinical drug development. Therapeutic confirmatory and therapeutic use trials are carried out in late clinical drug development. However, this serial approach does not impose a fixed order of studies, as for some drugs this may not be appropriate. Moreover, emerging results from an ongoing study may prompt a change in the development strategy or identify the need for additional studies from a previous category. For example, some specific human pharmacology trials, such as a QT interval study, are generally performed during late clinical development.

The scientific and functional disciplines that contribute to the clinical development stream are:

– clinical research that includes the clinical development strategy, the risk assessment of each study, the scientific input into the study protocols, the oversight and coordination of ongoing clinical trials and the interpretation of the results (all in collaboration with the investigators);

Table 3.2   Overview of types of clinical trials according to objectives.

Type of Study	Objective of Study	Study Examples
Human Pharmacology	– Assess tolerance – Define/describe PK and PD – Explore drug metabolism and drug–drug interactions – Estimate activity – Bio-equivalence – Explore other routes of administration	– Dose–tolerance studies – Single and multiple dose PK and/or PD studies – Drug–drug interaction studies – Comparative PK of drug formulations – Single and multiple dose PK with other route of administration (e.g. subcutaneous)
Therapeutic Exploratory	– Explore use for the targeted indication – Estimate dosage for subsequent studies – Provide basis for confirmatory study design, endpoints, methodologies	– Earliest trials of relatively short duration in well-defined narrow patient populations, using surrogate or pharmacological endpoints or clinical measures – Dose–response exploration studies
Therapeutic Confirmatory	– Demonstrate/confirm efficacy – Establish safety profile – Provide an adequate basis for assessing the benefit–risk relationship to support licensing – Establish dose–response relationship	– Adequate and well-controlled studies to establish efficacy – Randomised parallel dose–response studies – Clinical safety studies – Studies of mortality/morbidity outcomes – Large simple trials – Comparative studies
Therapeutic Use	– Refine understanding of benefit–risk relationship in general or special populations and/or environments – Identify less common adverse reactions – Refine dosing recommendation	– Comparative effectiveness studies – Studies of mortality/morbidity outcomes – Studies of additional endpoints – Large simple trials – Pharmaco-economic studies

PK: pharmacokinetics, PD: pharmacodynamics.
Source: Adapted from ICH E8 guideline [1], table 1, p. 3. Reproduced with permission of ICH.

– clinical operations that are responsible for the choice of participating countries and investigator centres, the central coordination of multinational studies, the proper monitoring of all clinical trials;

– data management responsible for the set-up of the case report form (CRF) and the clinical database wherein all individual study-specific data from all study participants are collected and stored, the regular blind reviews of the study data, the final 'freeze' of the database before transfer to the biostatisticians for blind analysis;

- medical review for a critical assessment of the medical data of the study participants, as well as the pharmacovigilance cases;
- study drug supplies for the management of study drugs (test drug, placebo, comparators, associated medication), from planning and manufacturing, over distribution to recovery and destruction;
- biostatistics: the development of the statistical analysis plan in the study protocol, possible intermediate analyses, as well as the final statistical analysis; and
- medical writing for the drafting of the final study reports in collaboration with the investigators.

3.4.4 Interaction between the development streams

The development of a new drug is a multidisciplinary process that engages experts with scientific and technical backgrounds that range from chemical engineering, medicine, pharmaceutical sciences, biochemistry to finance. There is constant exchange of data among the scientists who drive the chemical and pharmaceutical development, those who conduct the nonclinical safety evaluations and the scientists and clinicians responsible for the clinical development of the new drug. The communication between scientists involved in drug development is key to its success. Drug development experts do not work in a vacuum and their decisions and conclusions impact upon the work of their drug development team members. If, for example, chemical analysts observe a new impurity in a batch of an active ingredient during a chemical production process, they will report this to the toxicologists and to the clinicians who (plan to) run a clinical trial with the drug. The reason why analysts do so is because this new impurity may be toxic. Toxicologists may have to evaluate the toxicity of this new impurity and advise the clinical trial physicians to proceed with the clinical trial only if there is evidence that the new impurity is safe. Alternatively, if unexpected toxicity is observed in animal tests whilst clinical trials are ongoing, these should be taken into account and can lead to modifications in the clinical protocol. These modifications may be the introduction of warning signals that allow physicians to carefully observe and analyse the symptoms of the patients enrolled in the trials. Not only the scientists involved in a drug development project play an important role in the communication and exchange of observations, patients are also involved. If, during the conduct of a clinical trial, patients experience problems with swallowing a tablet, pharmaceutical formulation experts are involved to modify the pharmaceutical form to eliminate the problem. This can be resolved by applying a coating to the surface of the tablet or using appropriate formulation technologies to increase patient friendliness and compliance. Such changes to the formulation may have an impact on analytical development whereby new stability studies of the coated tablet have to be initiated. These examples illustrate that an observation made in one development stream (e.g. chemical and pharmaceutical development) may impact the course and rate at which another stream (e.g. clinical development) will proceed. The drug development team functions here as a platform for the exchange of information between the development streams and supporting functions. A drug development project is therefore not a linear process but one that is characterised by continuous feedback loops and reiterations.

3.5   Phases in drug development

The traditional approach in the development of a new drug consists in a stepwise increase in knowledge about the drug. It is a process that consists of two main parts: early development and late development. In this book early development is subdivided into a pre-clinical phase and a clinical phase and late development is subdivided in a pre-approval phase and a post-approval phase. There are 5 clinical phases in drug development, phase 0 for limited microdose exploratory studies, phase 1 for human pharmacology studies, phase 2 when primarily therapeutic exploratory studies are conducted, phase 3 when essentially therapeutic confirmatory studies are conducted and phase 4 when mainly therapeutic use studies are performed. Human pharmacology studies are also still possible in phases 2, 3 and 4, therapeutic exploratory studies in phases 3 and 4 and therapeutic confirmatory studies in phase 4. The relationship between the types of clinical trials according to objectives and the phases of drug development where they can be performed is illustrated in Figure 3.3.

The pre-clinical phase of early development and microdosing in human volunteers corresponds with phase 0, the clinical phase of early development with phase 1 and a part of phase 2 (phase 2a). The pre-approval phase of late development corresponds with phases 2b and 3, whereas the post-approval phase corresponds with phase 4.

3.5.1   Early development

Early development is essentially exploratory in nature, whereas late development is confirmatory. The pre-clinical phase of early development is a critical step because it provides the data that makes it possible to conclude whether the drug candidate is sufficiently safe and bioavailable to be administered to man. These pharmacokinetic and safety data have been generated in *in vitro* and *in vivo* experimental systems with the objective to estimate as good as possible a safe starting dose in man. In the traditional course of drug development the clinical phase of early development consists of a single and repeated ascending dose administration to healthy human volunteers (phase 1 trial) often immediately followed by a limited therapeutic exploratory trial (phase 2a) in patients when the results obtained in healthy volunteers

Relationship between clinical drug development phases and types of clinical trials by objective

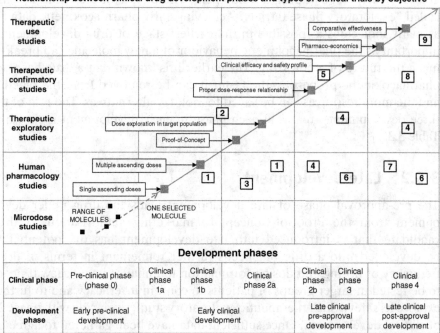

Figure 3.3 Clinical trials and their place in drug development.
1: Additional clinical pharmacology (e.g. biomarker exploration); 2: Integrated phase 1-2 study; 3: Additional pharmacokinetics (e.g. non-linear PK exploration); 4: Drug-drug interactions; 5: Seamless phase 2b-3 study; 6: Bioequivalence between new and former formulation; 7: New dosage form bioavailability; 8: Post-authorisation safety study (PASS); 9: Mortality/morbidity outcomes.
Source: adapted from ICH guideline E8 [1], Figure 1, p. 5. Reproduced with permission from ICH.

are encouraging. The phase 2a trial is performed to assess the therapeutic potential of the drug candidate in man for the first time (Proof-of-Concept). During recent years new approaches were explored to counter the increasingly reduced productivity in drug research and development organisations and proposals were made to use what has come to be called "phase 0" studies. In the "traditional" approach of new drug development, human pharmacokinetic data of a drug only become available after a phase 1 clinical trial is concluded. The amount of toxicology data that has to be produced in preparation of such a clinical trial with healthy volunteers is considerable. In order to improve the selection process of new drugs, regulatory authorities have introduced an alternative approach whereby the extent of toxicology testing required for an exploratory early phase study is reduced. In one approach a limited single-dose human trial can proceed with a very low subclinical starting dose of maximum 100 µg. This is already sufficient to characterise the pharmacokinetic behaviour of several compounds in man at a very early stage of drug development. These "microdose" trials are also called "exploratory phase 0 trials". Achieving early pharmacokinetic data for as many molecules as possible in the earliest stage of drug development is important as the pharmacokinetic behaviour of a new molecule can break or make the future of a new drug. The earlier it is known that a drug has poor pharmacokinetic properties, the faster it can be removed from the pipeline and the more resources can be saved to look for alternatives. The role of the three development streams at each phase in early development is shown in Table 3.3.

3.5.2   Late development

The pre-approval phase of late development leads the drug under development from the Proof-of-Concept to marketing authorisation. A drug candidate that is introduced into late development has the potential to be developed into a drug but needs further refinement in terms of dose, frequency of dosing and dosing formulation to enhance its efficacy. It needs to be tested in larger groups of patients to confirm its efficacy and to further explore its safety. Such therapeutic exploratory studies coincide with phase 2b of clinical development. Once sufficient data have been gathered to agree on a therapeutic strategy, the drug under development has still to be tested in therapeutic confirmatory trials with larger and diverse groups of patients. In the case of a drug developed to treat a chronic disease, treatment over longer periods of time is then envisaged. Such studies are conducted during phase 3 of drug development. The role of the three development streams at each phase in late development is shown in Table 3.4.

The post-approval phase of late development starts at the time of marketing authorisation and can continue until the end of the drug life cycle. Once the drug is approved for marketing, new data are collected through clinical practice. This phase coincides with phase 4 of clinical drug development. When unexpected safety problems arise during clinical practice they can also be addressed in additional nonclinical and clinical test programmes in this phase of development. These investigations are referred to as translational drug research.

Also during this phase, new drug formulations, different dosing regimens, different routes of administration, other indications and new drug combinations may be developed and tested in the clinic.

3.5.3   Milestones in drug development

A milestone is a time point in drug development where important decisions are taken to progress the drug further in development. Before such decisions are taken an internal review process is initiated to make sure that all data needed for the next step are available and that they are of the required quality. Such a data review is called a 'stage gate'. Although there are many

Table 3.3   Early development phases, milestones and stage gates.

Phase	Development streams			Approx. duration
	Chemical/pharmaceutical	Nonclinical	Clinical	
Pre-clinical	Tentative upscaling of chemical synthesis; development of a pharmaceutical formulation for animal testing to ensure high bioavailability and tolerability; development of an analytical method for the active ingredient and drug product; establishing of preliminary quality specifications; preparation of the IMPD, the investigator's brochure (IB) and IND/CTA dossier.	Pharmacokinetics, toxicology and safety pharmacology *in vitro* and in experimental animal species to assess bioavailability and safety in man after single and repeated exposure; identification of critical safety parameters to be followed up in the clinic; proposal of a safe starting dose and a ceiling dose for the First-in-Human clinical trial; preparation of the IMPD, the investigator's brochure (IB) and IND/CTA dossier.	Conduct exploratory phase 0 clinical trial in healthy volunteers (microdose studies); risk assessment in man based on nonclinical safety data. Development of the protocol and the working process for the First-in-Human clinical trial; preparation of the IMPD, the investigator's brochure (IB) and IND/CTA dossier.	9–12 months
Milestone/ stage gate	Internal review and decision to apply for approval to start clinical development (1a/b)			
Regulatory	Application to the authorities to request approval to proceed with a First-in-Human study by means of a clinical trial application (CTA, EU) or investigational new drug application (IND, US); approval from local regulatory authorities and local ethics committee to conduct a First-in-Human study			2–6 months
Clinical (1a)	Development of a pharmaceutical formulation that is safe and stable for phase 1 clinical trials; development of quality specifications and test methods appropriate for phase 1; update of IMPD and IB.	Repeated dose toxicology studies; further pharmacokinetic studies; studies to address specific toxicological endpoints of concern identified in nonclinical studies; update of IMPD and IB.	Single-dose study in healthy human volunteers with close monitoring of critical safety parameters; dose setting for a repeated dose clinical trial based on the first-in-human study; development of the protocol and the working process for the repeated dose clinical trial; update of IMPD and IB.	3–6 months

(Continued overleaf)

Table 3.3   (*Continued*)

Phase	Development streams			Approx. duration
	Chemical/pharmaceutical	Nonclinical	Clinical	
Milestone/ stage gate	Internal review and decision to enter Phase 1b			
Clinical (1b)	Further refinement of the pharmaceutical formulation based on clinical pharmaco-kinetic and tolerance data; development of pharmaceutical formulation for use in later phases of development; refinement of quality specifications; exploration and refinement of the validation of the analytical methods; update of IMPD and IB.	Fertility and embryo–fetal toxicology studies; extended repeated dose toxicology studies and resolution of safety issues identified in nonclinical and clinical studies; more advanced pharmacokinetic studies; update of IMPD and IB.	Repeated dose clinical trials in healthy volunteers; dose setting for a repeated dose clinical trial in patients based on the repeated dose clinical study; development of the protocol and the working process for the repeated dose clinical trial with patients; update of IMPD and IB.	3–9 months
Milestone/ stage gate	Internal review and decision to enter Phase 2a			
Clinical (2a)	Preparation of the upscaling of chemical synthesis; exploration of new formulations for late development; validation of QC and stability testing; update of IMPD and IB.	Extended repeated dose toxicology studies in rat and dog.; pre- and post-natal development study in rat; preparation of the nonclinical part of the risk assessment for transfer to late development; update of IMPD and IB.	Small-scale clinical trials in patients; preparation of clinical part of risk assessment and efficacy for transfer to late development; update of IMPD and IB.	6–12 months
Milestone/ stage gate	Internal review and decision to enter late development			

Table 3.4   Late development phases, milestones and stage gates.

Phase	Development streams			Approx. duration
	Chemical/pharmaceutical	Nonclinical	Clinical	
Pre-approval (2b)	Upscaling of the chemical synthesis beyond pilot-plant manufacturing scale; qualification of the active ingredient when new impurity profiles arise due to change in chemical synthesis; preparation of the end-of-phase 2 (EoPh2) dossier; update of IMPD and IB.	Repeated dose-toxicity studies; carcinogenicity studies; prenatal and post-natal development toxicity study; advanced pharmacokinetic studies; mechanistic toxicology studies *in vitro* and *in vivo*; preparation of the end-of-phase 2 (EoPh2) dossier; update of IMPD and IB.	Confirmatory phase 2b clinical trials in patients; development of the protocol and the working process for the phase 3 clinical trial; preparation of the end-of-phase 2 (EoPh2) dossier; update of IMPD and IB.	1 – 3 years
Milestone/ stage gate	Internal review and decision to start clinical phase 3 study (EoPh2 review)			
Regulatory	EoPh2 submission to authorities (US FDA) and approval from local regulatory authorities and local ethics committee to conduct a phase 3 study			
Pre-approval (3)	Upscaling of chemical synthesis and pharmaceutical manufacturing to full manufacturing scale; stability studies; definitive active ingredient and drug product specifications; preparation of chemical/pharmaceutical part of NDA and MAA dossiers.	Carcinogenicity studies; juvenile toxicology studies if paediatric indication; advanced pharmacokinetic studies; *ad hoc* mechanistic toxicology studies; preparation of nonclinical part of NDA and MAA dossiers.	Large-scale Phase 3 clinical trials in patients; specific human pharmacology studies; specific safety studies (e.g. thorough QT study); preparation of clinical part of NDA and MAA dossiers.	2 – 4 years

(Continued overleaf)

Table 3.4   (*Continued*)

Phase	Development streams			Approx. duration
	Chemical/pharmaceutical	Nonclinical	Clinical	
Milestone/ stage gate	Internal review and decision to submit dossier for marketing authorisation			
Regulatory	Compose registration dossier (NDA, MAA) and submit it to obtain marketing authorisation			
Post-approval (4)		Bio-equivalence studies in experimental animals; mechanistic toxicology and safety pharmacology studies *in vitro* and *in vivo* to respond to questions from translational medicine; pharmacokinetic studies when new routes of administration or fixed-dose combinations are explored; *ad hoc* juvenile toxicology studies to support paediatric development.	Post-approval efficacy/effectiveness studies; post-approval safety studies; comparative effectiveness studies; bio-equivalence studies; fixed-dose combination studies; morbidity/mortality studies; pharmacoeconomic studies.	Until withdrawal
Milestone/ stage gate	Internal review and decision to submit dossier on line extensions for marketing authorisation			
Regulatory	Compose registration dossier (NDA, MAA) and submit it to obtain marketing authorisation			

minor stage gates in drug development such as the availability of a validated analytical method for the quality control test of the active pharmaceutical ingredient, or the availability of a toxicology report, there are a number of formal and pivotal stage gates that are shared by all drug development organisations. A major stage gate in drug development is also referred to as a milestone. The phases in drug development together with the milestones in early and late development for all development streams are summarised in Tables 3.3 and 3.4. Milestones and stage gates will be discussed in more detail in Chapters 5 and 6.

3.5.3.1 First-in-Human clinical trial

The administration of a drug candidate to a healthy volunteer or a patient for the first time is an important step in drug development. The exploratory and experimental nature of a First-in-Human (FIH) clinical trial warrants particular attention from nonclinical and clinical experts and a thorough analysis of all the nonclinical data at hand is conducted before the decision is taken to start clinical research. The proposal to start a FIH clinical trial, the scientific data that support it and the clinical protocol for the FIH are submitted to the health authorities for approval. The determination of a recommended safe starting dose for a FIH clinical trial is discussed in detail in Chapter 5.

3.5.3.2 End of phase 2

Therapeutic exploratory trials (phase 2) are important clinical trials as they explore different dosing regimens from which one with the best efficacy and safety will be selected for the conduct of therapeutic confirmatory clinical trials in a large and more diverse population of patients (phase 3). The conduct and the successful outcome of a therapeutic confirmatory clinical trial depend on the quality of the data obtained from the phase 2 trials and the careful selection of the definitive dosing regimen. The time point at which the decision is made to start a phase 3 clinical trial is generally referred to as the 'end of phase 2'. The meeting at which the protocol of the phase 3 trial is agreed upon is the 'end of phase 2 meeting' or 'start of phase 3 meeting'. The proposal to move the drug to phase 3 in clinical development, the scientific data that support it and the clinical protocol are submitted to the health authorities for approval. The data required to start phase 3 in drug development are described in detail in Chapter 6.

3.5.3.3 Plant transfer

At a certain moment in time during drug development, the chemical and pharmaceutical manufacturing process is developed to a level that it is ready for transfer to a full-scale chemical and pharmaceutical manufacturing plant. This is a huge undertaking that involves different experts in chemical and pharmaceutical engineering, analytical chemistry, quality assurance, supply management, production management, pharmaceutical formulation, finance and investment. Once the transfer – which can take a full year or even more depending on the complexity of the project – is completed, a full-scale manufacturing campaign is planned to supply phase 3 clinical trials and the market.

3.5.3.4   Submission for marketing authorisation

Once the data from the phase 3 clinical trial(s) confirm that the selected dosing regimen is efficacious and safe and all the required chemical/pharmaceutical and nonclinical data are available, the decision is taken to prepare a regulatory dossier for submission to the health authorities to request marketing authorisation. The activities that lead to the composition of the dossier are coordinated by the drug development team and may take several weeks to months to finalise. During this process all data relating to the quality, safety and efficacy of the new drug are transferred into a preformatted file called a 'Common Technical Document' or 'CTD'. The 'CTD' constitutes the core database of the registration dossier. Once the dossier is complete and checked for quality and consistency it is submitted by the regulatory department of the drug development organisation to all relevant regulatory authorities.

3.5.3.5   Marketing authorisation and launch

The time at which marketing authorisation is granted to a new drug is a crucial moment for a drug development organisation and the patients who are waiting for treatment. As soon as marketing authorisation is received the manufacturer of the drug will start discussions with the health authorities about price and reimbursement. Once these discussions are successfully finalised, the drug manufacturer starts the shipping of the drug product to the wholesalers for distribution and sale (market launch). Further milestones in the post-approval phase are the request for variations in the marketing authorisation (new indication, new formulation), the timely submission of Periodic Safety Update Reports (PSUR), and the regular updating of the Risk Management Plan and the Benefit-Risk assessment of the drug on the market.

3.6   Regulatory environment

3.6.1   Legislation and guidelines

The development of new drugs is a highly regulated process. While the legal framework on medicines enforces the legislation on the development, manufacture and distribution of drugs, drug development guidelines offer a non-legally binding framework that drug development organisations are recommended to apply. To enable the development of a new drug and to ensure that all drug candidates proposed for the conduct of clinical trials and for commercialisation are safe and effective and can be produced with a high level of quality, national and international regulatory authorities have issued specific guidelines for the development of drugs. Each of these guidelines addresses the criteria of quality, safety or efficacy or a combination of these. Some aspects of drug development, manufacture and control can be legally enforced and are described in the US Code of Federal Regulations [2] and EU Legislation [3] such as Good Clinical Practices (GCP) [4, 5], Good Manufacturing Practices (GMP) [6] and Good Laboratory Practices (GLP) [7]. National health authorities also issue guidelines local pharmaceutical industry is advised to follow if it wishes to obtain authorisation for manufacturing and commercialisation of the drug. However, only a few countries have issued guidelines that are sufficiently detailed to support and guide the development of a new drug. These detailed guidelines address the various aspects of a drug development project such as laboratory experiments, clinical studies, chemical and pharmaceutical development and manufacturing projects, quality and data assessment and data reporting. Drug development processes, however, may deviate from guidelines in so far that it can be scientifically justified. The following sections address the regulatory authorities and international organisations that issue drug development guidelines, followed by a section on regulatory processes and documents.

3.6.2 Regulatory authorities and organisations

3.6.2.1 The European Medicines Agency (EMA)

The European Medicines Agency (EMA) is an agency of the European Union, located in London. The main responsibility of the EMA is 'the protection and promotion of public and animal health, through the evaluation and supervision of medicines for human and veterinary use'. As a result, the Agency is responsible 'for the scientific evaluation of applications for European marketing authorisations for both human and veterinary medicines (centralised procedure)' and also publishes scientific guidelines on quality, safety and efficacy testing requirements on its website. Besides, the agency offers 'multidisciplinary guidelines' that connect different disciplines such as paediatrics, cell therapy and tissue engineering, vaccines, biosimilars, gene therapy, herbal medicinal products and pharmacogenomics. It is the EMA's Committee for Medicinal Products for Human Use (CHMP) that prepares scientific guidelines after consultation with regulatory authorities in the EU member states to help applicants prepare marketing authorisation applications for human medicines. These guidelines provide the basis for the harmonisation of the interpretation and application of the detailed requirements to demonstrate the quality, safety and efficacy of the new drug. Although these guidelines offer guidance and cannot be legally enforced, the EMA encourages marketing authorisation applicants to follow them. The EMA strongly advises the applicants of a regulatory dossier – either a clinical trial application or a market authorisation application – to discuss deviations from its guidelines with EU regulators during the process of drug development following the procedures of scientific advice.

3.6.2.2   The United States Food and Drug Administration (US FDA)

The Food and Drug Administration (FDA) is responsible for 'protecting public health through the safety, efficacy and protection of human and veterinary drugs, biological products, food supplies, cosmetics and irradiated products, for protecting public health by fast-tracking innovations that make drugs and food safer, more effective and more available to the population and for communicating correct scientific information on drugs and food'. The agency issues 'guidances' or guidelines on very different topics of drug development and has a specialised department for new drug assessment. This division is the 'Center for Drug Evaluation and Research' (CDER). Every year it publishes new, revised and/or draft guidances. The CDER communicates with drug development organisations during the development of a new drug in relation to clinical trials, chemical and pharmaceutical development and the safety of a drug candidate. CDER is also responsible for the assessment of drugs submitted for registration of a clinical trial application and during the clinical trial in the form of an Investigational New Drug (IND) application and the application for marketing authorisation in the form of a New Drug Application (NDA). The Center makes use of "Scientific Advisory Committees" to assist in the assessment of a new drug.

3.6.2.3   The International Conference on Harmonisation (ICH)

The International Conference on Harmonisation of Technical Requirements for Registration of Pharmaceuticals for Human Use (ICH) is an organisation that was founded as a result of an international conference organised in Brussels in 1990 and that brought together representatives of the regulatory authorities and pharmaceutical industry in Europe, Japan and the United States to discuss scientific and technical aspects of drug registration. The mission of ICH is to achieve harmonisation among the regulatory guidelines that govern the development and registration of a new drug. Before ICH was founded, it was not uncommon that studies had to be repeated to comply with national requirements in different countries. The objectives of ICH are to:

- ensure the international harmonisation of the technical requirements for the safety, efficacy, and quality of drugs;
- allow the development and registration of drugs in an effective and cost-efficient way;
- promote public health, prevent duplication of clinical trials and minimise the use of animal studies without jeopardising the safety and efficacy of a new drug.

In order to reach these goals, ICH involves six parties during the process of harmonisation: the Japanese Ministry of Health, Labour and Welfare (MHLW), the Japan Pharmaceutical Manufacturers Association (JPMA), the European Union (EU, EMA), the European Federation of Pharmaceutical Industries Association (EFPIA), the US Food and Drug Administration (US FDA) and the Pharmaceutical Research and Manufacturers of America (PhRMA). ICH also invites three parties as observers: the World Health Organisation (WHO), the European Free Trade Association (EFTA) and Health Canada (HC-SC).

The activities of ICH are managed by the ICH Steering Committee and the harmonisation activities are conducted in ICH Working Groups. These are:

– the Expert Working group (EWG) that develops new (harmonised) guidelines and of which the members are appointed by the ICH Steering Committee;
– the Implementation Working Group (IWG) that facilitates the implementation of the guidelines in the ICH member states; and
– the Informal Working Group that develops concept papers on scientific topics which may be the subject of future harmonisation.

3.6.2.4   The Organisation for Economic Co-operation and Development (OECD)

The Organisation for Economic Co-operation and Development (OECD) is an intergovernmental organisation in which representatives of 34 industrialised countries in North America, Europe and the Asia Pacific region, as well as the EU Commission, meet to coordinate and harmonise policies, discuss issues of mutual concern, and work together to respond to international problems. The OECD secretariat is located in Paris, France. The guidelines of OECD that are of interest to drug development are the test and assessment guidelines (TG) and the guidelines on good laboratory practice (GLP) and compliance monitoring. These guidelines are issued by the division of the Environment, Health and Safety. The guidelines of OECD on test methods and GLP are accepted worldwide and referred to by all international and national regulations relating to the safety assessment of pharmaceuticals, veterinary products, foods, food and feed additives, cosmetics and industrial chemicals. The combination of the ICH and the OECD guidelines on the safety testing of drugs in development forms the basis of the mutual acceptance of safety data on drugs worldwide.

3.6.2.5   The European and US Pharmacopoeia

The mission of the European Pharmacopoeia is to 'promote public health by the provision of recognised common standards for use by healthcare professionals and others concerned with the quality of medicines, to facilitate the free movement of medicinal products in Europe, to ensure the quality of medicinal products and their components imported into or exported from Europe, to design European Pharmacopoeia monographs and other texts to be appropriate to the needs of regulatory authorities, those engaged in the quality control of medicinal products and their constituents and to the manufacturers of starting materials and their products'. The mission of the US Pharmacopoeia mirrors that of the European Pharmacopoeia and consists in 'improving the health of people around the world through public standards and related programmes that help ensure the quality, safety, and benefit of medicines and foods'. Both the European Pharmacopoeia and the USP are strongly involved in the fight against counterfeit drugs. With counterfeit and adulterated medicines posing an increasing risk to patients in the United States and worldwide, the U.S. Pharmacopeial (USP) Convention has issued standards for drug products that were subject to adulteration. For example, more than 200 patients worldwide reportedly died after batches of heparin were adulterated with oversulfated chondroitin sulfate that can be derived from the dietary supplement chondroitin and mimic heparin's blood-thinning properties.

It is beyond the scope of this book to present an exhaustive overview of all guidelines that are applied in drug development and have been issued by these organisations. A short overview with some examples and reference to the relevant websites are given in Table 3.5.

3.6.3   Regulatory processes and documents

In Section 3.5 on the phases in drug development an overview is given of the most important processes that take place during the development of a new drug. These processes result in scientific and technical data that are reported in documents and combined in a dossier that is submitted to the health authorities. These dossiers are used to convince the health authorities that the proposed drug is safe and efficacious to be developed or approved for marketing, and can be manufactured consistently with high quality. The processes that govern the interaction between the drug development organisation and the health authorities are 'regulatory processes'. In such a process, the drug development team has to follow a series of administrative steps imposed upon by the authorities for the submission of scientific and technical data. The authorities follow a set of administrative procedures to manage and review the data in a timely manner and visit and inspect the sites where the raw nonclinical, clinical and chemical and pharmaceutical data were generated and/or the product (active substance of medicinal drug product) is or will be manufactured. The authorities review the data to make sure that the claim made by the drug development organisation is justified. They can also raise questions

Table 3.5   International organisations issuing drug development guidelines.

Source	Website	Example of a guideline	Objective of the guideline
EMA	http://www.ema.europa.eu	Committee for medicinal Products for Human Use (CHMP) Guidelines on the limits of genotoxic Impurities (EMEA/CHMP/QWP/251344/2006).	Helps drug development organisations to deal with genotoxic impurities in active ingredients.
FDA	http://www.fda.gov	FDA Guidance for Industry estimating the maximum safe starting dose in initial clinical trials for therapeutics in adult healthy volunteers (US HHS, FDA, CDER, July 2005).	Provides advice and guidance on the estimation of a safe starting dose for first-in-man clinical studies.
ICH	http://www.ich.org	Harmonized Tripartite Guideline – general considerations for clinical trials (ICH-E8, 17 July 1997).	Describes internationally accepted principles and practices in the conduct of both individual clinical trials and overall development strategy for new medicinal products.
OECD	http://www.oecd.org	Principles of GLP and Compliance Monitoring, no 1 (ENV/MC/CHEM(98)17, Paris, 21 January 1998).	Assists drug development organisations in managing their laboratory practices such that the data retrieved can be used to apply for the start of clinical studies and marketing authorisation.
European/US pharmacopea	http://www.edqm.eu http://www.usp.org	Certification of suitability to the monographs of the European Pharmacopoeia (RESOLUTION AP-CSP (07) 1).	Allows active ingredient manufacturers to demonstrate that their products can be tested in accordance with a pharmacopeial monograph.

or request additional studies to obtain assurance that the claims are justified. These regulatory processes do not occur exclusively at the end of the drug development process when the team submits the regulatory dossier for market authorisation. On the contrary, the exchange of information and the review of scientific data already starts before the conduct of a phase 1 human pharmacology trial. The process of data submission, regulatory review and any communication between the sponsor and the regulatory authorities is called a regulatory process, see Figure 3.4. For each clinical study conducted during drug development, the authorities have to give their approval before a human pharmacology trial, a therapeutic exploratory trial or a therapeutic confirmatory trial can be initiated.

Before a clinical trial can proceed in a country, a dossier has to be submitted to the competent regulatory authorities of that country to obtain authorisation for the conduct of a clinical trial. This dossier contains country-specific administrative documents besides chemical, pharmaceutical, nonclinical and clinical

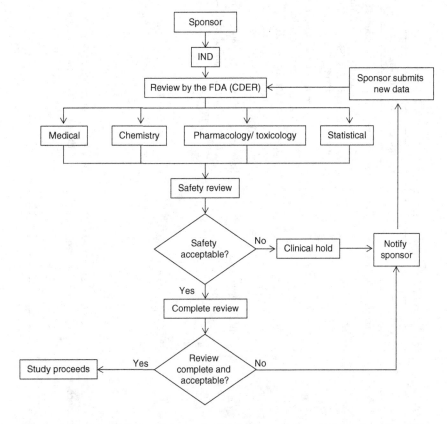

Figure 3.4   A regulatory process: a simplified representation of the review of an IND.

data. The authorisation is only granted when the dossier has been reviewed by the experts of the competent authorities and no objections are made to proceed with the clinical trial. For example, to conduct a clinical trial in the US, a regulatory dossier known as an 'Investigational New Drug'-application (IND) is submitted to the US FDA to start a clinical study in the USA. By analogy, a Clinical Trial Authorisation (CTA) is used in the EU. Other regulatory documents used during drug development are the Investigative Medicinal Product Dossier (IMPD), the Investigator's Brochure (IB) and the Request for a Special Protocol Assessment to start carcinogenicity studies in experimental animals. These dossiers are used at critical time points during the development of a new drug. At the end of the pre-clinical phase and before the start of phase 1, an IND, CTA, IMPD and IB are prepared and submitted to obtain an approval for the conduct of a human pharmacology clinical trial. When the decision is made to proceed to phase 2 or phase 3 clinical trials, the dossiers are updated with new knowledge accumulated since the last submission and submitted to obtain authorisation to proceed to the next phase of development. The IND, IMPD and IB are frequently updated as new scientific data become available during drug development. When the drug development process is completed, a dossier is prepared to apply for a marketing authorisation of the drug. This dossier is called a 'New Drug Application' (NDA) in the USA and a 'Marketing Authorisation Application' (MAA) in the EU. Table 3.6 gives an overview of the regulatory dossiers that have to be submitted at the various milestones of the drug development process.

Table 3.6 Regulatory documents to be submitted during drug development.

Phase in drug development	Milestone in drug development	Regulatory documents submitted to and reviewed by FDA	Regulatory documents submitted to and reviewed by EMA
Early development	End of pre-clinical phase/start of phase 1	IND, IB	IMPD, CTA, IB
	End of phase 1/ start of phase 2	Update of IND, IB	Update of IMPD, CTA, IB
	End of phase 2a/ start of phase 2b	Update of IND, IB	Update of IMPD, CTA, IB
Late development	End of phase 2b/ start phase 3	Update of IND, IB	Update of IMPD, CTA, IB
	End of phase 3	NDA	MAA
	Phase 4	Update of IB, update of NDA	Update of IB, IMPD, MAA, Five yearly revisions of the marketing authorisation

3.6.3.1   Clinical Trial Authorisation (CTA) application

Before starting a clinical trial in the EU with a drug candidate, a drug in development or a medicine, an application is filed with the national authorities of the member state where the study will be conducted. Prior to the submission of the application for a clinical trial authorisation a unique "EudraCT" number is obtained from the EudraCT Community Clinical Trial System [8]. The EudraCT database is a registry of interventional clinical trials in the EU and in the European Economic Area (EEA) countries for which a CTA has been granted. It provides an overview of all clinical trials but is only available to regulatory authorities (full access) and sponsors (only own information). Some of these data are available to the public through the EU Clinical Trials Register [9].

Besides administrative forms, a CTA application contains

- the clinical trial application form;
- the protocol of the proposed clinical trial prepared in line with the Community Guideline on Good Clinical Practice;
- the Investigator's brochure (IB) that gives a summary of the nonclinical and clinical data on the drug candidate and the drug product relevant to the planned clinical trial and provides guidance to the clinical investigator using all information that has been produced thus far in the drug development process;
- the Investigational Medicinal Product Dossier (IMPD) in which the investigational medicinal product or 'IMP' is defined as a pharmaceutical form of the active ingredient or placebo to be tested or used as a reference in a clinical trial, including products with a marketing authorisation but used or assembled (formulated or packaged) in a way different from the authorised form, or when used for an unauthorised indication, or when used to gain further information about the authorised form;
- an overview of noninvestigational medicinal products used in the trial;
- the labelling of the drug product (IMP);
- references to a Paediatric Investigation Plan (PIP), if applicable (see below and Chapter 7).

When the CTA dossier is submitted to the competent authority of an EU member state, a review of the data is carried out by experts of the authorities within a period of maximum 60 calendar days. This timeframe includes the validation of the request for authorisation. If the request is considered valid and there is no ground to refuse the clinical trial to proceed by day 60, the clinical trial is considered authorised. If an application is considered not valid, the competent authority informs the applicant of its decision within the first 10 calendar days following the review period and explains the reason for its decision.

3.6.3.2   Investigational New Drug (IND) application

An Investigational New Drug (IND) application is a regulatory document that is submitted to the US FDA to notify the US authorities of the intention of the drug development organisation to engage in the development of a new drug [10]. An IND application contains the following information:

- Nonclinical pharmacology, pharmacokinetics and toxicology data when an application is made for the conduct of a FIH clinical trial. When the IND application takes place later in development, all nonclinical and clinical data produced thus far are submitted.
- Data on the composition, manufacturing, quality control, quality specifications and shelf life of the active ingredient and the drug product.
- The protocol of the clinical trial for which the application is submitted and all relevant information on the clinical investigator and the institutional review board (IRB). The IRB is the US equivalent of the ethics committee in Europe.

There are 3 types of IND:

- an investigator IND that is submitted by a clinician in charge of the conduct of a clinical trial to study an unapproved or approved drug to explore new indications or new patient populations;
- an emergency use IND that allows the FDA to authorise the use of an experimental drug in an emergency situation. This may occur when there is not sufficient time for the sponsor to follow the normal regulatory process or when patients do not meet the inclusion criteria as stated in the clinical protocol, or when an approved clinical protocol is not available;
- a treatment IND is used for experimental drugs that show great promise in clinical testing for serious or immediately life-threatening conditions while the definitive clinical results are not available yet or the FDA review is still underway.

There are two categories of INDs, i.e. a commercial IND that is used when the sponsor is planning to put the drug on the marketplace and a research or noncommercial IND. The Center for Drug Evaluation and Research (CDER) offers a Pre-Investigational New Drug (IND) Application Consultation Programme to foster early communications between the drug development organisation and the drug review divisions of CDER to provide guidance on the preparation of an IND. IND applications are reviewed by scientific experts of the drug review divisions that are organised per therapeutic area. The review period of the IND application by CDER is 30 days. An IND is not formally approved by the FDA. Once the IND is submitted, the drug development organisation must wait 30 calendar days before initiating any clinical trials. During this time, the FDA will review the IND for safety to assure that participants are not subjected to unreasonable risk. A clinical hold can be issued by the US FDA to delay or to suspend a previously approved clinical trial. It may be either the complete interruption of the clinical trial or a part thereof. If a clinical trial is planned under an IND and the FDA has serious concerns about the safety of the clinical trial subjects, it notifies the drug development organisation of its concerns within a timeframe of 30 days and may prevent the clinical trial from proceeding. This is called a 'clinical hold'. It is an order issued by FDA to the sponsor to delay a proposed clinical investigation or to suspend an ongoing investigation. The clinical hold order may apply to one or more of the investigations covered by an IND. When a proposed study is placed on clinical hold, subjects may not be given the investigational drug. When an ongoing study is placed on clinical hold, no new subjects may be recruited to the study and placed on the investigational drug. Patients already enrolled in the study should be taken off therapy involving the investigational drug unless specifically permitted by FDA in the interest of patient safety. A similar 'clinical hold' approach is also applicable in the EU.

3.6.3.3   Investigational Medicinal Product Dossier (IMPD)

An Investigational Medicinal Product Dossier (IMPD) is an EU regulatory document that offers information related to the quality of the 'investigational medicinal product' (IMP), manufacturing, control, nonclinical and clinical data [11]. An IMPD contains:

- Chemical and pharmaceutical (quality) data on the composition, manu-facturing, quality specifications, quality control and proposed shelf life of the drug product. This information is required to ascertain that the drug development organisation is able to consistently produce a drug product with high quality.
- Nonclinical pharmacology, pharmacokinetics and toxicology data with a critical assessment of the efficacy and the safety of the drug product.
- Previous clinical trial and human experience data.
- An overall risk and benefit assessment providing an integrated summary that critically analyses all nonclinical and clinical data in relation to the potential risks and benefits of the proposed clinical trial.
- Noninvestigational medicinal products (NIMP) that are used in the trial should have been granted a marketing authorisation in the EU member state where the clinical trial is proposed to take place.

An IMPD is an integral part of a Clinical Trial Authorisation application. It is reviewed by the expert reviewers in the national member states' regulatory authorities and ethics committees.

3.6.3.4 Investigator's Brochure (IB)

Every request to obtain authorisation for a clinical trial is accompanied by an investigator's brochure (IB) [12]. This (ICH-based) document provides the clinical investigators and other personnel involved in the clinical trial with all the information that is necessary to understand the rationale behind the dose selection, dose frequency/interval, routes and methods of administration and the safety monitoring procedures contained in the clinical trial protocol. The IB is a document that reflects the state of knowledge on the drug candidate and is updated annually and as soon as new critical data on the drug become available. The content of an IB is discussed in more detail in the section on Good Clinical Practices in this chapter.

3.6.3.5 Paediatric Investigation Plan (PIP)

A paediatric investigation plan (PIP) is a drug development plan in the EU with the objective to gather and assess nonclinical and clinical data in preparation of clinical studies with children and data from paediatric studies to support the authorisation of paediatric drug products [13]. A PIP includes a 'description of the studies and of the measures to adapt the medicine's formulation to make its use more acceptable in children, such as use of a liquid formulation rather than large tablets'. If a proposed clinical trial is part or is intended to be part of a PIP then a reference to such plan is made. In the USA similar – but not identical – systems are in place to encourage R&D organisations to develop appropriate paediatric drugs under the FDA Amendments Act of 2007 (FDAAA), the Best Pharmaceuticals for Children Act (BPCA) and the Pediatric Research Equity Act (PREA) [14].

3.6.3.6 Marketing Authorisation Application (MAA) in the EU

When the data obtained from the clinical trials show that the drug under development is safe and efficacious in patients and that it can be manufactured with high quality, the drug development organisation may decide to seek marketing authorisation [15]. To this end a dossier is prepared that compiles all the data that address the quality, safety and efficacy of the drug. When such a 'regulatory dossier' or 'registration dossier' is filed in Europe it is called a 'Marketing Authorisation Application' (MAA). The MAA is accompanied by all relevant chemical/pharmaceutical, nonclinical and clinical data. A more detailed discussion on the content of a MAA is presented in Chapter 6.

3.6.3.7 New Drug Application (NDA) in the USA

The equivalent of a EU-based MAA in the USA is called a 'New Drug Application' (NDA) [16]. The NDA is the vehicle through which drug development organisations formally request the FDA to approve a new drug for marketing in the USA. The objectives of the NDA are to provide all required information to the US FDA to allow the reviewers to decide whether the new drug is sufficiently safe and efficacious and can be made available to American patients. The scientific data to be included in an NDA are essentially similar to those of the MAA. A more detailed discussion on the content of a NDA is presented in Chapter 6.

3.6.3.8   Drug Master Files (DMF)

In some cases an active or inactive ingredient from a third party may be used in drug development. For example, a drug development team that develops a formulation of a very poorly water soluble drug may need to introduce an excipient into the formulation to increase the bioavailability of the new drug. However, the use of this excipient is protected by intellectual property rights owned by a third party who is not willing to divulge confidential information about its synthesis, characteristics and properties. The team, however, is obliged to include information pertaining to the synthesis, quality and stability of the excipient used in the drug product in the New Drug Application (NDA). In order to solve this dilemma, the US FDA allows a manufacturer of an (in)active ingredient to submit confidential information about synthesis and manufacture directly to the US FDA in the form of a 'Drug Master File' (DMF) [17]. This prevents the exchange of confidential information that constitutes the intellectual property of the third party with the drug development organisation. This DMF contains information about the (in)active ingredient, its manufacture, quality specifications, in-process controls, release tests, analytical methods and stability data. When the drug development organisation submits a new drug application with the US FDA to obtain approval for the drug, it will insert a letter from the manufacturer of the (in)active ingredient stating that the confidential information was submitted by the manufacturer directly – but separately from the NDA – in the form of a Drug Master File. This letter authorises the drug development organisation to refer to the DMF. This letter is known as a "Letter of Access". The DMF system applies to active as well as to inactive pharmaceutical ingredients and to packaging materials.

3.6.3.9   Active Substance Master File (ASMF)

In analogy with the DMF procedure in the USA, a similar but not identical procedure was developed in the EU. In the EU, a qualified pharmacist who is appointed by the applicant or holder of the MAA is responsible for the quality of the active ingredient and drug product under development or on the marketplace. The qualified pharmacist needs to have access to data that are necessary to make a decision with respect to the safety (e.g. impurities) and quality (e.g. appropriate analytical methodology) of the active ingredient. Therefore, critical data on the synthesis and quality control of the active ingredient have to be shared with the qualified pharmacist. However, only critical data are shared with the drug development organisation, while confidential data that constitute the intellectual property of the active ingredient

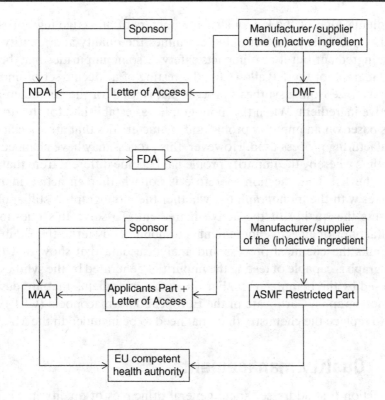

Figure 3.5   The US DMF (top) and EU ASMF (bottom) system.

manufacturer have to be submitted directly to the authorities (EMA or EU member states) by means of an 'Active Substance Master File' (ASMF) [18]. When a MAA is submitted to the authorities, a letter from the manufacturer of the active ingredient is added stating that the confidential information was submitted by the manufacturer directly – but separately from the dossier – to the authorities through an ASMF. This letter authorises the drug development organisation to refer to the ASMF and is known as the "Letter of Access". The section of the ASMF that is shared with the drug development organisation is referred to as the 'applicants part', while the section that is submitted directly to the competent authorities of the member state is called the 'restricted part'. A schematic overview of the US DMF and the EU ASMF system is presented in Figure 3.5.

3.6.3.10   Certificate of the European Pharmacopoeia (CEP)
Suppliers of established active ingredients generally make the claim that their active ingredients comply with the relevant monographs of the European Pharmacopoeia (EP). Although it offers a guarantee for high quality, it is not sufficient in view of the safety requirements that are required for active

ingredients. One of the key quality parameters of an active ingredient is its impurity profile since it not only determines the quality and identity of the active ingredient but it also impacts safety as some impurities may be toxic. A monograph of the EP allows for the testing of a specific set of impurities that may arise from a synthesis process that is used for the manufacturing of an active ingredient. When the monograph was established for the first time, it was based on an impurity profile and characteristics that are specific to the manufacturing process used. However, this process may have changed in the meantime whereby the impurity profile has become different from that tested for in the EP. The question therefore is not whether an active ingredient complies with the monograph but whether the monograph is still applicable to assess the quality of the active ingredient. To solve this question, the manufacturer of an active ingredient can submit a dossier to the EP in which it submits the chemical process and analytical data that show that the EP monograph is capable of testing the impurities generated by the synthesis process used by the manufacturer. For the active ingredients that are described in a monograph a Certificate of the European Pharmacopoeia (CEP) can be used to replace the chemistry data that need to be included in the MAA [19].

3.7   Quality management

This section first addresses some general principles of quality management followed by a discussion of important quality aspects that are relevant for drug development.

3.7.1   General principles

Quality management was initially developed to generate better products (or services) and was oriented towards the quality of products by means of testing and quality control. However, the focus gradually moved from product testing to the processes involved in its manufacture, the environment under which the manufacturing takes place and in the development of new products. The general principles of quality management are:

- The quality of a product implies conformity with the requirements imposed by regulations.
- Zero quality defects is the aim, but 'quality fit for purpose' is the standard.
- Proactive prevention of nonconformity (in-built quality by design) is preferable to reactive corrections (following audits or inspections). This is known as the 'Do it right the first time' approach.
- Higher level of quality has an incremental cost and top quality with zero error is very expensive.

Table 3.7 Quality management.

Quality planning	The process of building quality into the development or production processes and into the product. This includes more recent trends such as Quality by Design (QbD)
Quality control	The in-process efforts (incl. 'autoinspections' and 'monitoring') to improve the process output
Quality assurance	The systematic actions that provide confidence that a product satisfies (or will satisfy) given (regulatory) requirements. This includes the performance of audits, i.e. the systematic examination at a given point in time of (part of) a quality management system in an organisation by internal or external auditors. The findings give rise to 'Corrective And Preventive Actions' or 'CAPA' in order to prevent future errors. Inspections have a similar objective, but are performed by regulatory authorities and can be followed by regulatory actions
Quality improvement	The continuous effort to improve the quality, generally by implementing the classic 'plan-do-check-act' circles introduced by Deming and presented in the following website (http://www.balancedscorecard.org/thedemingcycle/tabid/112/default.aspx)

Together with the continuous focus on safety, the objective to guarantee medicines of top quality has been the main driver of the increased cost of drug development. The four elements of quality management are summarised in Table 3.7.

A quality management system (QMS) is defined as the 'legislation, organisational structure, procedures, processes and resources needed to fully implement these quality management elements'. In general a QMS includes a set of rules and regulations that are translated into operational procedures, monitored by quality control during operations and checked by audits and inspections. In the drug development process, QMS assures the quality of activities at all levels and steps in the process. An overview of the constituents of a QMS is given in Table 3.8.

3.7.2 Good Practices

The focus of this section is on quality requirements regarding the conduct of operations and tests in chemical/pharmaceutical, nonclinical and clinical development. They include a set of internationally agreed quality standards or Good Practices (GxP) according to the type of activities involved. Compliance with these standards provides public assurance that the quality of all the research performed and the data generated to support the marketing authorisation of a drug complies with current quality requirements and norms. An overview of these practices and the respective websites where they can be accessed is given in Table 3.9.

Table 3.8   Overview of the constituents of a quality management system.

Good Practices	A set of quality guidelines including Good Manufacturing Practices (GMP), Good Laboratory Practices (GLP), and Good Clinical Practices (GCP)
Standard Operating Procedures (SOP) & Operating Manuals (OPM)	A set of procedures and manuals tailored to each stakeholder organisation, describing how operations should be conducted to guarantee optimal quality
Quality control	In-process quality control by the operational teams
Audits	A form of quality assurance (QA) checks, performed by either internal auditors (but independent from the operational teams) or external ones
Inspections	With similar aims as audits, but performed by regulatory authorities

Table 3.9   Good practices.

Good Manufacturing Practices (GMP)	http://www.ich.org/products/guidelines/quality/article/quality-guidelines.html
Good Laboratory Practices (GLP)	http://www.oecd.org/chemicalsafety/testing/goodlaboratory practiceglp.htm
Good Clinical Practices (GCP)	http://www.ich.org/products/guidelines/efficacy/article/efficacy-guidelines.html

3.7.2.1   Good manufacturing practices (GMP)

Although good manufacturing practices (GMP) regulations were developed to steer the manufacturing of drugs intended for the market, they are also applied to candidate drugs during development. It is obvious that GMP requirements that apply to full-scale manufacturing can hardly be complied with in small-scale manufacturing of a drug candidate in phase 1 of development since during this phase no assurance can be given that the production process is fully reproducible. That is why the US FDA developed a separate GMP for phase 1 production. If GMP does not fully apply to the production of a phase 1 formulation certain requirements must be met such as the availability of documentation on the production, quality assurance and the performance of quality control checks. For formulations that are produced in phases 2 and 3, GMP can be expected to have an increasing impact, whereas the production of phase 3 formulations must be performed under the same GMP requirements as those that apply to commercial products. Good manufacturing practices are described in ICH guideline Q7 for active pharmaceutical ingredients and in a guideline from the EU Commission for finished products. Here, we only discuss the EU guidelines that apply to finished products.

Basic principles

Good manufacturing practices are an integral part of quality assurance in a drug development organisation. The application of GMP provides a guarantee that drug products are manufactured reproducibly and in accordance with the quality criteria in the approved registration dossier to ensure their safety and efficacy. Only when there is full compliance with GMP can a drug development organisation obtain a manufacturing authorisation.

Quality assurance

Quality assurance is a concept that is made up of all the factors that relate to the quality of a product or process. It encompasses all processes and procedures leading to the development or the manufacturing of a high-quality product. GMP regulations refer to the quality standards for manufacturing and quality control that must be met.

Quality control

Quality control is the part of GMP regulations that is concerned with sampling, specifications of a finished product, inspection and the organisation of manufacturing processes, documentation and release procedures. The finished drug product is not released for use or sale or dispensing unless it can be established that it meets suitable quality standards.

Product quality review

All test results for the release of various batches of a finished product must be evaluated on a regular basis to determine whether there is no tendency of the product to deviate from the defined specifications. Quality product reviews can be performed on test results obtained from the chemical analysis of starting materials, intermediates and the finished drug product.

Personnel

Employees of a drug manufacturing facility must have the necessary expertise to make sure that the quality of a production process and the product can be guaranteed. These employees have received training for their specific tasks in the drug manufacturing process and their level of expertise is increased whenever that is required to maintain the same quality level. In pharmaceutical manufacturing the function of a qualified person (responsible pharmacist) is crucial. To protect employees against health effects due to exposure to a drug and drug product in the manufacturing environment strict industrial hygiene rules must be followed.

Buildings and facilities, instruments and machinery

Buildings must be designed in such a way that the risk of contamination of materials and products is minimal and that infestation by insects or other vermin is kept to an absolute minimum. Buildings must be properly maintained and product quality must not be compromised by repair and maintenance operations. Regular cleaning and, if necessary, disinfection must be carried out in accordance with the applicable procedures. Lighting, temperature, humidity and ventilation must be such that product quality is not affected during production and storage and that the operation of machinery is not impaired. Access to production areas is only allowed by authorised personnel.

Documentation

Documentation is an essential part of the quality assurance system. A well-designed system with clearly written and legible documents helps in the prevention of mistakes and makes it possible to reproduce the history of a batch production. Specifications, production formulas and instructions, batch records and procedures must be without error and available for inspection.

Production

The manufacturing of a drug must be carried out in accordance with clearly described procedures. These procedures must be in compliance with GMP to ensure that the drug product is manufactured to quality standards and pursuant to the relevant manufacturing and marketing authorisations.

Contract production and analysis

When a drug development organisation decides to contract manufacturing and QC analysis out to a third party, the various activities involved must be clearly defined so that there is no misunderstanding about the responsibilities of both parties. This way the quality standards of the drug product and the manufacturing process can be met. The licensing out of pharmaceutical activities implies a written contract between the "contract giver" and the "contract acceptor" in which the responsibilities of each party are clearly defined and indicate the conditions under which the responsible pharmacist will release the drug product.

Complaints and recalls

All complaints and other information on drug products that might be indicative of a quality problem must be evaluated in accordance with written procedures. A system must be available through which a drug product that does not meet the necessary quality standards can be rapidly recalled from the market.

Self-inspection

Self-inspections must be carried out at regular intervals so that compliance with GMP principles can be assessed, and if needed, measures can be taken to ensure that these principles are adhered to.

3.7.2.2 Good laboratory practices (GLP)

The principles of good laboratory practices (GLP) for nonclinical laboratory studies were published for the first time by US FDA in 1976. This regulation served as a basis for the development of the principles of GLP by the Organisation of Economic Co-operation and Development (OECD) in 1978. The OECD principles of GLP were formally recommended for use in member countries by the OECD Council in 1981.

The principles of GLP were introduced to promote the quality and the validity of test data used for the determination of the safety of chemicals and chemical products. It is a managerial concept covering the organisational process and the conditions under which laboratory studies are planned, performed, monitored, recorded and reported. This set of rules is intended to make experimental testing more transparent and controllable with the objective to prevent any fraud in the setting up and reporting of test results for regulatory use. Although these rules improved significantly the reliability of such test results they don't provide assurance on the intrinsic scientific quality of the data. To ensure scientific quality additional quality systems have to be imposed by test facility management or in certain cases by national authorities. One example is the organisation of ring tests in hematology and serum biochemistry.

The principles of GLP apply to all nonclinical and environmental safety studies required by regulations for the purpose of registering or licensing of pharmaceuticals, pesticides, food and feed additives, cosmetics and veterinary products and for the regulation of industrial chemicals. The principles of GLP cover:

- test facility organisation and personnel;
- quality assurance programme;
- facilities;
- apparatus, material and reagents;
- test systems;
- test and reference items;
- standard operating procedures;
- performance of the study;
- reporting of study results; and
- storage and retention of records and materials.

Test facility organisation and personnel

GLP defines the responsibilities of test facility management, the study director, the principal investigator and study personnel. Responsibilities of the test facility are for example to ensure that there is sufficient and qualified personnel to perform the studies and that standard operating procedures with test conduct instructions are in place. The study director is the leader of the study in the test facility and one of his/her responsibilities is the approval of the study plan and amendments and to make sure that they are available to laboratory personnel. A principal investigator is appointed when several parts of a study are conducted in different test facilities. In each of the test facilities there is a study director in charge of the part of the study conducted in his/her laboratory. The principal investigator oversees the entire study and is responsible for the application of GLP in all study parts. All personnel involved in the conduct of the study must have received sufficient training for the conduct of their part of the study and be knowledgeable of the application of GLP.

Quality assurance programme

Each test facility should have a documented quality assurance programme and this should be carried out by one or more individuals (quality assurance unit, QAU) who are familiar with the test procedures and are directly responsible to management. One of the main tasks of the QAU is to conduct regular audits (study based, facility based and process based) to ensure that all tests are carried out in compliance with GLP and that the reported results accurately and completely reflect the raw data of the studies. The QAU also maintains copies of all approved study plans and standard operating procedures.

Facilities

The size, construction and design of the test facility should be such that it meets all the requirements necessary for the good conduct of studies. Storage rooms, rooms for receipt and storage of test and reference items, archives and waste-disposal rooms should be separated from the areas where tests are conducted.

Apparatus, material and reagents

All apparatus, including validated computerised systems used for the generation, storage and retrieval of data should be of a design and capacity that is appropriate for the studies normally conducted in the facility. The apparatus should be periodically inspected and calibrated according to the standard operating procedures. All chemicals used should be adequately labelled and stored and information about their source, preparation date and stability should be available.

Test systems

Appropriate conditions should be in place to store, house, handle and take care of biological test systems (e.g. rodents, dogs) and records of source, date of arrival and arrival conditions should be maintained. To maintain the integrity of a study test systems that become diseased or injured during the course of the study should be isolated and treated. Before the start of a study the biological test system should be acclimatised to the test environment for an appropriate period of time. Any material that comes into contact with the test systems during the course of the study should be free of contaminants at levels that would interfere with the study.

Test and reference items

Each test and reference item should be appropriately identified and the handling, sampling and storage procedures identified. The stability of the test and reference item under storage and test conditions should be known for all studies where they will be used. When the test item is administered to a biological test system using a vehicle (e.g. solvent, feed), the homogeneity, concentration and stability should be determined.

Performance of the study

For each study a study plan or study protocol has to be available prior to the start of the study. The study plan contains all elements that are necessary for the proper conduct of the study (e.g. test methods with reference to the OECD or ICH test guidelines, identity of test and reference items, test system and justification for its selection, characterisation of the test system, detailed experimental design). The study plan has to be approved by the study director, test facility management and the sponsor of the study and verified for GLP compliance by the QAU.

Each study should carry a unique identification number and all items and documents relating to this study should carry this number. The study should be carried out according to the study plan and any deviation thereof should be documented and acknowledged by the study director. All data generated during the conduct of the study should be recorded directly and signed and dated by laboratory personnel. Any change to the data should be signed and dated and the reason for the change given.

Reporting of study results

A final report should be prepared for each study and signed and dated for approval by the study director and/or the principal investigator. A statement of compliance with GLP and an overview of all GLP inspections that took place during the course and at the end of the study are added. Any change to the final report is made under the form of an amendment that clearly states the reason for change and is signed and dated by the study director.

Storage and retention of records and materials

The documents and items of each study that should be retained in archive are the study plan, the raw data, samples of test and reference items, specimens (e.g. tissues, histopathology slides) and the final report. Beside specific study-related items records of QAU inspections, personnel training records, apparatus maintenance and calibration records, validation records for computerised systems, SOPs and environmental monitoring records are also kept in archive. Only personnel authorised by management should have access to the archives and movement of material in and out of the archives should be recorded. Archives should be built and designed to optimally preserve the archived materials and protect them against fire.

3.7.2.3   Good clinical practices (GCP)

The currently applicable ICH E6 guideline 'Good Clinical Practice' (GCP) was finalised in May 1996, adopted in the EU in July 1996 and published in the US Federal Register in May 1997. It is 'an international ethical and scientific quality standard for designing, conducting, recording and reporting trials that involve the participation of human subjects'. The objective is to protect the safety, wellbeing, integrity and rights of clinical trial participants, and to make sure that the data generated are sound and credible to protect future patients treated with the drug. This guideline describes:

–   the general principles of good clinical *research* practices;
–   the responsibilities of the principal actors involved, i.e. the Institutional Review Board (IRB)/Independent Ethics Committee (IEC), the investigator and the sponsor;
–   guidance on the content and format of the clinical study protocol, the investigator brochure, and other so-called Essential Documents.

The guideline should be followed whenever performing clinical studies that are generating data to be submitted to regulatory authorities, but are recommended in other trials as well.

The principles of GCP

A good clinical study should be conducted in accordance with current regulations, GCP and the ethical principles laid down in the Declaration of Helsinki (see Section 3.9.3) guaranteeing the individual safety, wellbeing and rights of clinical trial participants. This includes a freely given informed consent to be obtained from every subject prior to its participation in the trial and involves respect to current privacy and confidentiality rules in handling the study participants' identity and personal data. Each study should be initiated only after a favourable opinion of an IEC/IRB and continued only if the anticipated benefits outweigh the foreseeable risks and inconveniences and should be supported by adequate nonclinical and clinical information on the drug(s) to be investigated. Each clinical study should be scientifically sound and described in a clear and detailed protocol that should be followed meticulously and each individual involved in conducting the study should be adequately qualified, trained and experienced to perform his/her respective task(s). Any medical decisions should always be the responsibility of a qualified physician. All information in relation to the trial should be recorded, handled and stored in a way that it can be easily retrieved, verified, interpreted and reported. Investigational drugs should be manufactured, handled and stored in accordance with GMP and used as prescribed in the study protocol.

Independent Ethics Committee /Institutional Review Board (IEC/IRB)

An Independent Ethics Committee /Institutional Review Board (IEC/IRB) is a committee of experts that reviews whether the proposed study is scientifically sound. Their evaluation is based on information provided in the study protocol and the investigator's brochure (IB) and the quality of the investigators. In accordance with the Declaration of Helsinki, they also assess whether the trial participants are sufficiently protected (rights, safety, wellbeing, informed consent procedure, recruitment procedure, payments, insurance). The decision of an IEC/IRB can either be favourable, be a request for clarifications such as a hearing of the investigator or modifications, or be negative. During the conduct of the trial, the IEC/IRB is also responsible for continuous monitoring of the study (progress, amendments, temporal suspension or preliminary end of the trial), at least on an annual basis or whenever considered appropriate according to the risks. The IEC/IRB should have a 'reasonable number of members, who collectively have the qualifications and experience to review and evaluate the science, medical aspects and ethics of the proposed trial'. It should be constituted of at least 5 members with at least 1 nonscientist and at least 1 member who is independent of the institution(s)/trial site(s). Only members who are independent of the investigator and the sponsor should be allowed to vote on a decision/opinion. The IEC/IRB should have written procedures for its functioning and should retain all relevant records in relation to its activities.

The Investigator
The investigator oversees a clinical trial and should be properly qualified by education, training and experience to conduct the study. He/she should be familiar with the study protocol and other study documents and should comply with applicable regulations and GCP. He/she should establish a list of coworkers to whom significant trial duties can be delegated. A qualified physician should be responsible for all trial-related medical decisions and the subject's primary physician should be informed about its participation in a clinical study. An investigator should:

- Have adequate time, resources and facilities available to conduct the study within the foreseen timelines.
- Obtain prior informed consent of every study participant, he/she is responsible for the communication with the IEC/IRB, he/she should conduct the study in compliance with the protocol, and he/she is also accountable for the correct use of the investigational drug(s).
- Complete the Case Report Forms (CRF), wherein all the study data of a trial participant are recorded, and maintain the Investigator Study File (ISF) with all the Essential Documents as required. He/she should give direct access to these documents as well as to trial-related source data to sponsor personnel (monitors, auditors) and inspectors.
- Report all Serious Adverse Events (SAEs) and all Suspected Unexpected Serious Adverse Reactions (SUSARs) immediately to the sponsor, who should pass them on to the Regulatory Authorities and the IEC/IRB.

– Provide the Regulatory Authorities and the IEC/IRB with the study report within set timelines.

The sponsor

A sponsor of a clinical trial should implement and maintain an adequate Quality Management System (QMS) and utilise adequately qualified staff members throughout all stages of the clinical trial process (design, protocol writing, statistical planning and analysis, supervision of the trial, medical review, interpretation of study results, report writing). In large multicentre trials, some of the supervising duties can be transferred to an independent Executive Committee and/or a Steering Committee that will only allow the presence of sponsor personnel in their meetings as non-voting members. The sponsor is also responsible for study data management and data analysis, which can be a huge undertaking in large clinical trials with a vast amount of data generated. Again, the sponsor can delegate the oversight of critical data as well as the data analysis to an independent Data Monitoring Committee (DMC) or Data Safety and Monitoring Board (DSMB). There is currently increasing pressure from society at large and regulatory authorities to require that data oversight and analysis be done by such bodies that are independent of the sponsor. Whenever trial-related duties are transferred to one or several Contract Research Organisations (CROs or service providers), the sponsor remains ultimately responsible. The sponsor is responsible for the selection of an appropriate investigator and the site where the trial will be conducted as well as for establishing a clinical trial agreement between the sponsor and the investigator. Such agreement includes all financial aspects of the trial conduct at the site (compensation for all investigations and other work done, compensation to subjects, insurance for product liability, etc.). The sponsor is responsible for the:

– manufacturing, supply and proper handling of all investigational products used in the trial, including the return of unused drugs from the sites and their destruction;
– updating of the IB on a regular basis for the ongoing safety evaluation of the investigational product(s) as well as for the safety reporting to the IEC/IRB and the regulatory authorities;
– monitoring of the clinical trial with a description of the purpose of monitoring (essentially an in-process quality control system), selection and qualifications of monitors (or Clinical Research Associates, CRAs), extent and nature of monitoring (frequency of on-site or remote monitoring), monitor's responsibilities (for more details, see the guideline), monitoring procedures and monitoring reports (post-monitoring letter to the investigator, visit report to the sponsor supervisor); and
– preparation of the study report and for providing it within the applicable deadlines to the IEC/IRB and regulatory authorities.

When sponsors perform audits, as part of implementing quality assurance, they should consider the purpose of the audit, the selection and qualification of auditors and the auditing procedures. Otherwise, some provisions are described in cases of non-compliance with the study protocol, GCP, regulations, premature termination or suspension of a trial or multicentre studies.

Clinical trial protocol

Besides general administrative information such as study title, sponsor, investigator sites, the background information about the drug product and the trial objectives and purpose, a clinical study protocol includes the following topics:

- trial design: type (e.g. parallel groups, double-blind, placebo-controlled), randomisation and blinding, study treatments and duration of study periods, stopping rules, etc.;
- approach in selection and withdrawal of subjects: inclusion/exclusion criteria, withdrawal criteria, etc.;
- treatment of subjects: study treatment(s), allowed/forbidden co-medications, treatment compliance monitoring, etc.;
- assessment of efficacy and safety: primary and secondary endpoints, procedures for safety reporting, etc.;
- statistical analysis: sample size calculation, statistical plan (methods, interim and final analyses), types of analyses (intention to treat versus per protocol), etc.;
- data management, the quality management system used, ethical considerations, direct access to source data/documents, financing and insurance, publication policy, legal provisions, and others.

The Investigator's Brochure (IB)

The Investigator's Brochure (IB) is a compilation of the available chemical/pharmaceutical, nonclinical and clinical data on the investigational drug product that are relevant for future clinical studies to be performed. This document is regularly updated at least once a year or when significant new information becomes available. This document is important for the investigator in view of his/her responsibilities regarding product safety monitoring, to understand the potential risks and anticipated adverse reactions of the drug product, to inform the investigator about specific tests, observations or precautions that may be needed, and to provide guidance on the recognition and treatment of possible adverse drug reactions.

3.7.3 Standard Operating Procedures (SOP)

Every stakeholder involved in drug development should have a set of written Standard Operating Procedures (SOP) and Operating Manuals (OPM) that describe, respectively, in general terms (SOP) or in more detail (OPM) the instructions needed to reach uniformity in the performance of specific operational activities or tasks. SOPs and OPMs translate how good practices (GMP, GLP, GCP) should be implemented within for example the drug development organisation or contract research organisations (CRO). The number of SOPs and OPMs varies according to the number of activities. In clinical drug development the number of SOPs and OPMs can be very high (>100). For example, SOPs describe the quality management system (QMS) of the drug development organisation, drafting and reviewing of essential study documents, selection of participating countries and centres in clinical trials, general principles of monitoring clinical trials, pharmacovigilance in clinical trials, initial and continuous training of staff members, etc. OPMs describe the content and format of an investigator brochure, study protocol, study report (detailing the SOP about study documents), content and format of the investigator manual (to fill out the case report form) or monitoring guide (to monitor the study) (detailing the SOP about monitoring clinical trials). SOPs and OPMs are generally drafted by specialists in quality management in collaboration with representatives from the operational functions. They should reflect current operations and should be updated whenever needed. The complete set should be reviewed at least annually in order to decide whether existing procedures should be updated or revised, and/or whether new ones should be added. SOPs also describe in detail the procedures that are necessary for the conduct of nonclinical safety studies. SOPs are generated by the test facility, approved by test facility management and made available to laboratory personnel at their work stations. Deviations from SOPs are possible but they should be documented and acknowledged by the study director or principal investigator. According to the growing experience of the test facility with certain test methods the SOPs can be amended and the amendments approved by test facility management. SOPs and OPMs are extensively used in chemical and pharmaceutical development and in major units the number of SOPs governing pharmaceutical development and manufacturing activities may be as high as several hundred to a thousand documents.

3.7.4   Quality control

During drug development, a quality control (QC) system monitors in real time the quality of the work and the study data. For example, according to GCP, implementation of a quality control system and the monitoring of clinical trials is explicitly stated as a responsibility of the sponsor. The purpose of clinical trial monitoring is to verify and make sure that:

- the rights and well-being of study participants are protected;
- the reported study data are accurate and complete, and can be verified with source data (i.e. data collected at the site of the clinical trial);
- the study is conducted in accordance with the study protocol and applicable SOPs, GCP and regulations.

Routine clinical trial monitoring is traditionally performed according to a standard strategy. For example, regular (every 6 weeks) on-site visits to the investigator centres are done by what are called clinical study monitors (CSM) or clinical research associates (CRA) who verify all source data (100% source data verification or SDV). The GCP guideline states that 'the sponsor should ensure that the trials are adequately monitored', leaving it to the sponsor to 'determine the appropriate extent and nature of monitoring' but in reality all too often the monitoring activity covers the full data set. This conservative approach ('when in doubt, monitor everything') stems from the fact that the GCP guideline lists more than 20 activities under the responsibilities of the clinical trial monitors appointed by the sponsor.

In 2013, the FDA and EMA issued guidance on risk-based approaches of clinical trial management and monitoring, promoting more flexible and targeted monitoring strategies based on prior risk assessment and risk mitigation [20, 21] (for more details, see Section 3.7.6). Monitoring as a quality control system during the conduct of clinical trials allows identification of problems early on and corrective actions and preventive actions (CAPAs) to be suggested in order to do better in the future. The most common deficiencies encountered are:

– failure to follow the protocol;
– failure to keep adequate and accurate records;
– problems with the informed consent form;
– failure to report adverse events; and
– failure to account for the disposition of study drugs.

Also, every drug development activity and every correction that is performed during quality control (QC) should be properly documented and filed, serving as an 'audit trail' in case of compliance checks by auditors or inspectors. The holder of a manufacturing authorisation to supply an active ingredient and drug product to a clinical trial, must have a quality control department. The quality control of a drug is not limited to the performance of release tests and laboratory activities but also includes aspects of product quality at the level of synthesis intermediates and in-process controls. To ensure that the activities of the QC department are carried out in compliance with GMP, accurate and complete documentation, availability of sampling procedures, written and validated test protocols and finally, a stability programme for the manufactured clinical trial batches (marketing stability) needs to be available and initiated.

3.7.5 Audits and inspections

During the development of a new drug the clinical, nonclinical and chemical and pharmaceutical activities are subject to audits and inspections.

3.7.5.1 Audits

Audits are an integral part of a quality assurance (QA) system and are critical evaluations of an organisation, a procedural system, a process, a study, a project or a product. These audits are conducted by the organisation in an attempt to assess whether the processes and procedures have been followed and data integrity can be guaranteed. They are either performed by specialised internal corporate audit teams that are independent from the operational teams and the routine monitoring or quality control functions, or can be delegated to external teams from QA service providers. The audit teams visit the premises and site of development and investigate laboratory notebooks, patient records, data management systems, availability of procedures, compliance with regulations, etc. These audits can take several days, can either be conducted before, during or after the end of a study or the submission of a clinical trial or marketing authorisation application, and can be performed routinely or 'for cause' (whenever a potential problem has been identified that warrants further checking). Auditors summarise their findings (critical, major or minor) in an audit report that is transmitted to the entity who requested the audit and its operational teams in order to correct the findings (whenever still possible) or to install measures to prevent them from recurring in the future.

3.7.5.2 Inspections

Inspections are quality assurance investigations that are similar to audits, but that are conducted by regulatory authorities, mostly FDA, EMA or national agencies. All stakeholders in the drug development process can be inspected, but most often sponsors, manufacturing sites, investigator centres, contract research organisations (CROs) and service providers are inspected, and much less frequently ethics committees and independent study committees. Inspectors summarise their findings in a report such as a 'form 483' report after an inspection of a manufacturing plant, and send it to the management of the inspected site that has to propose an action plan in order to improve its performance. Inspection findings can lead to sanctions such as putting non-compliant investigators or organisations on a 'black list', closing a drug manufacturing plant, excluding the data from an investigator centre from a study analysis, etc.

In the interest of public health and to assure that the drug product is manufactured in accordance with the data that have been submitted to obtain marketing authorisation, the authorities can inspect the manufacturing premises and quality control laboratories to verify if the procedures described in the regulatory dossier are acceptable for marketing authorisation. If it appears that there is no alignment between the submitted data and the findings of the inspection team, the marketing authorisation of the drug product may be delayed or even refused. These inspections are therefore called 'pre-approval inspections' (PAI). A PAI starts from the following premise that:

- the data introduced into a clinical trial or marketing authorisation application are an accurate reflection of all the original scientific data that have been collected during drug development;
- the data that describe the manufacturing processes for clinical or commercial supply is to be considered as a "binding contract" between the manufacturer and the authorities; and
- the results of the scientific studies and the clinical trials have been produced under GMP for chemical and pharmaceutical data, GLP for nonclinical data and GCP for clinical data.

3.7.6 Quality risk management

The traditional approach to quality management in drug development is rather reactive and retrospective because the quality of a product or the outcome of a study is only checked near the end of the process. It is also labour intensive and expensive and based on only a few findings. This approach is based on:

- a set of guidelines (without much updating);
- procedures (SOPs and OPMs);
- intensive monitoring as quality control;
- a limited number of audits and inspections to check for non-compliance; and
- corrective actions to remove the cause of non-compliance.

In spite of these efforts, however, the top 5 deficiencies in clinical trial quality management did not change much since the introduction of GCP in 1996 [22]. Less than 3% of entered data in case report forms (CRFs) are corrected afterwards [23] and findings of FDA inspections giving rise to significant changes in regulatory decisions are relatively rare [24]. In addition, serious drug quality issues have not been prevented, as is shown by the closure of some manufacturing plants and the resulting drug shortages in the USA. Therefore, a radical paradigm shift in approaches of quality management in drug development became inevitable.

A new approach introduces risk management principles in quality management, known as 'Quality Risk Management' (QRM). This approach was first introduced in the chemical and pharmaceutical streams of drug development with the publication of the ICH Q9 guideline on 'Quality risk management' [25]. The objectives of this guideline are to:

- shift from reactive issue correction to proactive risk-based issue prevention;
- implement Quality by Design (QbD) principles;
- use the wealth of existing data on quality more efficiently to identify systematic issues earlier.

A quality by design (QbD) approach is an 'enhanced' approach towards product development in that its focus is on determining not only the right parameters of the manufacturing process and the specifications of the drug product but rather to conduct an indepth investigation of each and every material introduced in a manufacturing step of the drug product. Quality by design is discussed further in Chapter 5.

In this guideline, QRM is defined as 'a systematic process for the assessment, control, communication and review of risks to the quality of the drug product across the product lifecycle'. However, QRM should not be limited to improve GMP, as was the intention of ICH guideline Q9, but the underlying principles should now also be applied to GCP and to Good Pharmacovigilance Practices (GVP) as demonstrated by the recent publications of several guidance documents in these fields:

– the FDA guidance 'Oversight of clinical investigations – A risk-based approach to monitoring' [20];
– the EMA 'Reflection paper on risk based quality management in clinical trials' [21];
– the EMA guideline 'Good Pharmacovigilance Practices (GVP)' [26]. This is a set of several modules and annexes, some already published, and others to be published later; a table of contents is kept updated on the GVP webpage [27].

The principles of QRM are effectively utilised in many areas of business and government including finance, insurance, occupational safety, public health, pharmacovigilance and by the respective regulatory agencies. The importance of quality systems such as QRM has been recognised in the pharmaceutical industry although their full application remains rather limited. It is commonly understood that risk is defined as the combination of the probability of occurrence of harm (or hazard) and the severity of that hazard if it is materialised. However, achieving a common understanding of the application of risk management among various stakeholders is often difficult because each of them might perceive different potential hazards, place a different probability of occurrence and attribute different severities to each of them. Although there are many stakeholders in the development of drugs including patients, medical practitioners, authorities and industry, the protection of the patient by good risk management should be considered of prime importance.

Risk-based approaches such as QRM and quality by design (QbD) are already well-established activities in chemical and pharmaceutical drug development, but are getting only slowly introduced in clinical drug development. Examples of activities in clinical development where risk management is applied are: risk assessment before starting FIH studies; risk-based clinical trial management; risk-adapted clinical trial monitoring; risk-based audits and inspections; and risk management plans in relation to drug safety; but there is still a long way to go.

3.8 Project risk management

Drug development projects may fail because of serious safety concerns, poor pharmacokinetics or insufficient therapeutic efficacy. Chemical and pharmaceutical issues are rarely the cause of a decision to stop a drug development project. However, this is changing because of the increasing number of molecules with (very) low water solubility that is introduced in drug development.

3.8.1 Nature of risk

The severity as well as the probability of harm to occur in a drug development project should be taken into account in risk assessment and risk management. Important questions that have to be asked when a new drug development project is initiated are whether:

- Scientists involved in a drug development project have a clear view of the potential issues that may arise in the course of the project. For example, are chemical process engineers and medicinal chemists aware of potential intellectual property (IP) issues when they implement and develop a particular route of chemical synthesis?
- The list of potential concerns is complete. Is the drug development team aware of all possible threats to the project, not only based on all available data but also based on theoretical considerations?
- The drug development team is capable of reducing or avoiding the risk.
- The risk associated with a given project impedes other development projects in the drug portfolio.
- The risk is evenly spread over the drug portfolio

Once the risk factors of a project have been identified at the start of a project, the team has to share these findings with the functional teams and departments and contractors supporting the drug development project. This generates awareness and commitment to the project and develops the right attitude and focus of all scientists involved. When all activities and tests are conducted with the risk factors and appropriate risk-mitigation measures in mind, there is a greater chance that the risk will be kept under control. The management of risk consists of the identification of the risk, the analysis of the risk, the identification of appropriate mitigation measures and the tracking of the risk. During the course of the project risk should gradually decrease as more information becomes available and experience increases. For example, the development of a new pharmaceutical manufacturing process selected for the formulation of a water-insoluble drug may prove to be quite risky at the time of initiation while no proof is available that the drug will be absorbed and consistent systemic exposures will be achieved in humans. Once the initial hurdles of preliminary manufacturing campaigns and development activities are taken, a more stable process can be installed that – although not yet validated – will reduce the risk of failed batches, unpredictable systemic exposures and increasing costs. Once the manufacturing process has been demonstrated to be reproducible and consistently yield a product of high quality, the risk is further reduced. A low and acceptable risk level is reached when the manufacturing process is considered mature.

Although a substantial reduction of risk of a manufacturing process during development may contribute to the reduction of the overall risk of the project this does not mean that the overall risk has been eliminated. The overall risk of the project is only reduced to an acceptable level when the final clinical data (phase 3 clinical trials) have shown that the drug is safe and efficacious in patients and a marketing authorisation has been granted by regulatory authorities.

3.8.2   Types of risk

The types of risks that may impede the success of a drug development project are:

- Technical risks that are associated with safety, efficacy and manufacturability (quality).
- Business risks that are not only associated with financial aspects but also with the safety and efficacy of drugs of the same pharmacological class from the competition already on the market or still in development. The risk in such a case may become so high that a drug development organisation may decide to abandon the project to prevent further costs and the drug to become third or fourth choice in the physicians' therapeutic arsenal. Also, the business/customer pool may change during the project or issues with respect to intellectual property rights may surface.
- Team risks that are associated with the capacity of a drug development team to manage the project from a technical point of view. The careful selection of team members is crucial not only in view of their functional expertise but also in view of their capabilities as a team player. Finally, team leadership is crucial in securing the timelines and the quality of R&D output.
- Management risks that are associated with interdependence with other projects, critical timelines and a limited amount of resources (budget, people, equipment, infrastructure). These types of risk may be mitigated by assigning the most experienced managers to the development team who were found to be stress resistant in critical times or by careful balancing availability of resources versus need for resources at critical time points.

–   Organisational risks that are associated with the coordination of drug
    development team members and supportive functions often employed
    and active at different locations in the world.
–   External risks that are associated with external factors such as business,
    markets, and finance. For example, the conduct of a clinical trial can be
    interrupted when a critical component of the synthesis of the drug prod-
    uct is no longer available on the market.

In summary, a drug development team should not only address the technical
risks associated with the development of a drug candidate but should also
take into consideration the risks associated with the team's composition and
effectiveness, the organisational support, the technical and functional support
and the business environment.

3.8.3   Analysis of risk and 'show stoppers'

The analysis of risk can be rationalised by asking the question: 'What can go
wrong if the decision is taken to follow a specific approach in a specific domain
of a drug development project?' Each risk analysis needs to address:

–   the approach that is followed and the concern that is associated with that
    approach;
–   the potential problem that can be caused by that approach;
–   the consequence of the risk associated with the problem.

The combination of the issue (what the problem is), the concern (why the
issue is considered to be important and therefore may develop into a major
problem) and the consequence (what will happen if the concern materialises)
is the 'risk topic'. For example, a sudden drop in the *in vitro* dissolution profile of a new HIV drug may point to a flawed manufacturing process and may
result in a reduced systemic exposure of the drug in patients. In other words,
the problem, i.e. a pharmaceutical performance indicator, generates the concern of reduced systemic exposure with the potential (and grave) consequence
of developing HIV resistance.

It is appropriate to attempt to quantify the risk to allow a ranking of potential problems. In order to rank risks, two parameters are considered, i.e. the
severity if the concern materialises and the probability that the concern will be
materialised. In our example, the probability that the sudden drop in *in vitro*
dissolution results (or 'materialises') in a lower systemic exposure is high and
the severity of a reduced systematic exposure, i.e. the development of resistance, is equally high. If one would rank probability and severity along a scale
ranging from 1 to 3 to 5, then, in our example, both probability and severity
would be ranked as high as 5. Multiplying probability and severity results in a
factor that is termed a 'risk score' or:

$$\text{Risk score} = P\,(\text{probability}) \times S\,(\text{severity})$$

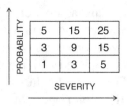

Figure 3.6   Risk score matrix.

In the example, the risk score is 25 ($P=$ 5 and $S=$ 5) which is the highest risk score that an 'issue' may entail, see Figure 3.6.

From this risk matrix, it can be inferred that risk levels may be as low as 1, because the probability that the concern is materialised is low and because the severity if the concern is materialised is low as well. In this case, the risk is considered acceptable. Risk scores that range between 1 and 3 are considered generally acceptable. Risk scores ranging between 5 and 9 are risks that should be addressed and every measure should be taken to reduce them further. The risk is only tolerable if it can be considered 'residual risk', i.e. if efforts have been made to remedy the risk but they all have failed. This is what is called the ALARP principle that means that the risk is 'As Low As Reasonable Practicable'. A risk, however, that ranges between 15 and 25 is considered unacceptable and must be reduced to a lower level. An issue that has a risk score of 25 and cannot be remedied is considered a "show stopper" and the project may be aborted. In our example, the sudden drop in *in vitro* dissolution is a 'show stopper' and everything needs to be done to remove the risk.

Although the actual number assigned to a risk score in itself has no meaning, the relative risk scores do because they allow the efforts to be prioritised in view of the overall project risk. Other aspects are also important when screening and ranking risks. These are the time and effort required to reduce the risks and the attention of the team to prevent risks to appear or develop. It is also important to weigh risks versus benefit. If benefit clearly outweighs the risk then it may be appropriate to accept the risk as such, but it is clear that this decision should be based upon facts, logical argumentation and the safety of the patient in mind. In all cases, the approach consists of reducing the severity of the risk and then identifying actions to reduce the probability with which the event may (still) occur. It is important to increase the detectability of the event causing the risk to prevent it re-appearing and causing harm.

3.9   Ethical considerations

This section focuses on ethics associated with biomedical research in drug development. First, some general aspects are discussed such as the responsible conduct of scientific research, the problem of conflicts of interest, and the issue of confidentiality versus transparency. Then, the use of experimental animals is considered, as well as the bioethics of experiments involving human subjects.

3.9.1 General aspects

3.9.1.1 Scientific research integrity

When researchers are under competitive pressure ('publish or perish') and the emphasis in their work is sometimes more focused on quantity than quality, irresponsible practices in research may result. An irresponsible form of misconduct in scientific research is fraud, which can be either due to fabrication, falsification or plagiarism of research data, results or publications. Milder types of misconduct are nevertheless unacceptable such as inappropriate use of statistical methods. Because there is currently no global standard code or guideline about the conduct of responsible research, the international organisations of science academies IAC (InterAcademy Council) and IAP (formerly InterAcademy Panel) published a joint policy report 'Responsible conduct in the global research enterprise' (October 2012) offering guidance on the basic responsibilities and obligations of researchers and research institutions [28]. The fundamental scientific research values are honesty, fairness, objectivity, reliability, scepticism, accountability and openness.

3.9.1.2 Conflicts of interest

In the case of drug development, conflicts of interest play an important role. Frequently this is associated with financial interest, but inappropriate use of influence, undue pressure or abuse of power may play a role. During drug development, potential conflicts of interest exist between the sponsor of the research (e.g. a commercial drug development organisation or a noncommercial research foundation) and other actors in the field. Actors such as the investigator, the contract research institute, members of the Independent Ethics Committee (IEC) or Institutional Review Board (IRB), members of a Data Monitoring or other study committees, decision makers in regulatory agencies, reimbursement committees, and committees responsible for editing clinical practice guidelines, as well as scientific/medical journal editors and peer reviewers may become subject of conflict of interest. Some, if not most, organisations develop a code of conduct to prevent improper influence, guided by the following principles: independence whenever possible (although expertise is sometimes concentrated so that key positions are often occupied by the same experts), a balanced composition of committees, and transparency when conflicts arise. Examples of disclosure policies for potential conflicts of interest are the financial disclosure forms completed by clinical investigators and used by NDA applicants, by external experts participating in EMA or FDA meetings, and by authors who wish to publish their research in a journal belonging to the International Committee of Medical Journal Editors (ICMJE).

3.9.1.3 Confidentiality versus transparency

All data collected during development are confidential and constitute the intellectual property of the drug development organisation. This applies for example to the chemical manufacturing process, the drug delivery technology, the animal toxicology data and the clinical research data. However, there is an increased pressure on the drug development organisation to be transparent about its clinical development data. Currently, drug development organisations are required to communicate the results of their clinical trials, the observed adverse effects and pharmacovigilance data and make them publicly available. This requirement for public transparency is not applicable to nonclinical experimental data and data on chemical and pharmaceutical production processes and drug products. There is also an increased pressure to make available the data obtained during the clinical trial to the clinical research participants. Finally, evaluations carried out and decisions made by the drug agencies are to be made publicly available as well. The interested reader can find a lot of information on this topic on the website of the AllTrials initiative 'All trials registered | All results reported' (www.alltrials.net).

3.9.2   Use of experimental animals

It is not possible to conduct a safety assessment project in drug development without the use of live animals. Considerable progress is being made in the reduction of the use of experimental animals, the replacement of *in vivo* systems by equally valid *in vitro* test systems and the refinement of test methods and test strategies to reduce pain, suffering and distress in experimental animals (principle of the three Rs). In drug discovery and early drug development *in vivo* testing in toxicology and safety pharmacology is replaced as much as possible by *in vitro* alternatives (e.g. bacteria for the detection of mutagens, microsomes for comparative drug metabolism, genetically engineered cells for cardiovascular safety). Later in drug development *in vivo* systems are required to obtain more accurate data on the possible toxic effects of the drug candidate in humans. For some toxicological endpoints such as skin corrosion, skin and eye irritation and skin sensitisation progress has been made to reduce or eliminate animal suffering. Animal testing can be adequately replaced by well-validated *in vitro* test systems such as the bovine corneal opacity and permeability assay (BCOP, Section 4.3.3.3) in eye irritation testing and the local lymph node assay in the mouse (LLNA, Section 4.3.3.3) for skin sensitisation testing. For some aspects of local tolerance testing such as tolerance for intravenous applications most alternative *in vitro* systems are not fully predictive of the *in vivo* situation. When there is no alternative to *in vivo* testing the experiment should be performed in such a way that unnecessary pain, suffering, distress or lasting harm in the test animals is avoided or minimised as much as possible. The use and care of experimental animals are regulated and compliance of any breeder, supplier or testing laboratory with these regulations is imposed by the authorities. These regulations apply to:

-   the replacement and reduction of the use of experimental animals and further refinement of test procedures and living conditions;
-   breeding, care, accommodation and sacrifice;
-   operations of breeders, suppliers and users;
-   evaluation and authorisation of projects;
-   all live non-human vertebrate animals including larval and fetal forms and live cephalopods.

The facilities that handle and use experimental animals should be accredited for that purpose and compliance with animal welfare regulations is ensured by regular inspections of the facilities by the national competent authority. In choosing between procedures of animal testing, the procedure should be selected that uses a minimum number of animals and causes minimal pain, suffering, distress or lasting harm to the animals without compromising the objective of the study. Death as the endpoint of a procedure should be avoided as much as possible. When this cannot be avoided the number of animals dying should be kept as low as possible and the duration and intensity of the suffering as minimal as possible. Painful procedures should only be carried out under local or general anaesthesia or analgesia. The management of facilities handling and using experimental animals should appoint a doctor in veterinary medicine with experience in laboratory animal sciences and medicine to be in charge of the animal welfare programme. Laboratory staff should be adequately trained to carry out experimental procedures on animals, taking care of animals and sacrificing animals humanely.

Each breeder, supplier or test laboratory must install an internal ethics committee (animal welfare body in the EU, institutional animal care and use committee in the USA) that is composed of a doctor in veterinary medicine, at least one practicing scientist of the facility and at least one member representing general community interests and not being affiliated with the facility. It is the responsibility of this committee to:

-   advice laboratory staff on matters relating to animal welfare;
-   advice laboratory staff on how to apply as much as possible the principles of replacement, reduction and refinement;
-   inspect the facilities for compliance with animal welfare regulations and policies;
-   submit reports to facility management;
-   prepare and review animal care and use protocols;
-   monitor and report on procedures relating to animal welfare;
-   review and authorise animal studies.

One of the major responsibilities of the ethics committee is the review and the approval of animal studies that are to be performed in the facility.

To this effect the following aspects of the experiment are taken into consideration:

- rationale and purpose of the study that justifies the use of animals;
- justification of the selection of the species and number of animals requested;
- availability of alternatives (less invasive techniques, other species, *in vitro* testing);
- adequacy of training of personnel to conduct the study;
- housing and husbandry requirements;
- methods proposed for sedation, analgesia and anaesthesia;
- unnecessary duplication of experiments;
- multiple major operative procedures;
- criteria to reduce suffering of the animals (removal, sacrifice);
- methods for euthanasia and disposition of animals;
- methods of physical restraint (devices, duration, training, veterinary intervention).

All animals should be provided with appropriate accommodation, environment, food, water and care. Restrictions of the animal's physiological and ethological needs should be kept to a minimum and animals should be transported under appropriate conditions. Guidelines covering animal experimentation are available at several websites [29–31].

3.9.3   Experiments involving human subjects

This section deals with ethical aspects of biomedical research involving human subjects in general, and more specifically with ethical considerations related to clinical drug development.

3.9.3.1   Brief historical background
Since the Hippocratic Oath in ancient Greek times, *primum non nocere* (first, do not harm) has been the basic ethical principle of western medicine. It wasn't until 1949 that the Nuremberg Code defined legitimate experiments in humans. This Code includes principles such as informed consent, scientifically sound experiments, absence of coercion, and beneficence to participants. In 1964, the World Medical Association published the Declaration of Helsinki, the cornerstone of current thinking about the ethical conduct of biomedical research that involves human subjects. In the meantime it has been revised several times [32, 33]. The Declaration of Helsinki has been incorporated in the ICH E6 Good Clinical Practice guideline (1996) and has since then been the legal basis of the ethical standard for clinical studies.

3.9.3.2   Basic principles and the Declaration of Helsinki
The 3 basic principles of bioethics in human experiments are explained in Table 3.10.

Table 3.10   Principles of bioethics in human experiments.

Respect for research subjects	Recognising that they are autonomous human beings, thus implicating that their informed consent should be obtained before starting the trial. Equally, less autonomous subjects (e.g. young children, unconscious patients, patients with dementia) should be maximally protected
Beneficence	The welfare of the research participant is of primary importance. Hence, the obligation to do no harm and to maximise the benefit/risk ratio for the subjects and society
Fairness	A fair and right treatment of the study participants. Their altruism should be no blank cheque

The Declaration of Helsinki combines both ethical and operational principles in relation to the conduct of biomedical research in humans. The most important principles are cited in Table 3.11.

3.9.3.3   Ethics review of clinical research

Before the start of a clinical trial, the study should be approved by an Independent Ethics Committee (IEC) or Institutional Review Board (IRB) that will review whether the rights, safety and wellbeing of the participants are sufficiently guaranteed and the study is scientifically sound. The IEC/IRB should review the protocol, the Investigator Brochure, the informed consent form, the curriculum vitae of the investigators, subject recruitment procedures (e.g. advertisements), and payments to study participants; all within a certain time limit (different from country to country). It can ask questions and can request the investigator to give verbal explanation about certain aspects of the trial.

After approval and during the conduct of the trial, the IEC/IRB monitors the study on a regular basis, according to the risks involved and the safety

Table 3.11   Ethical and operational principles in human experiments.

Ethical principles	Respect for the individual and their right to make informed decisions (refusal to participate in a trial may not jeopardise the patient–physician relationship and the medical care of a patient), the subject's welfare must always take precedence over the interests of science and society, increased vulnerability of research participants calls for special vigilance
Operational principles	Research in humans should always be science based (scientifically unsound research is by definition unethical), there should be a reasonable belief of benefit for the study population, the protocol should be approved by an IEC/IRB and the study executed by qualified investigators, the trial should be registered in a public data base before its start and a fair account of the results should be published, new interventions should be tested against the best current treatment, one should be extremely careful about the use of placebo, and research participants should have post-trial access to the best intervention studied

information received. Substantial amendments to the study protocol should also receive approval before they are implemented. The organisation of IEC/IRB reviews of clinical trials differs from country to country. In some countries, the review is done by the Ethics Committee (EC) of the institution where the study is conducted, but in others it can be done by an EC that is independent of the trial site. For multicentre and multinational trials in the EU, the review is centralised in a single Ethics Committee per country, and again depending on the country, either in one of the participating centres or by an independent EC. In some countries, the reviewing Ethics Committees needs to be 'accredited', while in others this is not the case. Similarly, Independent Ethics Committees can be commercial or non-for-profit organisations, both performing in accordance with the same standards. Information regarding the composition of an IEC/IRB and its functioning can be found in the GCP guideline.

3.9.3.4   Use of placebo

Although there are ethical concerns about the use of placebo in human experiments (see the Declaration of Helsinki), many placebo-controlled clinical trials are still conducted during drug development. The main reason is that it is the only practical way to determine the true specific effects of a drug, independent of other non-specific effects. Non-specific effects can be study effects (the result of merely participating in a study and being particularly well monitored) and placebo effects (positive or negative effects due to disease regression/progression or impact of other extrinsic factors). Including a control arm in the study treated with placebo (therapeutically inactive formulation similar to the active formulation), and assuming that the non-specific effects will be the same in the active (or 'verum') and the control arms (in a randomised and blinded design), allows determination of the true drug effect by comparing the results in the placebo arm with the results in the active arm.

The importance of the placebo effect (measured by the percentage of placebo responders) varies greatly as a function of the pathology and is more pronounced in symptoms where psychological factors play a role, e.g. in depression, angina pectoris, pain, etc. The ethical problem of placebo treatment lies in the fact that a proven effective medicine might be withheld from these patients. The use of placebo in these circumstances can be acceptable provided that certain precautions are taken such as:

– using an add-on design, i.e. all study groups receive the best available treatment and 'on top of' the active test drug or placebo;
– accepting that the test drug is individually stopped prematurely in case a problem arises according to escape criteria described in the study protocol (the percentage of 'stoppers' can even be an outcome measure);

- accepting individual rescue medication in case of problems (again according to pre-specified criteria);
- providing extra monitoring and follow-up of patients (e.g. in the case of depressive patients with suicidal ideation);
- foreseeing an independent Data Monitoring Committee (DMC) or Data and Safety Monitoring Board (DSMB) to manage stopping rules.

3.9.3.5 Informed consent

Before being enrolled in a clinical trial, study participants must consent to participate after having received all necessary information to freely decide autonomously to participate or not. The information should be given orally, by the investigator or a team member, with sufficient time for questions and explanation. A detailed written information form, approved by the IEC/IRB, should also be available and the subject should receive ample time to discuss his/her participation with relatives. When ready, the participant signs and dates the Informed Consent Form (ICF), which is countersigned by the investigator and filed in the Investigator study file. The GCP guideline foresees at least 20 items to be included in the ICF adapted to the trial, e.g. study objectives, treatments (maybe placebo), procedures, benefits, risks and inconveniences, payment and compensation, that participation is voluntary, may be refused or withdrawn without consequences for the subject, that sponsor personnel and inspectors may have direct access to the original medical records, that the subject's identity will be kept confidential, and the contact details of a contact person in case of need for additional information. Special attention should be paid to informed consent in vulnerable subjects. When the participant is unable to give informed consent himself (e.g. children or demented patients), the legal representative can sign the ICF. In emergency situations or with unconscious patients, where prior consent is impossible, a legal representative should consent when available. Once the study participant is again able to consent himself, his proper consent should be requested to maintain him in the study.

A valid informed consent from the study participant supposes that he/she:

- is sufficiently knowledgeable about the study, i.e. that he/she can easily understand and read the given information, which assumes the use of simple lay language;
- is sufficiently competent to comprehend the given information and to assess the consequences (particularly tricky in vulnerable subjects);
- consents out of free will, without coercion or outside influence.

With the ascent of modern media, the information process of study participants is no longer limited to oral and written information, but includes the use of pictures, (animated) cartoons, films and videos (especially in the case of children).

3.9.3.6   Payments

Clinical trials can be very demanding of the participants because many visits to the investigational centre are necessary, or multiple or lengthy exams and procedures causing discomfort, as well as lifestyle restrictions. Therefore, payments of study subjects, healthy volunteers or patients, are sometimes justified. Extra expenses (e.g. travel costs) can be reimbursed and payments for trial participation may be considered, provided that they remain reasonable and related to the inconvenience and discomfort incurred. Payment should never be related to risk. The amount of payment should be stated in the informed consent form and approved by the IEC/IRB.

3.9.3.7   Confidentiality

In a sensitive area such as drug development, where competition is fierce and considerable personal medical data are handled, it is no surprise that confidentiality plays an important role.

Commercially sensitive information about the drug and the studies should be kept confidential. In particular, investigators and their staff should be aware of the confidentiality rules laid down in the study protocol and/or the contract between the sponsor and the site. Investigators who perform clinical drug trials for different sponsors should see to it that the different study data and files are kept apart from one another.

Protection of the privacy of study participants is important in relation to their identity, their personal data, and their biospecimens (e.g. blood, urine, tissue biopsies, isolated stem cells, genetic material, etc). Most of these aspects are currently regulated in legislation addressing privacy, data protection and the storage and use of biological specimens, which may differ among countries.

The full identity of study participants should be kept confidential. A unique identifier should be used when collecting, handling, storing and reporting study related data. Personal data (sensitive data such as ethnic descent or sexual orientation, and health data) should be handled with special care. Different rules apply when the data are identifiable (directly or indirectly), coded (with a unique identifier only available to the investigator), anonymised (non-identifiable retrospectively), or anonymous (collected as such). These should be clearly specified in the study protocol. Tissue sampling and biobank storage requires even stricter rules, especially when genetic testing is included in the study protocol. Whenever a genetic signature of a subject is requested for current or future research, it should be clearly stated as such in the informed consent form. If the genetic test is done on coded biospecimens, then the protocol should foresee if and how the subject should be informed about the result. If it is decided that it should be performed on an anonymized sample, and the result is only available for current and future research, then the subject should be equally well informed via the informed consent form.

3.10   The global nature of drug development

The pharmaceutical business, like many other businesses today, is a global enterprise. Many pharmaceutical companies are large multinationals that operate worldwide. The main drivers of globalisation are an open economy, economies of scale and operational efficiency gains. The major advantage of this approach is that innovative medicines can reach more patients faster worldwide, although this 'access to all' principle remains a challenge, as illustrated by the limited availability of high-priced anti-HIV and targeted anti-cancer drugs in developing countries. A disadvantage of this evolution is criminal abuse, such as the worldwide distribution of substandard and counterfeit medicines.

Within this context, the development of new drugs has also become a global enterprise. The globalisation of drug development has largely been facilitated by the creation in 1990 of the International Conference on Harmonisation (ICH), with the objective to harmonise regulatory requirements for drug registration in the USA, Europe and Japan (soon extended to other countries as well). Global harmonisation of regulatory guidelines and requirements avoids duplication of drug testing, allows that clinical data from one region are used for Marketing Authorisation (MA) applications in other regions, and enables worldwide MA applications on the basis of a common technical dossier, ultimately leading to reduced development times and costs.

Other supra-national organisations or projects, such as the World Health Organisation (WHO), the Organisation for Economic Co-operation and Development (OECD), the agreement on Trade-Related aspects of Intellectual Property Rights (TRIPS), the Pharmaceutical Inspection Co-operation Scheme (PIC/S), and the European Union (EU), have also developed harmonised standards or taken initiatives to stimulate regional and global co-operation on regulatory processes (e.g. mutual recognition of drug authorisations) and practices (e.g. sharing review and inspection reports between regulatory authorities). All together, these measures contributed to the increasingly global nature of drug development.

Despite all these efforts for worldwide regulatory convergence that should make life easier for drug development organisations, there is still a lot of disparity, variance or disagreement between regions and countries when it comes to certain issues related to drug development and approval. For example, China, Taiwan and South Korea still require some clinical trials to be performed locally, and there is not always agreement between the EMA and the FDA on drug approval and labelling on the basis of the same MA application. There are many reasons for this, to name but a few: (real or perceived) differences in target patient populations, different patterns of medical practice, disagreement on clinical study endpoints, national protectionist measures, while some authorities are just more risk averse than others. Therefore, any global drug development strategy should also respect these local specificities ('think global, act local').

In applying a global approach to new drug development, a lot of attention should go to the identification and control of ethnic factors that may influence the drug's effectiveness and safety. Therefore, ICH has issued a guideline on 'Ethnic factors in the acceptability of foreign clinical data' [34], later complemented by a 'Questions and Answers' document to clarify key issues [35], while the EMA released a 'Reflection paper on the extrapolation of results from clinical studies conducted outside the EU to the EU-population' [36]. Ethnic characteristics that might influence drug effects are classified as intrinsic (related to the drug recipient, such as patient, pathogen or tumour genotype) or extrinsic (related to the environment or culture). As part of a global development strategy, it is recommended to verify whether the new drug is sensitive to (some of) these ethnic factors (e.g. is less efficacious in black as opposed to white people, or has specific side effects in Asians as opposed to Caucasians) and to suggest how to control these different effects (e.g. by adapting the drug dosage or dosing regimen). Some of these factors are not only important to explain inter-regional drug differences, but may also play a role within one region. In practice, extrinsic characteristics are the most problematic to deal with, i.e. differences in medical practice (e.g. use of different comparator drugs or co-medications), in disease definition (e.g. heterogeneous medical conditions, different interpretation of scores/scales), or in study population (e.g. different life style, medical and social environment). The guideline also introduces the concept of a 'bridging study' that a new region may require in order to determine whether clinical data from a foreign region are acceptable for its own population (only if the results are demonstrated to be similar in both regions).

Two different development strategies can be applied to study (and cope with) these regional or population differences. Either the clinical development plan explores these differences from the start with specific studies in early drug development, followed by multi-regional clinical trials in late development, or alternatively, the clinical development is conducted entirely in one region or population, and is later supplemented with a bridging study in (each of) the new region(s) or population(s) in order to verify whether the initial results can be used to substantiate worldwide drug approval.

There are numerous operational and logistic challenges to conduct a global drug development programme, especially with regard to large multi-regional clinical trials, such as:

– sufficient knowledge of region- or country-specific regulatory requirements;
– identification and choice of participating countries and investigator sites;
– production of study drugs and management of the drug-supply chain (including customs clearance);

- document handling in different languages; and
- monitoring or auditing of sites all over the world.

Therefore, most (even large multinational) pharmaceutical companies tend to outsource all or part of these activities to large full-service Contract Research Organisations (CROs) that operate worldwide, but without delegating either their responsibility or their accountability.

Finally, the globalisation of drug development has had a profound impact on the geographical distribution of locations where clinical trials are performed. Until two decades ago, almost all clinical trials were conducted in developed or mature areas such as the USA and Western Europe, but today, an ever-increasing part of these studies is carried out in emerging or developing regions such as Eastern Europe, Asia (especially China, India, and Asia Pacific), Latin America, and the Middle East. In the beginning there was some concern about the quality of clinical studies performed in these emerging countries. However, a comparison of the quality of data from a large number of clinical trials conducted across the globe revealed no significant differences in trial quality between different emerging and mature regions or countries [37].

References

[1] ICH Guideline. General considerations for clinical trials (E8), 17 July 1997.
[2] http://www.gpo.gov/, Accessed: July 8th, 2013.
[3] http://ec.europa.eu/health/index_en.htm, Accessed: July 8th, 2013.
[4] Directive 2001/20/EC of the European Parliament and of the Council of 4 April 2001 on the approximation of the laws, regulations and administrative provisions of the Member States relating to the implementation of good clinical practice in the conduct of clinical trials on medicinal products for human use.
[5] Commission Directive 2005/28/EC of 8 April 2005 laying down principles and detailed guidelines for good clinical practice as regards investigational medicinal products for human use, as well as the requirements for authorisation of the manufacturing or importation of such product.
[6] Commission Directive 2003/94/EC of 8 October 2003 laying down the principles and guidelines of good manufacturing practice in respect of medicinal products for human use and investigational medicinal products for human use - Replacement of Commission Directive 91/356/EC of 13 June 1991 to cover good manufacturing practice of investigational medicinal products.
[7] OECD Series on Principles of Good Laboratory Practice and Compliance monitoring (1998), Number 1, OECD Principles on Good Laboratory Practice (as revised in 1997), ENV/MC/CHEM(98)17, OECD, Paris.
[8] https://eudract.ema.europa.eu/, Accessed: July 8th, 2013, 2013.
[9] https://www.clinicaltrialsregister.eu/, Accessed: July 8th, 2013.
[10] http://www.fda.gov/drugs/developmentapprovalprocess/, Accessed: July 8th, 2013.
[11] http://ec.europa.eu/health/documents/eudralex/vol-10/, Accessed: July 8th, 2013.
[12] http://www.ich.org/products/guidelines/efficacy/article/efficacy-guidelines.html, Accessed: July 8th, 2013.

[13] Regulation (EC) No 1901/2006 of the European Parliament and of the Council of 12 December 2006 on medicinal products for paediatric use and amending Regulation (EEC) No 1768/92, Directive 2001/20/EC, Directive 2001/83/EC and Regulation (EC) No 726/2004.

[14] http://www.fda.gov/Drugs/DevelopmentApprovalProcess/DevelopmentResources/ ucm049867.htm, Accessed: July 8th, 2013.

[15] http://ec.europa.eu/health/documents/eudralex/, Accessed July 8th, 2013.

[16] http://www.fda.gov/Drugs/DevelopmentApprovalProcess/HowDrugsareDeveloped andApproved/default.htm, Accessed July 8th, 2013.

[17] http://www.fda.gov/Drugs/DevelopmentApprovalProcess/FormsSubmissionRequire ments/DrugMasterFilesDMFs/UCM2007046, Accessed July 8th, 2013.

[18] Committee of Human Medicinal Products CHMP/QWP/227/02 Rev 3 and Committee of Veterinary Medicinal Products EMEA/CVMP/134/02 Rev 3, Guideline on Active Substance Master File Procedure, 31 May 2013.

[19] http://www.edqm.eu/en/certification-new-applications-29.html, Accessed July 8th, 2013.

[20] FDA Guidance for Industry. Oversight of clinical investigations – A risk-based approach to monitoring, August 2013.

[21] EMA Guidance. Reflection paper on risk based quality management in clinical trials, 18 November 2013.

[22] http://www.fda.gov/AboutFDA/CentersOffices/OfficeofMedicalProductsandTobacco/ CDER/ucm256374.htm, Accessed July 11th, 2013.

[23] http://www.mdsol.com/About Us/Resource Library/White Papers (Adopting Site Quality Management to Optimize Risk-Based Monitoring), Accessed July 11th, 2013.

[24] Meeker-O'Connell A & Ball L K (2011) Current trends in FDA inspections assessing clinical trial quality: an analysis of CDER's experience. *FDLI (Food and Drug Law Institute) Update* **2:** 8–12.

[25] ICH Guideline. Quality risk management (Q9), 9 November 2005.

[26] EMA Guidelines on good pharmacovigilance practices (GVP), 8 January 2014.

[27] http://www.ema.europa.eu/ema/index.jsp?curl=pages/regulation/document_listing/ document_listing_000345.jsp, Accessed 10th February, 2014.

[28] http://www.interacademycouncil.net/24026/GlobalReport.aspx, Accessed July 8th, 2013.

[29] http://www.aphis.usda.gov/animal_welfare/awr.shtml, Accessed July 8th, 2013.

[30] http://grants.nih.gov/grants/olaw/olaw.htm, July 8th, 2013.

[31] http://eur-lex.europa.eu, Accessed July 8th, 2013.

[32] http://eur-lex.europa.eu/LexUriServ/LexUriServ.do?uri=CELEX:31999D0575:EN: NOT; Accessed July 8th, 2013.

[33] The World Medical Association (2013). WMA Declaration of Helsinki – Ethical principles for medical research involving human subjects, WMA Inc., Fortaleza, Brazil.

[34] ICH Guideline E5(R1). (February 1998) Ethnic factors in the acceptability of foreign clinical data. ICH, Geneva.

[35] ICH Guidance document E5 Q&As (R1). (June 2006) Questions and Answers: Ethnic factors in the acceptability of foreign clinical data. ICH, Geneva.

[36] EMA-CHMP Guidance document. (October 2009) Reflection paper on the extrapolation of results from clinical studies conducted outside the EU to the EU-population. EMA, London.

[37] Desai PB, Anderson C, Sietsema WK. (2012) A comparison of the quality of data, assessed using query rates, from clinical trials conducted across developed versus emerging global regions. *Drug Information Journal*, **46** (4), 455–463.

4

Methods and Techniques Used in Drug Development

4.1 Introduction

To facilitate the reading of Chapters 5 and 6 that address the processes of early and late development, this chapter describes a selected number of methods and techniques used in drug development. It is not the objective of this chapter to provide the reader with detailed information on the conduct of laboratory and clinical tests. The intention is rather to explain why these methods and techniques are used and on what principles they are based. When needed, a summary is given of the conduct of tests. The methods and techniques described in this chapter constitute the toolbox of drug development and are organised according to the three main drug development streams: chemical and pharmaceutical development, nonclinical development and clinical development. Some of the methods and techniques described in one development stream are equally applied in others, although most of the time in a different form.

4.2 Chemical and pharmaceutical development

A vast number of methods and techniques are used in chemical and pharmaceutical development. They range from analytical chemistry to full-scale drug manufacturing. Since it is impossible to describe all of them, the methods and techniques selected in this section refer to the physicochemical characterisation of the active ingredient, the formulation of the active ingredient and the determination of the quality of the active ingredient and the drug product [1, 2].

Global New Drug Development: An Introduction, First Edition.
Jan A. Rosier, Mark A. Martens and Josse R. Thomas.
© 2014 John Wiley & Sons, Ltd. Published 2014 by John Wiley & Sons, Ltd.

4.2.1   Physicochemical characterisation of the active ingredient

4.2.1.1   Introduction

The methods described below constitute an important part of early chemical and pharmaceutical drug development activities. They are used to determine the physicochemical characteristics of the active ingredient that may have an impact on the performance of the drug product. The performance of the drug product is the extent by which a drug product (e.g. oral tablet) is capable of making the active ingredient systemically available. Since the performance of a drug product is not only driven by the pharmaceutical technology used to develop the dosage form, but also by the physicochemical characteristics of the active ingredient, the following methods and techniques constitute a pivotal part in the development of the active ingredient and the drug product [2].

4.2.1.2   pK and solubility testing

One of the main objectives of early formulation research is to develop oral solutions of the drug candidate with sufficient bioavailability. In recent decades the number of molecules that entered the development pipeline with poor aqueous solubility has increased considerably. Therefore, the determination of the solubility of new active ingredients is performed as one of the first tests in drug development. Solubility determinations are conducted by exposing an excess of solid to a given solvent for about 60–72 h at a given temperature with stirring. Once equilibrium is attained, the concentration of the active ingredient in the solvent phase is determined after separation by filtration or centrifugation. Active ingredients can be subdivided into two major categories: ionisable substances and non-ionisable substances. In case of ionisable compounds such as carboxylic acids and amines the pK value can be determined. The pK value is used to express the extent of dissociation or the strength of weak acids. The dielectric constant is also a key parameter to study the solubility of non-ionisable compounds. For ionisable compounds acid–base titrations are used to determine their solubility as a function of the pH. Solvent(s) and mixtures thereof are used for the determination of the solubility of non-ionisable compounds. More detail on these techniques can be found in textbooks on physicochemistry.

4.2.1.3   Polymorphic modifications

Polymorphism is an important aspect of the physical properties of a drug. Because of the complexity of the chemical structure of most drugs many different polymorph forms can exist. They can be either amorphous or crystalline. In crystalline compounds individual molecules are positioned in lattice sites or three-dimensional arrays. Each polymorphic form may have different physicochemical properties such as solubility, melting point, plasticity and hygroscopicity, and as a consequence may affect the technological and biopharmaceutical properties of the active ingredient and the drug product. The knowledge of the polymorphic form of a drug candidate is important for the development of the first formulations to be used in nonclinical testing. Stable polymorphs have a lower solubility than metastable polymorphic forms and thus have poorer biopharmaceutical properties [1,3]. When metastable forms of drug candidates are to be selected to enhance bioavailability, the metastable form has to be shown to be sufficiently stable during the processing and storage of the drug product. It is therefore essential to select the most suitable polymorphic form in the early stage of drug development. Different polymorphs can be made by means of appropriate recrystallisation techniques using different solvent systems and the selection of the polymorphic form for further development drives the selection of the manufacturing process. Only one polymorphic form is thermodynamically stable and the other metastable forms will convert, eventually, to the more stable form. Thus, transformation towards a more stable polymorphic form can occur as a result of pharmaceutical processing such as milling, grinding, tabletting, spray drying and granulation. Early detection and quantification of these transformations is important to ensure the quality of the finished drug product. An analytical method to study polymorphic behaviour of drugs is differential scanning calorimetry (DSC). DSC is a thermoanalytical technique in which the difference in the amount of heat required to increase the temperature of a sample and reference is measured as a function of temperature.

4.2.1.4 Partition coefficient

The partition coefficient of a drug is a physicochemical parameter that is determined in late discovery or early development. It represents the partition of a drug molecule between an aqueous phase and a lipid phase. The lipid phase most used for the determination of the partition coefficient is 1-octanol. The partition coefficient is expressed as the log of the concentration of the drug in 1-octanol divided by its concentration in water when in equilibrium ($\log P_{ow}$ with 'o' for oil or octanol and 'w' for water). The partition coefficient of drugs can be determined according to the HPLC method, the shake flask method or the slow stirring method. The $\log P_{ow}$ provides a first indication on how easily the drug can reach the systemic circulation and the intended target in the body. It is also used to get an idea of the tendency of the unchanged drug to accumulate in the body. A drug with a relatively high $\log P_{ow}$ (e.g. 3.5) does not necessarily accumulate in the body when it undergoes extensive metabolism. The $\log P_{ow}$ is a selection criterion that is used (among many others) to assess the 'druggability' of a molecule. For a drug to be orally absorbed, it should first pass through the lipid bilayers of the membrane of the enterocytes in the intestinal epithelium. For an efficient passage through these layers, the drug must be hydrophobic enough to 'partition' into the lipid bilayer, but not to the extent that once it is in the bilayer, it remains there and does not distribute into the systemic circulation.

4.2.1.5 Surface characteristics

For active ingredients to be processed in drug product manufacturing such as the filling into capsules, surface characteristics may play an important role. Particles may appear in different forms such as plates, needles and cubes that greatly influence their flowing behaviour during handling in pharmaceutical production. Therefore, photomicrographs are taken to observe the surface characteristics of the active ingredient and used as a reference during later processing experiments.

4.2.1.6 Compatibility testing

One of the first experiments that are conducted in the early phases of pharmaceutical development is compatibility testing. Compatibility testing identifies the excipients that cannot be used in combination with the active ingredient because they may interact and lead to a change of the composition of the drug product. Some excipients may chemically react with the active ingredient and cause its degradation. Others may cause liquefaction, a phenomenon whereby a mixture of the active ingredient with an excipient results in eutectic formation as is observed in caffeine combinations. Eutectic formation takes place when compounds come into intimate contact with each other in the solid state (e.g. during compaction) and when they are mutually soluble in each other in the liquid state.

4.2.1.7 Decomposition

A broad screen of stability testing is performed during early development to assess the stability of the active ingredient. These studies are also referred to as 'forced decomposition studies' whereby the compound is exposed to acid degradation, alkaline degradation, aqueous degradation, dry powder degradation, degradation under the influence of light and oxidative stress degradation by, for example, an oxidising substance such as hydrogen peroxide.

4.2.2   Formulation of the active ingredient

4.2.2.1 Introduction

At this stage it is appropriate to explain the difference between terms such as 'pharmaceutical formulation', 'dosage form' and 'finished drug product' as these are frequently used in the development of a drug. The term pharmaceutical formulation or formulation refers to the quantitative and qualitative composition of a drug product and the formulation technologies that are used to produce such a formulation. A dosage form relates to the route of administration such as the oral, parenteral or transdermal route and to its physical appearance. The finished drug product is the combination of a pharmaceutical formulation that consists of an active ingredient and excipients introduced in an appropriate dosage form to be administered to patients and of the packaging. The packaging consists of the outer packaging such as a carton box and the inner or immediate packaging such as a blister or a bottle. The term 'formulation' is thus used to focus on the changes that occur in the composition of a drug product during development. The term 'formulation change' refers to the changes in the quantitative composition. A 'phase 1 formulation' is the term assigned to the drug product used in a human pharmacology trial. A 'phase 2 formulation' is the term assigned to the drug product used in a therapeutic exploratory trial.

Pharmaceutical or drug formulation is the scientific discipline that transforms active ingredients into a 'form' (a *dosage* form) that can be administered to experimental animals or to humans (healthy volunteers and patients) to make the drug molecule systemically available [4]. The science of drug formulation can be divided into two major parts: classical and high-tech formulation. There are various types of dosage forms such as oral tablets, intravenous solutions, inhalation formulations and implants and their selection is driven by the therapeutic indication of the active ingredient. In pre-clinical toxicology studies, for example, the dosage form has to be kept simple because it needs to be prepared in a laboratory environment from small quantities of active ingredient. At the same time it has to assure sufficient bioavailability for proper toxicology testing. In general, at this stage in development the oral formulations for toxicology are solutions or suspensions. When dosage forms are developed for patients, they should be patient friendly, ensure compliance, be stable for many years and manufacturable at large scale with an acceptable cost of goods structure. The following section presents an – oversimplified – overview of the major pharmaceutical dosage forms that can be developed.

4.2.2.2 Enteral and parenteral formulations

Enteral formulations are dosage forms that are developed for oral administration. Typical examples are tablets and capsules. In both cases the active pharmaceutical ingredient is mixed with a number of inactive ingredients, also called excipients. Excipients are used to ensure the stability and manufacturability of the dosage form and to enable the absorption of the active ingredient from the gastrointestinal tract.

A tablet is a mixture of the active ingredient and excipients that is compressed into a predetermined shape. Generally, it contains approximately 5-10% of the active ingredient and the remaining material consists of fillers, disintegrants, lubricants, glidants and binders. For example, fillers are used to make sure that the tablet is sufficiently large to be handled in case of low dosage strengths (microgram or milligram range). Disintegration excipients aid in the disintegration of the tablet once it is introduced into the gastrointestinal tract. The time needed for a tablet to disintegrate is the disintegration time and it is used as a quality control test to measure the speed by which an active ingredient is released from the dosage form. The time that is required to release and to dissolve the active ingredient from an oral dosage form can be measured *in vitro* at body temperature using solutions simulating gastric and intestinal content and is called the *in vitro* dissolution time.

A capsule is a simple gelatinous envelope that consists of a body and a cap. The drug and the excipients is present in the capsule as a powder. Capsule contents – in contrast with tablets – are not compressed. Tablets as well as capsules can be coated – for example – to make them resistant to the acid medium of the stomach and to ascertain that the active ingredient is only released in the small or large intestine. Both formulations can contain slow- and fast-release particles in which the active ingredient is formulated in such way that it generates rapid and sustained absorption. Oral dosage forms can also be liquids such as solutions, suspensions and emulsions. Liquid formulations contain the active ingredient and a number of excipients such as stabilisers to ensure the stability of a suspension and/or emulsion, buffers to ascertain a specific pH region, bulking agents to ensure a specific texture of the liquid, viscosity enhancers or reducers, surfactants to solubilise the active ingredient and adjuvants to protect the liquid formulation from microbial growth.

Parenteral formulations are sterile solutions, emulsions or suspensions that can be used for intravenous, subcutaneous, intramuscular or intra-articular administration. They are generally stored in liquid or lyophilised form at lower temperatures to ensure their stability. Lyophilisation or freeze drying is a process that removes water from a liquid formulation, thereby creating a powder that is stable for extended periods of time and that allows storage at normal (ambient) temperatures. Sometimes, injectable solutions are diluted before administration, whereby the active ingredient is transferred from a vial into a bag for IV infusion to which other drugs can be added.

In the development of formulations for intramuscular injection poorly water soluble drugs can be administered as nanosuspensions from which the drug molecule is slowly released from the injection site (depot) to ensure a steady plasma concentration over an extended period of time. To obtain a slow and steady release from an intramuscular depot with drug molecules with a relatively good water solubility they can be transformed into so-called 'pro-drugs'. Pro-drugs are chemical derivatives of the drug molecule (e.g. ester) that are more lipophilic and from which the drug molecule is slowly released into the blood stream through the action of metabolising enzymes (e.g. plasma esterases).

4.2.2.3   Other formulations

There are different topical formulations possible but the most commonly used are creams and ointments, gels and pastes. Depending on the lipophilic

fraction of the formulations, they are known as creams or ointments. Pastes
are mixtures of oil, water and powders.

Besides the classical formulations such as tablets, capsules, parenteral formulations, creams and ointments there is a myriad of dosage forms that can
be developed and they range from titanium-based implants to combinations
of drugs and devices (e.g. drug-releasing stents). However, it is beyond the
objective of this book to address all these dosage forms in detail.

4.2.2.4 Approaches for poorly soluble drugs

Modern drugs are complex molecular entities of high molecular weight that
require special technologies to make them 'work', i.e. to become therapeutically active. Drug molecules that were developed in the 1960s to the 1980s
proved to be active 'on their own', i.e. they exhibited intrinsic bioavailability
and when ingested as such showed therapeutic activity. During the more
recent decades it became clear that formulation technologies had to be
developed to make new active ingredients bioavailable by using salt or pH
modifications and the use of solvents or lipids (mixtures). However, today's
drug molecules are not active 'on their own' and need high-tech technologies
to make them active. This means that the research for appropriate formulation technologies constitutes an important part of the drug development
process. What follows is an overview of the technologies that can be used to
make these complex molecules systemically available.

There are different formulations possible in early development for administration to experimental animals to assess the toxicity and the pharmacokinetics of a drug candidate [1].

One of the simplest approaches to enhance the bioavailability of active
ingredients is the use of pH adjustments by means of buffers. The pH at
which an active ingredient is introduced into a formulation is dependent upon
its solubility and its stability in solution. It is therefore important to study
the stability of the active ingredient under different pH conditions. Besides,
extreme pHs can cause tissue inflammation or precipitation preventing the
active ingredient from local absorption. The most commonly used buffering
agents are maleic acid, tartaric acid, glycine, lactic acid, citric acid and
acetic acid.

Another approach is the use of what are called co-solvents. Co-solvents
increase the solubility of the active ingredient in water. In some cases, mixtures of co-solvents are used to reduce the toxicity of one of the co-solvents.
A typical co-solvent is dimethylsulfoxide that facilitates the penetration of
the drug molecule through the skin and cell membranes. However, its use is
mostly limited to dermatological preparations. A risk inherent in the use of
co-solvents is the precipitation of the active ingredient once the drug enters
a biological medium. For example, pain or thrombophlebitis can occur at the
injection site after IV bolus injections.

Cyclodextrins are cyclic oligosaccharides with a hydrophilic outer surface and a lipophilic central cavity. They have been shown to increase the aqueous solubility of many poorly water soluble drugs by forming a water-soluble drug ligand. Both hydroxypropyl and sulfobutylether cyclodextrins have been used in different formulations for various routes of administration in experimental animal species. For example, 20-40% (w/v) aqueous solutions of cyclodextrins are frequently used in single-dose applications for either the oral or the IV routes of administration. Cyclodextrins can be used in combination with pH-adjustment approaches.

Surfactant and micellar systems can enhance the solubility of an active ingredient and can also improve the wetting and dissolution characteristics of drug particles. Surfactant systems are used in many dosage forms such as solutions, colloidal systems (e.g. emulsions, microemulsions), capsules and tablets. Some conventional surfactants, however, may generate systemic toxicity including histamine release and adverse cardiovascular effects. For example, histamine release in dogs was observed after using Cremophor EL, a commonly used surfactant in drug formulation. Surfactant systems are particularly well suited for low-dose formulations in early formulation development. Typical surfactants are polysorbates (e.g. Tween 80, Tween 20) or polyoxyl castor oil (Cremophor EL, Cremophor RH40, Cremophor RH60). They can be used with or without pH adjustment. Alternatively, bile salt and lecithin based micelles can be used such as taurocholate (TC), taurodeoxycholate (TDC), and deoxycholate (DC). Egg or soy phosphatidylcholine, soy phosphatidylethanolamine and oleic acid monoglycerides are frequently explored to increase the bioavailabilty of a new active ingredient. Suspensions are broadly used in all experimental animal studies because their preparation is quite straightforward and can be combined with hydrophilic polymers or surfactants. Examples of suitable polymers are methyl cellulose (MC), hydroxylethyl cellulose (HEC), or hydroxypropyl cellulose (HPC). A typical suspension may contain 0.5% (w/v) HEC and 0.2% (w/v) tween 80. A problem with suspensions is that the particles in suspension may aggregate and their physical stability compromised. A change in particle morphology, aggregation and sedimentation impacts the dissolution of the active ingredient and consequently its bioavailability.

Nanosuspensions may improve the dissolution and as a consequence the systemic availability of the active ingredient. With particles in the nanometer range and with a narrow size distribution, nanosuspensions also proved to have a good physical stability. With the increasing number of poorly water soluble drugs being introduced in drug development, nanosuspensions are now also frequently used in early development formulations.

Emulsions are colloidal systems that contain oil-in-water (o/w) or water-in-oil (w/o) droplets stabilised by surfactants. For nonclinical toxicology studies emulsion formulations can be selected based on the solubility of the active ingredient in lipids and surfactant solutions. Microemulsions are an improved version of emulsion formulations and self-(micro)emulsifying drug delivery systems (SEDDS, SMEDDS) are increasingly applied in the development of early formulations. The advantages of microemulsion systems are the generation of small particles in the nanometer range (often <150 nm), thermodynamic stability and the potential to improve bioavailability. A large group of excipients, including GRAS (generally regarded as safe) compounds, can be used to produce SEDDS and SMEDDS formulations.

Liposomes are concentrically arranged phospholipid bilayers whereby the hydrophilic part of the phospholipid molecule is directed towards the aqueous phase (internal or external), while the lipophilic parts are directed to each other (as in the structure of cell membranes). Liposomes can be used to deliver a wide variety of drug compounds such as hydrophilic compounds in the internal aqueous core and lipophilic compounds in the lipidic bilayer. Amphiphilic compounds can be adsorbed onto the double lipidic membrane. Liposomes are generally considered biocompatible and are well tolerated.

An interesting approach in formulation technology is thin-film hydration, but its usefulness is limited due to the difficulties associated with the introduction of the concept in full-scale pharmaceutical manufacturing. Thin-film hydration consists of dissolving the active ingredient and lipids (e.g. phospholipids, cholesterol, other lipids) in organic solvents such as chloroform, ethanol, methanol or a mixture of chloroform and methanol. The solvent is then removed, which leaves a thin film containing the active ingredient in the lipids. The thin film is then hydrated with aqueous buffers by which milky-like suspensions are produced.

Finally, solid dispersions are frequently used. A solid dispersion is a dispersion of the active ingredient in an inert carrier in the solid state. They appear as 'solid solutions' where the active ingredient is molecularly dispersed in a hydrophilic polymer. This is achieved by solvent evaporation or hot-melt extrusion. Solid dispersions can be used to stabilise the polymorphic character of a drug, which is a major advantage of this formulation technology. Examples of polymers that are used to act as solid dispersion vehicles are polyvinylpyrrolidone (PVP), hydroxypropylmethylcellulose (HPMC), HPMC phthalate, HPMC acetate succinate, PEG4000, Pluronic F68, PEG3350 and Gelucire 44/14.

4.2.3 Determination of the quality of the active ingredient and the drug product

In drug development, the determination of the purity and stability of the active ingredient and the *in vitro* performance, purity and stability of the drug product are essential components of the assessment of the quality of the drug. Analytical chemistry techniques are indispensable tools to test the compliance of the active ingredient and the drug product with the quality specifications assigned to them and to allow the drug candidate to be released to the next phase in drug development and finally the market place. The following sections give an overview of the most important and widely used analytical methods.

4.2.3.1   Spectrometry

UV and visible spectrometry

There exist various spectrometric methods that are applied in analytical chemistry. Spectrophotometric analysis is based on the light-absorbing properties of chemical substances. Ultraviolet (UV) spectrophotometry operates in the UV region of the electromagnetic spectrum (190–400 nm) and is most used for the quantitative analysis of molecules eluting from a liquid chromatographic system (LC). Visible-light spectrometry or colorimetry operates in the visible region of the electromagnetic spectrum (400–700 nm) and is most used for the quantitative analysis of coloured chemical substances or chemical substances that can be reacted to form a chromogen. This analytical technique is most used in automated analysis in clinical biochemistry.

IR spectrometry

Infrared (IR) spectrometry operates in the IR region of the electromagnetic spectrum (0.8–1000 μm). This region is divided into the near-(0.8–2.5 μm), mid-(2.5–15 μm) and far-(15–1000 μm) infrared spectrum, named for their relation to the visible spectrum. Each of the molecular functions in a chemical substance have a specific absorption band in the IR spectrum, for example OH- and NH-groups absorb between 2.3 and 3.2 μm, while aldehydes, ketones and acids absorb IR light between 5.7 and 6.1 μm. IR spectrometry is used for the identification of drug molecules and their synthesis intermediates in medicinal chemistry, chemical and pharmaceutical development and is a reference method for the identification of an active ingredient in combination with high-pressure liquid chromatography. Regulatory authorities generally require two methods, each of them based on a different physical principle (e.g. IR and NMR, IR and mass spectrometry) to unequivocally identify an active ingredient. An example of an IR spectrum is given in Figure 4.1.

The major advantage of IR spectrometry is that it produces a 'fingerprint' of a drug molecule that is specific to its molecular structure (stretching vibrations and bending vibrations).

Fluorometry

Fluorometry is based on the principle that a molecule emits light when it is irradiated with light of a shorter wavelength. Fluorometry is an accurate and very sensitive technique that is used in quantitative analytical chemistry and applied in liquid chromatography as a detection device.

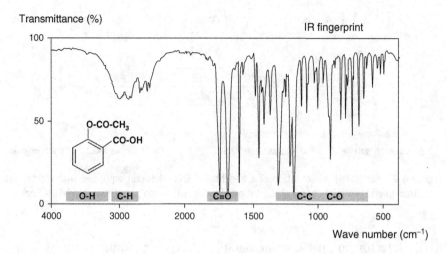

Figure 4.1 Infrared spectrum of aspirin.

Mass spectrometry

The principle of mass spectrometry is based on the ionisation and fragmentation of the molecule with subsequent separation of the ions and fragments formed based on their mass-to-charge ratio (m/z). There exist many approaches to form ions. Electron ionisation (EI) and chemical ionisation (CI) are used when the analytes are introduced in the ion source in the gas phase, as used in the coupling of gas chromatography and mass spectrometry (GC-MS). When the analytes enter the ion source dissolved in a liquid eluent, techniques such as electrospray ionisation (ESI), sonic spray ionisation (SSI) and atmospheric-pressure chemical ionisation (APCI) are used. Other ionisation techniques are matrix-assisted laser desorption ionisation (MALDI), which is used for the identification of peptides and fast atom bombardment (FAB). The ions and fragments formed in the ion source are then separated either in an electric and magnetic sector or a quadrupole mass filter. For the identification of proteins the fragments formed in the MALDI ion source are separated according to the time-of-flight principle (TOF). With this technique, the mass of the fragments is recorded according to the time they take to pass the mass filter, in this way a full mass spectrum is obtained as a snapshot rather than by sweeping through a sequential series of m/z values. Electron multipliers are used for the detection of the ions. A mass spectrum is represented by the relative abundance of each ion as a function of its mass-to-charge ratio (m/z) and is highly specific for each chemical substance.

Since the pathways of fragmentation of ionised molecules are well understood it is possible to reconstruct the molecular structure of the analyte based on its pattern of ion fragments. When a mass spectrometer is used

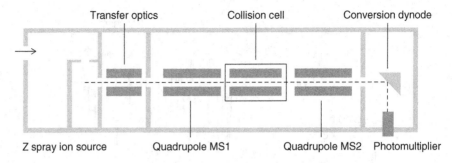

Figure 4.2 Schematic presentation of a benchtop MS/MS detector equipped with electrospray and atmospheric pressure chemical ionisation (Source: with kind permission of Waters Benelux).

as a detector in gas chromatography (GC) or liquid chromatography (LC) it provides structural information on the analytes when they exit the chromatography column. The sum of all ions produced in the mass spectrum of every molecule that exits the gas chromatograph yields a total ion chromatogram that is used for quantitative analysis. When the mass spectrometer is set to a specific m/z ratio only the molecules producing fragments with that m/z value are shown in the ion chromatogram. This allows for the analysis of compounds in complex media (e.g. plasma, urine, tissues). A very high sensitivity and selectivity is obtained by tandem mass spectrometry (MS/MS) using triple quadrupole technology. In this technique, two quadrupole mass filters are separated by a collision cell (Figure 4.2). The first quadrupole (MS1), is used to select ions of a given m/z value that are characteristic of the analyte and are referred to as 'precursor ions'. The selected precursor ions are broken down by collisionally induced dissociation (CID) with a reagent gas such as argon to form the so-called 'product ions'. The second quadrupole (MS2) is then used to select one or several product ions. These MS/MS transitions are highly compound specific and have a higher selectivity than single stage MS. This technique, which is also referred to as multiple reaction monitoring (MRM), is used for quantitative analysis in chemical and pharmaceutical development and in bioanalysis in combination with high-pressure liquid chromatography (HPLC).

Nuclear magnetic resonance spectrometry (NMR)

NMR is a radio-frequency spectroscopy method based on the magnetic field that is generated by the spinning of electrically charged atomic nuclei (e.g. protons, ^{13}C, ^{19}F, ^{31}P). The nuclear magnetic field of the nuclei interacts with the very large magnetic field (10 000–50 000 G) of the instrument whereby the nuclear magnetic field can reach a number of quantum states. The spin states that are oriented parallel to the external magnetic field are lower in energy than the spin states opposing the external field. A transition between the various spin states can be induced by irradiating the nuclei with radio-frequency photons (60–1000 MHz). The absorption of energy during this transition is the basic principle of NMR. When the radio-frequency pulse is discontinued, some of the spins that transitioned to a higher energy state return to their lower energy state. The energy that is released is recorded as the NMR signal. Since the molecular environment of the protons can produce characteristic shifts in the proton NMR spectrum, NMR is a powerful tool in the identification of molecules in medicinal chemistry and chemical development. A good example to show how a proton NMR spectrum is interpreted is that of aspirin (Figure 4.3). From the spectrum it can be derived that there are 6 types of protons (a, b, c, d, e, f) with each of them in their specific molecular environment. The signal on the right of the spectrum (smallest shift) comes from the hydrogens of the acetyl function (f), the four signals in the middle come from the hydrogens of the aromatic ring (b, c, d, e) whereas the signal at the left of the spectrum (greatest shift) comes from the hydrogen (a) of the carboxylic acid function and that is closest to an electronegative atom, i.e. oxygen. The splitting of the peaks indicates the number of neighbouring hydrogen types. For example, the triplet in the aromatic region indicates that the hydrogen generating the signal is surrounded by two types of hydrogens. A singlet shows that the hydrogens producing the signal are not surrounded by hydrogens of a different type.

4.2.3.2 Chromatography

Chromatographic techniques are used to separate the chemical constituents of a mixture or an active ingredient from its impurities and to quantify them. The components of a chromatographic system are an injection port, a chromatographic column and a detection system. Chromatography is based

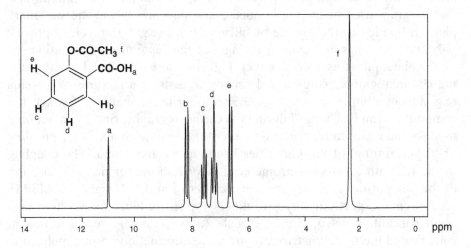

Figure 4.3 NMR spectrum of aspirin (reconstruction).

on the interaction of chemical substances present in a mobile phase (gas or liquid) with a stationary phase. This interaction can be adsorption, repartition, ion exchange, size exclusion or affinity. The differences between the structural and physicochemical characteristics of chemical molecules (e.g. polarity, lipid solubility, molecular weight) influence their interaction with the stationary phase. The different interactions with the stationary phase result in the separation of the mixture components when the mobile phase wherein they are dissolved is forced along the stationary phase. The stationary phase may consist of small-diameter particles (μm range) that are packed into a tube or the stationary phase can be coated on the inner surface of the tube. The mobile phase can be a gas (gas chromatography, GC) or a liquid (high-performance liquid chromatography, HPLC or LC). The mobile phase leaves the column and passes through a detector or a series of detectors. The detection system can be flame ionisation (for all chemicals), electron capture (for halogenated compounds) or mass spectrometry for GC and UV spectrophotometry, fluorometry or mass spectrometry for LC. The electronic signals from the detection system are plotted against volume or time, resulting in a graphical display that is called a 'chromatogram'. The first peaks of the chromatogram correspond with the components of the mixture that have the weakest interaction with the stationary phase. The time at which the components of a mixture exit the chromatographic column is the retention time and is specific for each substance under the given chromatographic conditions. The surface of the area of the electronic signal versus time is proportional to the amount of chemical that passed the detector. The analytical technique that is most used today in drug development is high-pressure liquid chromatography (LC) (Figure 4.4).

In LC, the chromatographic column (diameter of 2–5 mm and length 30–250 mm) is packed with particles of approximately 2–5 μm in size. The packings used in LC are bonded phase packings where the stationary phase is bonded to the surface of silica particles (e.g. C18 reversed phase), polymeric packings and chiral packings for the separation of enantiomers. The mobile phase is forced under high pressure (50–350 bar) through the chromatographic column and usually consists of a mixture of solvents (e.g. aqueous buffer solution, water, acetonitrile, methanol) of which the composition can be changed during the chromatographic run. LC is not only used for the quantitative determination of the analytes but also for profiling or 'fingerprinting' of the impurities in the active ingredient. The coupling of the LC with a mass spectrometer (LC-MS) allows for the identification of these impurities and very specific quantification. LC-MS and LC-MS/MS (tandem mass spectrometry) is routinely applied in bioanalysis where very small concentrations of drug molecule (ng/mL range) are quantified in complicated biological matrices. Some more information on the application of LC in bioanalysis is provided in the section on nonclinical development of

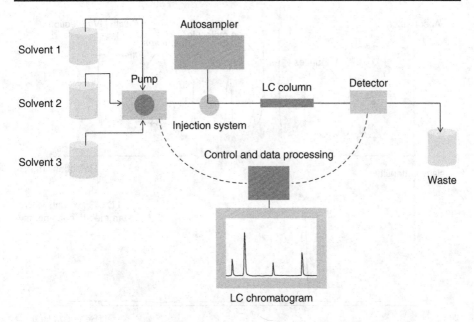

Figure 4.4 Schematic presentation of an LC system.

this chapter. More details on the performance and applications of LC can be found in textbooks on analytical chemistry and instrumentation. Figure 4.5 compares two LC runs of an active ingredient with its impurity profile, one with UV spectrophotometry and a second with MS/MS.

4.2.3.3 Melting point

The melting point of a solid is the temperature at which it changes from the solid to the liquid state at atmospheric pressure. Different methods exist to determine melting points. A classical Kofler bench consists of a metal strip in which a temperature gradient (from room temperature to 300°C) is generated. When an active ingredient substance is placed on a specific section of the metal strip the substance will melt and the melting point can be identified. Another method involves the use of a melting point apparatus for the analysis of crystalline solids and consists of an oil bath with a transparent window. Solid particles of a substance are introduced into a thin glass tube and immersed in the oil bath. The oil bath is heated and with the aid of the magnifier and a light source the melting process of the substance particles can be observed. At a certain temperature the particles will change their (crystalline) appearance and the melting process starts. Although melting-point determinations are simple and rather straightforward they are still widely used as part of the identification of a compound, but only in combination with other analytical techniques such as IR, MS, NMR or LC. Melting-point determinations are described in the official monographs of the European and the US Pharmacopoeia.

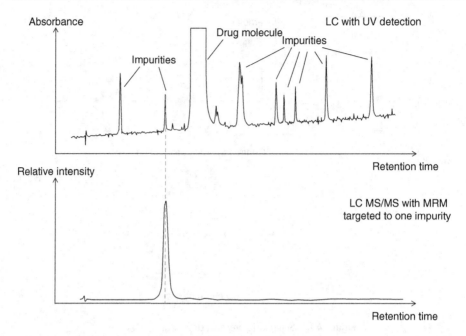

Figure 4.5   LC of an active ingredient with its impurities (hypothetical) using two detection systems (UV and MS/MS).

4.2.3.4   Stereochemical purity of the active ingredient

When a single enantiomer is selected as the active ingredient in a drug product, then, according to the European note for guidance 'Clinical Investigation of Chiral Active Substances/ III/3501/9', the other enantiomer has to be considered an impurity. It is therefore important that special attention is given to the identity and the stereoisomeric purity of the active ingredient. There are several methods that can be used to determine the identity and quality of a single enantiomer. These are for example optical rotation, melting-point determination, LC with a chiral stationary phase, optical rotary dispersion, circular dichroism and NMR using chiral shift reagents. These techniques are either used as research tools in drug development or as quality control techniques to test the stereochemical purity of an active ingredient.

4.3   Nonclinical development

The variety of test methods that are used in nonclinical drug development to assess the bioavailability and the safety of drug candidates is enormous and undergoes continuous evolution as new techniques in bioanalysis, cell biology, biochemistry, molecular biology, imaging, biomarkers and new (transgenic) test models *in vitro* and *in vivo* are introduced. The intention of this chapter is not to provide a complete overview of all the test methods that are used in drug development but to give a general idea of the experimental approaches that are currently most applied. The test methods and techniques are arranged according to their use in pharmacokinetics, safety pharmacology and toxicology.

4.3.1 Pharmacokinetics

Pharmacokinetics is the study of the absorption, distribution, metabolism and excretion of a drug (ADME). The term toxicokinetics is often used when the evolution of blood or plasma concentrations of the drug molecule and/or its metabolites are studied as a function of time in toxicology studies. Metabolism is the study of the enzymatic and non-enzymatic biotransformation of the drug in various organs/tissues and is an important factor in the elimination of the drug molecule from the body. There are numerous methods and techniques that are used to study pharmacokinetics. The most commonly used methods are described here and are grouped in absorption *in vitro*, plasma kinetics, mass-balance studies, metabolism, tissue distribution, bioanalysis and physiologically-based pharmacokinetic modelling. A more detailed description of these test methods can be found in appropriate textbooks on test methods in pharmacology and toxicology [5–9]. The basic principles of the analysis of pharmacokinetic data explained in this section are equally of application to human pharmacokinetics.

4.3.1.1 Absorption *in vitro*

Parallel artificial membrane permeation assay (PAMPA)
PAMPA is the first test that is carried out in drug discovery to obtain an idea about the capacity of the drug molecule to be absorbed passively from the gastrointestinal tract without any interaction of active transport systems. In this test, the permeation of the drug molecule is measured in a system where two compartments are separated by an artificial membrane. Solutions of the drug molecule in buffers of different pH are placed on top of the membrane and permeation is assessed by the determination of the concentration of the drug molecule in the receiving compartment. The analytical techniques used range from UV-spectrometry to LC-MS/MS. The results are reported as apparent permeation (P_{app}) and recovery.

Caco-2 assay
In this *in vitro* model, the drug molecule is assessed for its passive and active absorption from the gastrointestinal tract. The test system consists of two compartments that are separated by a monolayer of cells (Caco-2 cells) derived from human colon carcinoma cells grown onto a cell culture filter. The Caco-2 cells have a phenotype and function that is close to that of the enterocytes of

the small intestine and constitute an ideal barrier to investigate the transep-
ithelial transport characteristics of the drug molecule in both the absorptive
(apical to basolateral) and the secretory (basolateral to apical) directions. To
study the role of P-glycoprotein (P-gp) in drug transport, the test can be carried out in the presence of a P-gp inhibitor (e.g. verapamil). Possible inhibition
of P-gp transport by the drug molecule is studied using the P-gp substrate
taxol and is important to understand drug–drug interactions at the level of
gastrointestinal absorption.

4.3.1.2   Plasma kinetics

To characterise the pharmacokinetic profile of a drug candidate single-dose
pharmacokinetic studies are conducted in the animal species that will be used
in pharmacology and toxicology studies (e.g. mouse, rat, rabbit, dog). The
routes of exposure are those that are relevant for the intended therapeutic
use (e.g. oral, dermal, intravenous, subcutaneous, intramuscular, inhalation)
of the drug. The animals receive a single dose of the drug via the oral route
by gavage or any other appropriate route of administration. Blood samples
are taken pre-dosing and, for example, at 0.5, 1, 2, 4, 8, 12, 24 and 48 h after
administration. The selection of the sampling times at this stage is preliminary since it is not known when the plasma concentrations will reach the
maximum and how long it will take before the drug is completely eliminated
from the body for each of the animal species studied. Once the pharmacokinetic profile of the drug candidate is characterised a more tailored sampling
schedule can be applied in the following studies. The number of animals that
are required for blood sampling depends on the volume of blood needed for
bioanalysis and the size of the animal. For the dog, blood samples can be
drawn at all time points for each of the animals, whereas for rodents, more
animals are required to collect a sufficient blood volume for each time point
(e.g. 3 rats/sex/sampling point and each rat can be sampled maximum 3 times
during the same day). Plasma is separated from the cellular fraction of blood
by centrifugation and stored at −20°C pending analysis. The plasma concentrations obtained at each of the time points are then analysed by means of
standard models for pharmacokinetic analysis (e.g. WinNonlin).

The parameters that can be derived from the plasma concentration versus
time curves after single exposure and that are most used in pharmaceutical
development are elimination half-life ($t_{1/2}$), maximum plasma concentration
(C_{max}), time at which C_{max} is reached (t_{max}) and the area under the plasma
concentration versus time curve (AUC) calculated for different time periods
(from 0–24 h to 0–∞ h). In the interpretation of pharmacology, safety
pharmacology or toxicology data the AUC is often referred to as 'systemic
exposure' or just 'exposure'. The time to reach C_{max} (t_{max}) is used as an
estimate of the absorption rate. Other parameters such as the volume of
distribution (V_d) is derived from the absorbed dose and the initial plasma

concentration and whole-body clearance (Cl_{tot}) is derived from the volume of distribution and the rate of elimination that in turn is derived from the plasma half-life. When the drug is evenly distributed over the entire body then it is said to behave according to a one-compartment pharmacokinetic model. When it is retained at higher concentrations in different parts of the body then it behaves according to a multicompartment pharmacokinetic model. Each compartment represents an organ/tissue or group thereof where the drug is retained in a similar way. In the case of a two-compartment model (e.g. central and peripheral compartment) two rates of elimination can be derived from the plasma concentration versus time curve. These are referred to as the fast and the slow elimination rates or the distribution and elimination phase (α and β phase). The absolute oral bioavailability (F_{abs}) of a drug after single dosing is determined by comparing the dose-corrected AUCs obtained after intravenous and oral administration. An example of a plasma concentration versus time curve for a single oral administration is given in Figure 4.6.

Once the pharmacokinetic profile is characterised after a single exposure it is studied after repeated exposure. Depending on the elimination half-life and drug metabolism phenomena such as enzyme induction, an equilibrium is achieved between the rates of absorption and elimination at a given time after the start of administration. The drug has then reached its maximum plasma concentration, which is referred to as the steady-state concentration (C_{ss}). The time needed to reach steady state is specific for each drug and depends on the elimination half-life. The pharmacokinetic parameters that are derived from repeated-dose plasma concentration versus time curves are the C_{max} (maximum plasma concentration in one dosing interval), C_{min} (minimum plasma concentration in one dosing interval), C_{av} (average plasma

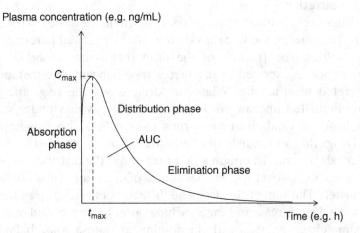

Figure 4.6 Plasma concentration versus time curve after single oral administration.

Plasma concentration (e.g. ng/mL)

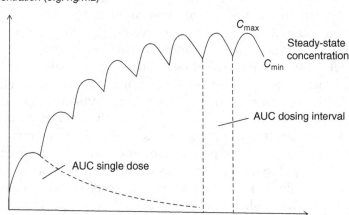

Figure 4.7 Plasma concentration versus time curve after multiple oral administration.

concentration of one dosing interval), the degree of fluctuation within a dosing interval $((C_{max} - C_{min})/C_{av})$ and the AUC of a dosing interval at steady state. An example of a plasma concentration versus time curve for multiple oral administration is given in Figure 4.7.

The pharmacokinetic profile of a drug candidate in plasma is normally first studied in single-dose and multiple-dose pharmacokinetic studies designed for that purpose. Once the critical parameters are known for each of the animal species that are used for toxicology testing, optimal blood sampling schedules can be applied to all toxicology studies.

4.3.1.3 Excretion

Once drugs are absorbed into the systemic circulation they can be excreted in urine, bile, faeces and in exhaled air as the unchanged parent drug and/or as metabolites. The fraction of the drug that is not absorbed after oral administration is excreted in the faeces together with the metabolites that are excreted via the bile. When the drug is volatile (e.g. anesthetics) it can be eliminated unchanged via the lungs. Drugs that undergo extensive metabolism and catabolism can form CO_2, which is also eliminated via the lungs. Drugs that accumulate in tissues over time are retained in the body for long periods of time. To obtain a first idea about the distribution of the drug and its metabolites over the various routes of excretion a mass-balance study is conducted. The sum of the drug and its metabolites recovered from all excreta, exhaled air, carcass and cage washings after a given period of time should approximately correspond with the administered dose. Mass-balance studies are usually performed with the drug molecule labelled with a radio-isotope

Table 4.1 Typical example of a mass balance after administration of a single oral dose to male and female rats.

	% of dose	
	Male	Female
Urine	52	65
Feces	37	27
Cage washings	1	2
Carcass	5	4
Total recovered	**95**	**98**

(e.g. ^{3}H, ^{14}C) in a metabolically stable position. The total radioactivity measured in the excreta and the carcass represents the parent compound and all metabolites combined. The duration of a mass-balance study depends on the elimination half-life of the drug and may vary from 48 h to 120 h or even longer. Mass-balance studies are performed on each animal species that is projected to be used in toxicology studies and the excreta recovered are often used for the isolation and identification of drug metabolites. An example of a mass balance is given in Table 4.1 where the excretion of total radioactivity in urine and faeces and the retention in the carcass is compared between male and female rats after a sample collection time of 120 h.

The radioactivity that is excreted in faeces can be a combination of drug substance that is not absorbed from the gastrointestinal tract and metabolites that are excreted via the bile (e.g. glucuronic acid and glutathione conjugates). To determine the extent of biliary excretion a mass-balance study can be conducted where the bile duct of the experimental animal is cannulated and the radioactivity excreted from the bile determined separately. With some drugs biliary metabolites are transformed by enzymes in the gut (e.g. glucuronidases) and reabsorbed from the gastrointestinal tract. This phenomenon is referred to as 'enterohepatic recirculation'. This can be explored in mass-balance studies with two animals where the bile duct of the first animal is cannulated and the bile is led into the intestine of a second animal. The animal species that is most used for this purpose is the rat.

4.3.1.4 Drug metabolism
The detailed knowledge of the biodegradation of a drug in nonclinical animal species and in man is very important for the understanding of the pharmacokinetic differences that may exist between experimental animals and man and of the relevance to man of certain mechanisms of toxic action operative in certain experimental animals (e.g. interpretation of tumours in rodent cancer studies). The biodegradation of a drug is generally based on the conversion of the relatively lipophilic drug molecule into a more water-soluble form that can be more readily excreted in urine or bile. Although drug

biotransformation generally leads to molecules that are pharmacologically and toxicologically less active and that are rapidly eliminated from the body, also more active molecules can be formed that are more toxic than the parent compound (bioactivation). Many bioactivation products are responsible for tumour production in rodents. Biodegradation of a drug can already take place in the gastrointestinal tract by the action of digestive enzymes (e.g. lipases) and the enzymes present in the epithelial cells (enterocytes) of the intestinal wall, but is largely dominated by the liver when administered orally. Other tissues where drugs can be metabolised are, for example, the kidneys, the lungs and the brain. The metabolism of a drug by the liver after absorption from the gut is referred to as the first-pass effect and is illustrated in Figure 4.8.

Metabolic transformation reactions can be grossly subdivided into Phase I and Phase II reactions. Phase I reactions relate to the chemical transformation of the parent molecule by oxidation, reduction, hydroxylation and dealkylation. Phase II reactions concern most of the time the conjugation of the parent drug molecule or its metabolites with larger molecules such as glucuronic acid and glutathione but also with smaller molecular groups such as sulfate and acetate.

The enzymes involved in Phase I metabolism reactions are either cytochrome P450 or non-cytochrome P450. The latter group concerns, for example, alcohol dehydrogenase, monoamino oxidase, esterases and amidases. Cytochrome P450 enzymes are localised in the endoplasmatic reticulum (ER) of the cell and are present in the highest concentrations in liver (all isoforms), intestine (CYP3A4), brain (CYP2D6), kidney and lungs. The study of cytochrome P450 enzymes is important in drug development because they drive most of the drug metabolism pathways and allow the explanation

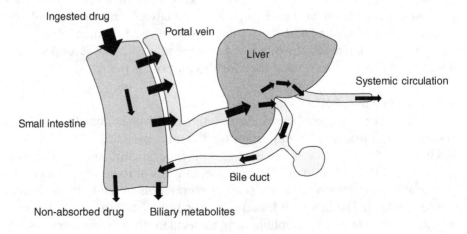

Figure 4.8 First-pass effect.

of pharmacokinetic differences between animals and man, interindividual differences in sensitivity to drugs in man and the relevance or not to man of some toxic mechanisms of action detected in experimental animals. Since their activity can be altered by other drugs they are essential in the assessment of drug–drug interactions. The cytochrome P450 isoforms that are most involved in drug metabolism (most of them in hydroxylation reactions) are CYP1A2, CYP2C9, CYP2C19, CYP2D6, CYP2E1 and CYP3A4 of which CYP2D6, CYP2C9 and CYP2C19 are susceptible to genetic polymorphism. Genetic polymorphism of metabolising enzymes is the causative factor of a different metabolic handling of drugs between ethnic groups (e.g. slow and fast metabolisers).

Metabolism in vitro
To obtain a first idea about possible differences in liver metabolism between animal species and man *in vitro* tests are performed where the metabolic profile is determined using post-mitochondrial (S9) fractions, microsomes or hepatocytes from various animal species and man. Liver microsomes are derived from subcellular fractions of liver cells (hepatocytes) and carry key drug-metabolising enzymes such as cytochrome P450 enzymes and glucuronyl transferases. The use of a radio-labelled drug not only facilitates the extraction and the separation of the metabolites formed but also permits the quantification of each of the metabolites. The identification of the molecular structure of the metabolites already permits a first idea of the metabolic pathways of the drug in liver to be obtained. The immediate result of such an approach is that the experimental species for nonclinical development can be selected on the basis of a metabolism pattern that is similar (or most similar) to that of man. The limitation of this *in vitro* approach is that it only reflects liver metabolism and does not take into account further metabolism of liver metabolites in other organ systems (e.g. kidneys, nasal epithelium). *In vitro* tests can also be performed with the S9 fraction or microsomes from other tissues such as epithelial cells from the small intestine or tubular cells from kidneys. However, to obtain a complete picture of all the metabolic pathways in the body *in vivo* metabolism studies are required.

Metabolism in vivo
In most cases, the excreta collected during mass-balance studies are used for the extraction, separation and identification of the metabolites present in urine and faeces. Also, isolation and identification of metabolites is done on plasma samples collected at different time points. The use of a radio-labelled drug allows for the determination of the amount of metabolites excreted over time. Metabolism studies can be performed after single dosing at different dose levels and after repeated dosing. The techniques that are employed to extract and isolate the metabolic fraction are very diverse and depend

on the type of metabolites formed and the concentrations present. In most instances the extracts (of which the recovery can be monitored by measuring the radioactivity present) are purified and the metabolites present separated and identified by LC-MS/MS. This can be very tedious when the number of metabolites formed is very large and when each of them is present in very low concentrations ($< 5\%$ of total radioactivity). Also, the presence of many conjugates (e.g. glucuronides) may constitute a hurdle to pass. Often, not all metabolites that are excreted in faeces get identified because their isolation is difficult due to binding to faecal material. The metabolic pathways of paracetamol are shown in Figure 4.9 as an example. The phase I reaction in the metabolism of paracetamol is N-hydroxylation that ultimately leads to the formation of an iminoquinone, which is a toxic metabolite. Imino-quinones are reactive molecules that readily bind to the cystein residues of proteins in the cell that are functionally important (e.g. components of the cell skeleton). The disturbance of the structure of these proteins may lead to cell death. Iminoquinones can also be detoxified by conjugation with glutathione. The formation of extensive amounts of iminoquinones can exhaust the cellular pool of glutathione and produce oxidative toxicity due to the loss of the capacity of the cell to eliminate reactive oxygen species (ROS).

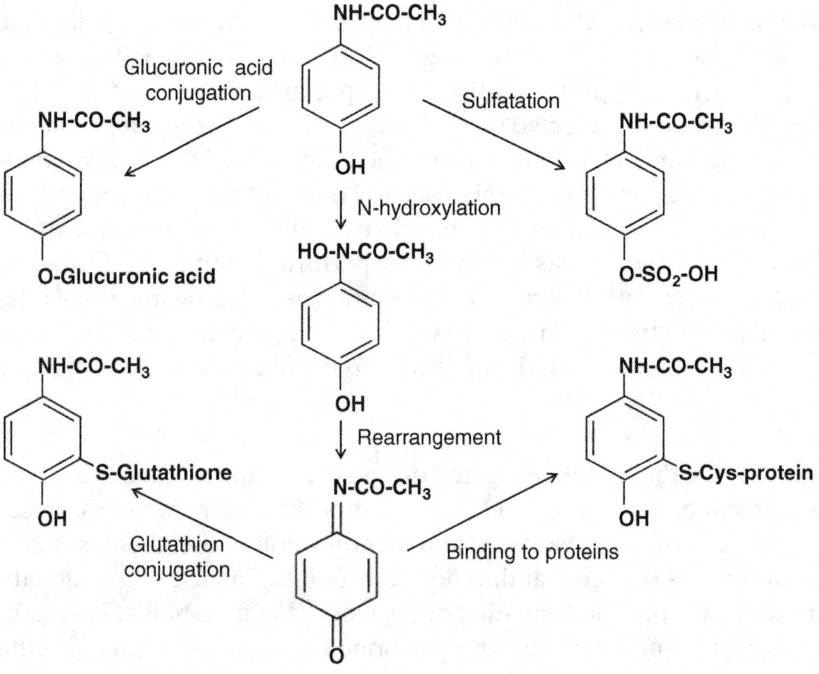

Figure 4.9   Metabolic pathways of paracetamol.

Paracetamol can be readily eliminated from the body through phase II reactions such as conjugation with glucuronic acid and sulfate.

Liver enzyme inhibition and induction

Repeated dosing of a drug may lead to the increased transcription of one or more of its metabolising enzymes. This results in a progressive decrease in plasma concentrations of the drug over time with reduced pharmacological activity as a consequence. This is referred to as liver enzyme induction. Liver enzyme induction is reversible upon cessation of treatment. When the drug inhibits an enzyme that is essential to the metabolism of another drug that is taken concomitantly, then the plasma concentration of that drug increases with higher pharmacological activity or toxicity as a result. This is referred to as liver enzyme inhibition. Often, this characteristic is used to 'boost' the plasma concentrations of drugs that otherwise undergo extensive metabolism. A classic enzyme inhibitor is grape fruit juice that inhibits the activity of CYP3A4 that is involved in the metabolism of many drugs. The capacity of a drug to induce or inhibit metabolising enzymes is determined by measuring the extent of metabolism of substrates typical for each of the enzymes studied. Some examples of substrates that can be used for the determination of the hydroxylation activity of a number of cytochrome P450 isoforms are given in Table 4.2. Apart from the measurement of the activity of cytochrome P450 enzymes the study of the induction of glucuronic acid transferase (UDP-GT) may be important in drug development. The induction of this enzyme increases the conjugation of the drug or its metabolites with glucuronic acid and subsequent biliary excretion. In such cases the excretion is increased of not only drugs that are conjugated before excretion but also of essential endogenic molecules such as growth and sex hormones.

Table 4.2 Substrates for the determination of the activity of CYP isoforms.

CYP isoform	Substrate
1A2	3-cyano-7-ethoxycoumarin
2C9	7-methoxy-4-trifluoromethyl coumarin
2C19	3-cyano-7-ethoxycoumarin
2D6	3-[2-(N,N-diethyl-N-methylamino)ethyl]-7-methoxy-4-methyl coumarin
3A4	7-benzyloxy-trifluoromethyl coumarin

4.3.1.5 Tissue distribution

Protein binding

In plasma, most drug molecules are bound to proteins such as albumin and α1-acid glycoprotein. Only the free (unbound) molecule is available for uptake in tissues where it can exert its pharmacological or toxicological activity at the target. It is therefore important to know the protein binding of the drug at various plasma concentrations in all relevant nonclinical animal species and in man. Knowledge of the extent to which a drug is bound to protein helps in the explanation of differences between *in vitro* and *in vivo* effects, the prediction of pharmacokinetic profiles and differences in sensitivity to toxicity of nonclinical animal species and man. Protein binding is measured *in vitro* by equilibrium dialysis at body temperature and at several drug concentrations. The concentration of the free drug fraction is usually measured by LC-MS/MS or by radioactivity detection when a radio-labelled drug molecule is used.

Whole-body distribution

The distribution of the drug and its metabolites over the entire body as a function of time is important in the interpretation of toxicology studies. Often toxicological effects are observed in organs/tissues where the drug or one of its metabolites is present at higher concentrations and has the longest residence time (e.g. due to tissue binding). Besides the study of the distribution of the drug and its metabolites in adult animals, tissue distribution studies are also carried out in pregnant animals to assess accumulation of the drug molecule and its metabolites in the fetus and in pigmented animals to investigate the binding to melanin in tissues that are sensitive to light. The techniques commonly used for the study of tissue distribution using radio-labelled drugs (e.g. ^{3}H, ^{14}C) are whole-body autoradiography (WBA) and the quantitative determination of the radioactivity in biological fluids and tissues by liquid scintillation counting (LSC), directly or after combustion. In WBA the animals are given the radio-labelled drug and are sacrificed at given time points after administration and then frozen in liquid nitrogen. The whole body is cut sagittally in slices and the distribution of the radioactivity visualised by exposure to a radiographic plate. In quantitative whole-body radiography (QWBA) the concentration of radioactivity in various tissues is measured by either densitometry of the exposed X-ray film or radioluminography (RLG). Radioactivity can also be determined in tissues and biological fluids by radio-activity detection LC after extraction. A more specific and quantitative method is the bioanalytical determination of the parent compound and its metabolites (in so far they are all known) in isolated tissues and body fluids at several time points after administration. More advanced techniques in the determination of the distribution of parent compound and metabolites in tissues are matrix-assisted laser desorption ionisation mass spectrometry (MALDI-MS imaging) and secondary ion mass spectrometry (SIMS). With MALDI-MS imaging the animals are treated with the drug molecule *in vivo* and are sacrificed at several time points after administration. The tissues are isolated and tissue slices transferred onto a carrier plate on which a matrix is applied by airspray. The surface of the matrix-treated tissue is then scanned with a laser beam that evaporates the matrix molecules and transfers electrons and protons to the drug and metabolite molecules. The protonated sample and matrix molecules are then analysed by MS/MS. Through the scanning of the laser beam over the sample surface a 2D image is created where the distribution of drug or metabolite fragment ions of a selected m/z value is visualised. The spatial resolution of this technique is about 100 μm [10]. In SIMS the tissue section is placed in a high-vacuum chamber and bombarded with a primary ion beam (e.g. Cs^+). Molecular fragments are ejected from the sample surface and the ionised secondary particles that are formed are analysed by MS/MS.

Bioanalysis

Bioanalysis is the quantitative determination of the parent drug molecule and its metabolites in body fluids (e.g. blood, plasma, urine, saliva) and in tissues. The analytes are present in very complex biological matrices and their concentrations are usually very small (ng/mL range). This means that for every drug molecule and metabolite quantitative and very selective analytical methods have to be developed and validated for all possible biological matrices and all relevant animal species and man. The analytical method should be sensitive, accurate, reproducible and have a sufficiently large dynamic range with the determination of the lower limit of quantification (LLOQ) and the upper limit of quantification (ULOQ). Prior to the application of the analytical method in nonclinical and clinical studies, the stability of the analyte in biological as well as solvent media has to be established for the temperatures and time periods that are relevant for the analytical procedures and the storage of spare samples. Often, an internal standard is used (e.g. deuterated drug molecule in the case of MS analysis) to compensate for possible losses during extraction and purification steps and the establishment of the calibration curve. The selection of extraction and purification procedures depends on the nature of the analyte and the biological environment from which it needs to be isolated. Some biological fluids such as saliva only need dilution in a solvent, whereas tissues such as adipose and brain tissue or specimen such as faeces need substantial clean-up before injection in the analytical apparatus. The analytical method that is most applied for the detection and identification of small molecules is high-performance liquid chromatography (HPLC or LC) coupled to tandem mass spectrometry (MS/MS). This method is very sensitive and can be made very selective by selecting only those ion fragments that are specific for the drug or metabolite to be analysed. During the extraction and purification steps, the bond between the drug molecule and proteins is destroyed, so that the quantitative data provided refer to total drug present in the biological sample. Data on protein binding for the respective species and biological medium are required to calculate the concentration of free drug.

4.3.1.6   Pharmacokinetic modelling

Besides the models that are routinely used for the characterisation of the pharmacokinetic profile of drugs from plasma concentrations as a function of time, there are more complex models that allow for the prediction of pharmacokinetic parameters in humans based on physicochemical, physiological and nonclinical pharmacokinetic data. These models are referred to as physiologically-based pharmacokinetic models (PBPK). PBPK models consider an integrated body model with a gastrointestinal tract (stomach, small intestine, large intestine), biliary tract, the most important organs (pancreas, spleen, liver, kidney, lung), a portal vein system and an arterial and venous blood pool (e.g. PK-SIM, SIM-Cyp, Gastroplus, ACSL). For each of the organ systems a minimum data set of the activity of metabolic enzymes and transporter peptides should be available. The minimal physicochemical characteristics that are needed to run such a model are molecular weight, acidity, water solubility, lipid solubility and the octanol–water partition coefficient ($\log P_{ow}$). The nonclinical pharmacokinetic parameters needed are the tissue–blood partition coefficients for every organ system, permeability, protein binding, hepatic clearance and renal clearance. The most important physiological parameters are the organ-specific blood flows. The results of PBPK modelling are calculated drug or metabolite concentration versus time curves and pharmacokinetic parameters for each organ or tissue. A typical presentation of a PBPK model is shown in Figure 4.10.

When the models are used to scale adult human pharmacokinetic data to children (age-dependent scaling) to help in the design of paediatric studies,

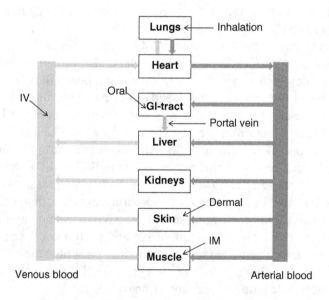

Figure 4.10   Example of a PBPK model.

then more physiological data are needed besides organ specific blood flows such as body and organ weights, organ composition, blood volume, cardiac output, total body water, extracellular water and body fat.

4.3.2 Safety pharmacology

In this section, an overview is given of some experimental methods that are currently most used in safety pharmacology but should by no means be considered as complete. Safety pharmacology is one of the three main scientific disciplines in nonclinical sciences. The difference between safety pharmacology and primary pharmacology (on-target) and secondary pharmacology (off-target) is that it does not study the effects of the drug candidate on pharmacological endpoints but on essential physiological functions in the body. In the safety screening of drug candidates in late discovery and early development most attention is paid to the cardiovascular function, respiratory function and central nervous system (CNS) function. Tests in relation to gastrointestinal function are not discussed in this section since observations of effects on liver and kidney function are integrated in toxicology testing. The only tests in safety pharmacology that should be performed in accordance to GLP [11] are the in vivo cardiovascular and respiratory safety test in the conscious dog and the in vivo CNS safety test in the rat. Guidance to the testing strategy to be followed and the conduct of the tests is provided in the ICH safety guidelines S7A and S7B [12]. More detail on the conduct and interpretation of safety pharmacology tests can be found in textbooks and the literature on safety pharmacology [13–21].

4.3.2.1 Cardiovascular safety

Cardiovascular safety screening is by far the most important activity in safety pharmacology in early drug development since the heart is vulnerable and critical to survival. Cardiovascular safety testing is mainly based on the study of the effect of drug candidates on the normal functioning of ion channels in the cell membranes of the cardiac muscle cells (cardiomyocytes) that is essential for normal heart contraction. The tests are first directed towards interaction with ion channels *in vitro* followed by test systems at the cell, tissue and whole-organ levels and ultimately in experimental animals.

hERG binding assay

In this *in vitro* assay, the possible interaction (binding) between the drug molecule and the human potassium ion channel is investigated. The potassium ion channel is a protein with a tubular structure that is produced in cardiomyocytes and is nested in the cell membrane. It plays an important role in the repolarisation of the cardiac ventricular muscle. When repolarisation is delayed by inhibition of the delayed rectifier potassium current there is an increased risk of heart arrhythmias and ultimately of

Torsade(s) de Pointes (TdP) that may lead to sudden death. A delay of ventricular repolarisation is characterised in the electrocardiogram (ECG) by the prolongation of the QT interval (see section on clinical development, Figure 4.14).

The effect of ion currents (Na^+, Ca^{2+}, K^+) on the polarisation and repolarisation of the heart muscle is explained in more detail in Section 5.2.2.2. In the hERG binding assay, either cells or cell membranes are used of a type of human embryonic kidney (HEK 293) cells, transfected with a gene (the human ether-à-go-go related gene, hERG) that encodes for the delayed rectifier potassium current (I_{Kr}) channels. The channels are first saturated with a radio-labelled ligand (e.g. ^{3}H-astemizole) and then the cells or cell membranes are incubated with the drug at various concentrations in a buffer solution. The displacement of the ligand by the drug molecule is determined by measurement of the released radioactivity after filtration. The results are expressed as the concentration at 50% inhibition (IC_{50}). This test is performed in drug discovery and can be adapted for high-throughput screening.

hERG patch clamp assay

The hERG patch clamp assay is the first *in vitro* cardiovascular functional test that provides an indication whether the drug molecule is capable of inhibiting the potassium ion current through the potassium ion channels. The patch clamp assay is performed on cells (e.g. Chinese hamster ovary cells (CHO), HEK293 cells) that are transfected with hERG. The cells are plated on glass coverslips that are continuously wetted with physiological saline and only one cell is selected for patch clamping (Figure 4.11). A patch clamp is a micropipette that is attached to the cell surface by suction and serves as an electrode. The tip of a patch clamp can cover ("patch") a membrane surface containing several ion channels at the same time. Since the HEK293 cells are

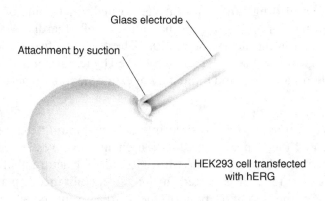

Glass electrode

Attachment by suction

HEK293 cell transfected with hERG

Figure 4.11   Single cell selected for patch clamping.

only transfected with one type of ion channel there is no interference from other confounding ion currents.

Through the patch clamp, the cell membrane is depolarised and then step-wise repolarised. During this voltage cycle, the hERG current (tail current) is recorded. After establishment of the background tail current, the drug is added at different concentrations to the perfusion solution and the tail currents recorded and compared against those induced by reference substances that are known to block the ion channel, such as astemizole or terfenadine. The results of the hERG patch clamp assay are expressed as the maximum concentration of the drug at which no effect on tail current is recorded.

Purkinje fibre assay

This *in vitro* tissue culture assay is closer to the *in vivo* situation than the hERG patch clamp assay. The hERG assay only evaluates effects on the potassium (K^+) channel, whereas in tissues, the effect of the drug candidate on all ion channels (Na^+, Ca^{2+}, K^+) involved in the depolarisation and repolarisation of the cardiac ventricular muscles is investigated. This test allows the evaluation of the propensity of a drug candidate to delay the conduction of the heart ventricular action potential that may lead to arrhythmias and ultimately to sudden death. Purkinje fibres are the prolongation of the conductive tissue of the heart ventricles and lead the cardiac action potential from the bundle of His to the cardiac ventricular muscles. In this assay, the left ventricular Purkinje fibres can be used from the heart of dog, sheep or rabbit. They are isolated from the heart and put in a tissue culture bath with continuous perfusion under physiological conditions. Depolarisation of the fibre is triggered by a stimulating electrode and the transmembrane action potentials are recorded by means of a glass microelectrode (Figure 4.12). The drug is dissolved in the perfusion medium at different concentrations and its effect on the action potential duration (APD) compared against base line and reference compounds. A prolongation of the APD (Figure 4.13) is indicative of the arrhythmogenic potential of the candidate drug. The results of the Purkinje fibre assay are expressed as the maximum concentration of the drug at which no effect on APD is recorded.

Isolated rabbit heart assay

In this tissue culture assay, the whole ventricular part of the heart of a rabbit is used to investigate the possible effect of drug candidates on action potential duration (APD), electrocardiogram (ECG) and hemodynamic parameters [22, 23]. The heart is isolated from the rabbit, the atria removed and mounted in an organ culture system with continuous perfusion at physiological conditions. This assay system is also referred to as the Langendorff perfused heart model. The advantage of a whole heart assay is that all interdependent physiological functions of the heart are present. The heart is implanted with

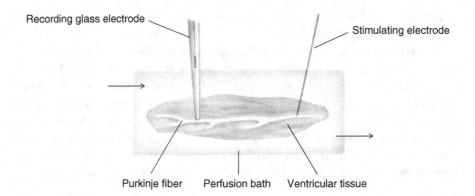

Recording glass electrode

Stimulating electrode

Purkinje fiber   Perfusion bath   Ventricular tissue

Figure 4.12 Experimental setup of a Purkinje fibre assay.

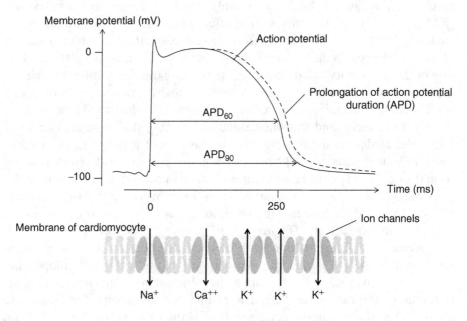

Figure 4.13 Prolongation of the action potential duration (APD).

stimulating electrodes, ECG electrodes, a flow probe, a pressure transducer, a temperature probe and a pH probe. The drug is added to the perfusion medium at different concentrations and for different time periods. The output of this test is the APD at, for example, 60% and 90% of depolarisation, QRS interval, QT interval, total coronary artery flow, intraventricular conduction, ventricular tachycardia, ventricular fibrillation, early after depolarisation (EAD), T-wave duration and Torsade(s) de Pointes (TdP). The highest concentration of the drug in the perfusion medium without any effect on cardio-electrophysiological and hemodynamic parameters is used in cardiovascular risk assessment. Although *in vitro* testing has its advantages, such as high throughput, lower cost and shorter screening timelines, it also has limitations.

A problem that is inherent to all *in vitro* and tissue perfusion systems in cardiovascular safety assessment is that there is always the risk that lipophilic drugs have the tendency to get adsorbed onto the materials that are used in the culture or perfusion apparatus. It is therefore important to determine the real concentration of the drug in the culture or perfusion medium after equilibration. Another hurdle in the interpretation of these tests is that the perfusion media used don't always contain protein so that drugs, which are otherwise bound to protein in *in vivo* situations, become more accessible to the heart tissue with a risk of tissue accumulation, which normally does not take place in *in vivo* situations. To overcome the limitations of *in vitro* testing cardiovascular safety testing must also be conducted in intact animals, either anesthetised or conscious.

Cardiovascular safety in anaesthetised animals

Before a cardiovascular safety assay is carried out on conscious dogs often the drug candidate is first evaluated in anaesthetised dogs for its possible cardiac and hemodynamic effects. Since anaesthetised dogs have a much more regular ECG pattern it is easier to detect any drug-related cardio-electrophysiological or hemodynamic effect when the drug is tested for the first time in an *in vivo* setting. As anaesthetised dogs cannot swallow drugs, the route of administration in this case is the intravenous route. Different dose levels of the drug are slowly injected to achieve plasma concentrations that are a multiple of the projected therapeutic levels. The cardio-electrophysiological and hemodynamic parameters are similar to those recorded in telemetered conscious dog studies described below. During this assay also blood samples can be collected for toxicokinetic analysis. The findings of this assay provide guidance to the dose selection and design of the conscious cardiovascular safety assay in the dog where the drug can be administered via the intended route of administration. Besides the dog Guinea pigs and sometimes monkeys are also used in this type of assay.

Conscious telemetered dog assay

In this assay, the cardiovascular effects of drug candidates are evaluated in conscious dogs that can freely move around in their pens without any restraint and thus with minimal stress [24]. Male dogs are implanted with telemetry transducers that can record continuously systolic and diastolic blood pressure, heart rate, cardiac output, left ventricular pressure and lead II ECG parameters such as PR, RR and QT intervals and QRS duration. After recovery from surgery, the animals are placed in pens that are equipped with a receiver that is connected with a telemetry recording system. The drug is administered to the dogs by gavage at different dose levels producing plasma concentrations that are a multiple of the intended therapeutic level. The dogs are observed for general clinical signs. Cardiovascular data are collected between 30 min and 12 h after dosing. During the experiment blood samples can also be collected at pre-dose and at several time points after oral dosing for toxicokinetic analysis. The highest dose or the highest C_{max} at which no cardio-electrophysiological or hemodynamic effects are observed is used for cardiovascular risk assessment. Telemetry studies can also be carried out in rabbits and monkeys.

4.3.2.2 Respiratory safety
The evaluation of the effect of the drug candidate on respiratory parameters is usually combined with the cardiovascular safety test in the conscious dog. For the measurement of the tracheal air flow a sealed mask is applied onto the animal's snout that is attached to a pneumotachograph and a pulmonary monitoring system. Data are collected at different time points from 1 up to 4 h after dosing and the parameters recorded are respiratory rate, tidal volume and minute volume. Also, blood samples can be taken for the measurement of the blood oxygen concentration [25].

4.3.2.3 CNS safety
The central nervous system (CNS) is a tissue of critical importance and the absence of any effects of the drug candidate on its normal functioning should be confirmed before clinical testing is performed.

Modified Irwin's test
This test is designed to investigate the acute and delayed neurotoxicity effects of a drug candidate after single exposure [26, 27]. The species of choice is the rat. The drug is administered once by gavage at different dose levels producing plasma concentrations that are a multiple of the intended therapeutic level. The dose range is based on findings from acute toxicity tests in the rat conducted in drug discovery to avoid mortality as much as possible. After dosing, the animals are observed during a week for mortality, general clinical signs, body weight and body weight gain. Neurobehavioural observations are made within the first 24 h after dosing for acute neurotoxicity effects and after 1 week for delayed neurotoxicity effects. Neurobehavioural observations are made in the cage and during manipulation of the animals. An overview with examples of the type of neurotoxicity effects that can be observed is given in Table 4.3.

During the experiment, blood samples can also be collected at pre-dose and at several time points after oral dosing for toxicokinetic analysis. The highest dose or the highest C_{max} at which no neurobehavioural effects are observed is used for CNS risk assessment.

Table 4.3 Some examples of neurobehavioural observations that can be made in a modified Irwin's test in the rat.

Behavioural	Spontaneous activity	Abnormal biting
		Restlessness
		Abnormal licking
	Motor-affective responses	Sedation
		Excitement
		Vocalisation
	Sensoro-motor responses	Tail pinch
		Corneal reflex
		Startle response
Neurologic	Muscle tone	Body tone
		Grip strength
	Equilibrium and gait	Righting reflex
		Ataxia
		Paralysis
	CNS excitation	Tremors
		Convulsions (clonic, tonic)
Autonomic	Eyes	Pupil size
		Light response
		Exophthalmia
	Secretions and excretions	Salivation
		Lacrimation
		Diarrhea
	Other	Body temperature
		Piloerection
		Respiratory rate

4.3.3 Toxicology

In contrast to safety pharmacology studies nearly all standard toxicology studies conducted in drug development have to be in compliance with internationally agreed test guidelines [12, 28] and good laboratory practices [11]. Tests that have to be tailored towards particular questions to be answered in drug development such as the elucidation of mechanisms of toxicity or carcinogenicity are not included in the test guidelines but need to be executed in compliance with GLP. The overview of toxicology tests given in this chapter is not exhaustive but representative of the tests that are currently most used in the safety assessment of drugs during development. More detail on the conduct and interpretation of toxicology tests in drug development can be found in textbooks on toxicology [29–34].

4.3.3.1 Acute toxicology

The first test that is carried out to assess the toxicity of a drug candidate *in vivo* is the acute toxicity test. In this test, a single dose of the drug is administered orally by gavage or by intravenous injection in one or several animal species. The first dose range used is to get a first idea about the no-observed-adverse-effect-level (NOAEL) after single dosing. The endpoints of this test are not mortality and morbidity but signs of acute toxicity. To that effect, the animals are observed for clinical signs, body weight, body weight gain and blood samples are drawn for hematology and serum biochemistry evaluation. The animals are sacrificed after the period of observation that may range from 1 day up to 2 weeks after administration of the drug. At necropsy, organ weights are recorded and gross pathology observations made. If necessary, tissues showing gross pathology effects can be examined histopathologically. The result of acute toxicology tests serves as a basis for the dose selection of the first *in vivo* single-dose safety pharmacology tests and the repeated-dose range finding tests later in early drug development.

4.3.3.2   Genotoxicology

There exist a vast number of assays that can be used in the genotoxicity testing of drugs. The tests described in this section are part of the so-called core battery for the first evaluation of the genotoxic potential of drugs in development. These tests address gene mutations as well as chromosome aberrations and aneuploidy (abnormal number of chromosomes).

Ames assay

This bacterial reverse gene mutation assay is the first test that is carried out to assess the mutagenic potential of a drug molecule in drug discovery and development. The assay is based on the conversion, by mutation, of a histidine-requiring bacterium (*Salmonella typhimurium*) into an histidine-independent bacterium that can grow in culture media that are poor in histidine. Histidine is an amino acid that is essential for the growth of the bacteria. Besides the mutation that makes the bacterium histidine dependent, other mutations have also been introduced that increase the sensitivity of the bacteria for mutagens such as the increase of the permeability of the bacterial wall for large molecules and a decrease in the efficiency of the DNA excision repair system. The Salmonella strains that are used in the Ames test are TA1535, TA100 and TA102 for the detection of base-pair substitutions and TA98 and TA1537 for frame shifts. Of the bacterial strains used, TA102, TA100 and TA98 have an increased sensitivity to chemical and spontaneous mutations of which TA102 is very sensitive to oxidative and crosslinking mutagens. The test substance is dissolved in the culture medium at different concentrations in the presence or absence of an external bioactivation system. This is referred to as S9-mix that is composed of the post-mitochondrial fraction of Arochlor- or phenobarbital-induced rat livers and a NADPH-generating system. The S9-mix has cytochrome P450 enzyme activity and mimics to some extent the bioactivation of pro-mutagens *in vivo*. The solutions of the drug with and without S9-mix are added to a biotin–histidine supplemented top agar, mixed and then poured onto glucose agar for incubation. A minimal amount of histidine is necessary to allow the bacteria to start growing. An Ames test is considered positive if the mean number of revertants per plate has increased at least 2-fold for one of the strains TA98, TA102 or TA100 or has increased at least 3-fold for one of the strains TA1535 or TA1537 and when a clear concentration-related effect is observed. Limitations to this test are precipitation of the drug because of low water solubility and toxicity to the bacteria (e.g. antibiotics).

Mouse lymphoma assay

The mouse lymphoma assay is a mammalian cell test and therefore more predictive of the possible genotoxic potential of a drug candidate in man. It detects gene mutations as well as chromosome aberrations in mouse lymphoma (L5178Y) cells. The principle of the test is based on the mutation of the gene encoding for the enzyme thymidine kinase ($TK^{+/-}$) that is active in the phosphorylation of thymidine before it can be incorporated in DNA. When this gene is wiped out by a mutation, phosphorylation of thymidine or thymidine analogs such a trifluorothymidine (TFT) does not take place. TFT is toxic and produces cell death when incorporated in the DNA of the cells. This means that when the cells are exposed to TFT after incubation with the drug and that gene mutation has taken place so that TFT cannot become incorporated in DNA the cells will continue to grow. The drug candidate is dissolved in the culture medium containing the mouse lymphoma cells and is combined with S9-mix or not as an external source of bioactivation. Treatment is 3 h with S9 and 24 h without S9 and the mutated cells are allowed to grow in a selective medium containing TFT. The result is positive when the mean mutant frequency of any test concentration exceeds the sum of the mean concurrent vehicle control mutant frequency taking into account the global evaluation factor (GEF) [35]. In the case of a positive response, colonies can be scored using the criteria of large and small colonies. Small mutant colonies are indicative of slow growth and are associated with chemicals that induce gross chromosome aberrations.

Micronucleus assay

This is the only *in vivo* assay that is part of the core battery of genotoxicity testing of drugs in development. The end points of this assay are chromosomal aberrations and aneuploidy. The principle of this test is based on the appearance of a chromosome fragment in polychromatic erythrocytes (PCE) in the bone marrow of the mouse. When a drug candidate produces chromosome damage in the early stages of the development of the erythrocyte, when the nucleus is still present, chromosome fragment(s) produced as a result of chromosome damage stay behind when the nucleus is expelled during maturation of the erythrocyte. That fragment is referred to as the micronucleus. When it can be demonstrated that the micronucleus contains a centromere, then this is an indication of aneuploidy. The advantage of this test over the other *in vitro* genotoxicity tests is that the drug can be administered via the intended route of treatment and that it undergoes the pharmacokinetics (absorption, metabolism, distribution, excretion) of an integrated biological system. For the conduct of a micronucleus assay in the mouse, 1 control, 3 dose groups and 1 positive control group are used with 5 males and 5 females each. The animals receive a single dose via the intended route of administration of the drug and are observed for mortality, body weight and clinical signs up to 48 h after dosing. The animals are sacrificed at 24 or 48 h after dosing and the bone marrow is collected from the femur. Bone marrow slides are prepared and polychromatic (PCE) and normochromatic (NCE) erythrocytes counted for the evaluation of bone marrow toxicity and the micronucleated PCEs counted for mutagenicity. The test is considered positive if the incidence of micronucleated PCEs is statistically significantly different from controls and shows a dose–response relationship. To make sure that there is enough systemic exposure to the drug candidate, often blood samples are collected for toxicokinetic analysis. The micronucleus test can also be integrated in subacute toxicology (2 weeks, 4 weeks) studies in the rat where bone marrow is collected for evaluation at the necropsy of the animals. There also exists an *in vitro* version of the micronucleus test where the micronuclei are recorded in human TK6 cells in culture.

4.3.3.3   Local tolerance

Bovine corneal opacity and permeability (BCOP) assay
The BCOP assay is used to identify the potential of chemical substances to irritate eyes and mucous membranes. The isolated corneas from the eyes of freshly slaughtered cattle are mounted in corneal holders that consist of anterior and posterior compartments that interface with the epithelial and endothelial sides of the cornea, respectively. The corneas are first allowed to equilibrate with medium to resume normal metabolic activity before a baseline opacity measurement is performed. The drug candidate is applied onto the epithelial surface of the cornea, whereas the posterior compartment is filled with medium. After incubation, the drug residue is removed and corneal opacity measured as the amount of light transmission through the cornea. Subsequently, corneal permeability is determined using sodium fluorescein. The *in vitro* ocular irritation score is calculated from the mean corrected opacity value and a mean corrected permeability value.

Hen's egg chorio-allantoic membrane (HET-CAM) assay
The HET-CAM test is used to identify the potential of chemical substances to irritate eyes and mucous membranes with the difference that with the BCOP assay a vascular system is involved. The target tissue in this test is the chorio-allantoic membrane (CAM). The CAM is composed of three

layers of which the inner layer (mesenchyme) contains blood capillaries and sinuses that are easily visible when the tip of the egg shell is removed. Fresh fertile White Leghorn chicken eggs are incubated until 9 days old. The egg shell of viable eggs is removed at the level of the air cell and the drug candidate is placed onto the CAM after removal of the inner membrane. The endpoints are hemorrhage, vascular lysis and coagulation. The time of appearance of any of these effects is recorded. The irritancy potential of the drug candidate is calculated on the basis of the time of appearance of each of the endpoints. A variety of methods of analysis is available but the one that is used extensively is the irritation score (IS) [36].

In vitro phototoxicity assay
This assay is performed when there are indications that the drug candidate is able to absorb UV or visible light and has the tendency to accumulate in skin or eye tissue. In the *in vitro* phototoxicity assay, mouse embryo fibroblasts (BALB/c 3T3 c31 cells) are incubated with several concentrations of the drug candidate and irradiated or not with artificial sunlight (270–800 nm). The cytotoxicity observed (e.g. neutral red uptake inhibition) of the drug with and without irradiation is then compared. There is an indication of phototoxicity if cytoxicity is increased upon irradiation with artificial sunlight.

Local lymph node assay (LLNA)
When it is the intention to apply the drug on the skin it has to be evaluated for possible skin sensitisation (skin allergy). Such a test can also be carried out for reasons of occupational health when there is a risk of skin exposure during the handling of the drug candidate in the laboratory or during manufacturing. The principle of the local lymph node assay is the observation of cell proliferation of T-lymphocytes in the draining lymph node of the ear of the mouse after contact with a potential skin allergen. In this assay the drug is applied topically at different nonirritating concentrations on the dorsal side of the ears of mice for three consecutive days. Five days after the first application the animals are injected with a fluorescent (BrdU) or radioactive (^{3}H-methyl thymidine) DNA tag and sacrificed 5 h later. The draining auricular lymph nodes are excised and pooled per treatment group. The proliferating capacity of the T-lymphocytes is then quantified by fluorimetry or liquid scintillation counting (LSC) and is proportional to the sensitising potential of the drug molecule. The result of the test is considered positive when at least one concentration of the drug candidate applied onto the ear leads to an incorporation of the DNA-tag that is 3-fold greater than that of the controls.

In vivo vascular tolerance assay
When a drug is intended to be administered via intravenous injection or infusion it is important to evaluate its potential to produce inflammation of

the vascular wall. This can be done *in vivo* in the vascular tolerance assay in the dog. Several concentrations of the drug candidate in an intravenous formulation are infused for a period of 2 h in 3 dogs per dosing group using a catheter inserted in the vena cephalica or vena saphena. During a period of 7 days after dosing, the dogs are observed for mortality, clinical signs with investigation of the sites of injection and body weight. After 7 days, blood samples are taken for the determination of hematology, coagulation and serum biochemistry parameters including parameters indicative of systemic inflammatory responses such as C-reactive protein (CRP) and tumour necrosis factor α (TNF-α). Since the composition of the infusion formulation (concentration of the drug as well as the concentration and nature of excipients used) plays an important role in intravenous tolerability, this type of *in vivo* tests is used to optimise infusion formulations. When swelling or hardening of the veins is observed upon clinical examination or when one of the parameters indicative of systemic inflammation is increased, the development of that intravenous formulation is stopped and new research started to resolve the problem.

4.3.3.4   Repeated-dose toxicology

Repeated-dose toxicology studies can be roughly subdivided into subacute studies (2 weeks, 4 weeks), subchronic studies (3 months), chronic studies (6 months in the rat, 9 to 12 months in the dog) and carcinogenicity studies in rodents that can last as long as 24 months.

Before repeated-dose toxicology studies can be started, dose range finding studies need to be performed to explore the optimal dose range for the next longer-term toxicology study to be carried out. Small groups of rats are treated for a short period of time with three dose levels of the drug. The limit dose is 2000 mg/kg body weight for rodents and 1000 mg/kg body weight for non-rodents. The first indications for a range of doses to be explored are provided by the acute toxicity tests that have been conducted already in drug discovery. Limitations for the administration of high-dose levels are saturation of absorption or the physicochemical properties of highly concentrated dosing solutions or suspensions (e.g. too high a viscosity for administration by gavage). The animals are observed for mortality, clinical signs and body weight and are sacrificed at the end of the exposure period. Blood samples are collected for limited hematology and serum biochemistry analyses. Gross necropsy is performed and a limited number of tissues examined for histopathological changes.

For dogs, first a single-dose escalation explorative toxicology study is performed by only using a couple of animals. The dogs are treated with successive escalating single doses of the drug each time separated by a wash-out period. The animals are observed for mortality and clinical signs and blood is drawn for limited hematology and serum biochemistry analysis. Based on the findings of this first experiment three dose levels are selected for a dose range finding study over a short time period (e.g. 5 days). The observations made are similar to those of the rat dose range-finding studies. During these studies blood samples are also collected for toxicokinetic analysis to obtain a first idea about the relationship between systemic exposure to the drug candidate and some of its metabolites and toxicity.

Once a dose range has been identified, the test protocol for subacute toxicity studies can be designed. The most important elements of the test protocol for these studies are summarised in Table 4.4.

Important parameters that can be derived from subacute toxicology studies in rodent and non-rodent species are the maximum dose without adverse findings (NOAEL), the maximum tolerated dose (MTD) and the dose–response and systemic exposure–response relationships. With these data at hand the dose range of the next longer-term toxicology studies to be carried out can be proposed. Normally, 3 dose groups and 1 control group are used but additional

Table 4.4 Test protocol elements for 14/28-day oral toxicology studies in rat and dog.

	Rat	Dog
Test article formulation	Solution, suspension	Solution, suspension, capsule
Number of dose groups	4–5 (including control)	4–5 (including control)
Number of animals/sex/ group	5	3
Mode of administration	Gavage	Gavage, capsule application
Duration in vivo phase	2 weeks	2 weeks
Observations	Mortality	Mortality
	Clinical signs	Clinical signs
		Electrocardiography
	Ophthalmologic exam	Ophthalmologic exam
	Body weight	Body weight
	Body weight gain	Body weight gain
	Food consumption	Food consumption
	Hematology	Hematology
	Serum biochemistry	Serum biochemistry
	Urinalysis	Urinalysis
	Organ weights	Organ weights
	Gross pathology	Gross pathology
	Histopathology	Histopathology
Toxicokinetics	Blood samples taken on day 1 and day 14 from 2–4 animals/sex/satellite dose group	Blood samples taken on day 1 and day 14 from all animals of all dose groups
Toxicological parameters	NOAEL (mg/kg body weight)	NOAEL (mg/kg body weight)
Toxicokinetic parameters	t_{max}, C_{max}, AUC, $t_{1/2}$	t_{max}, C_{max}, AUC, $t_{1/2}$
Recovery group	Ad hoc	Ad hoc

Table 4.5   Test protocol elements for subchronic and chronic oral toxicology studies in the rat.

	3-months	12 months	18–24 months
Groups	1 control, 3 test	1 control, 3 test	1 control, 3 test
Species	Mouse, rat, hamster	Mouse, rat, hamster	Mouse, rat, hamster
No animals/group	10/sex	20/sex	50/sex
Administration	Gavage	Gavage, diet	Gavage, diet
Clinical observations	1/day + 1/week (detail)	1/day	1/day
Ophthalmological exam	Start and end of study	As clinical observations	No
Neurobehavioural testing	End of study	As clinical observations	No
Body weight	1/week	1/week (first 13 weeks)	1/week (first 13 weeks)
Food/water consumption	1/week	1/week (first 13 weeks)	1/week (first 13 weeks)
Hematology	End of study, all	3 m, 6 m, end of study	12 m,18 m, end of study
Biochemistry-urinalysis	End of study, all	6 m, end of study	No
Gross pathology	End of study, all	End of study, all	End of study, all
Histopathology	End of study(C, H, lesions)	End of study (C,H, lesions)	End of study, C, H, lesions

C: controls; H: high dose group

dose groups can be considered if the extrapolation of the doses to longer periods of treatment is uncertain. When there is only borderline toxicity at the highest dose level in the subacute toxicology tests then the same dose level can be maintained for a 3-month test. If distinct toxicity is present at the highest dose level and some indications thereof at the mid-dose level in subacute toxicology tests the mid-dose level can be chosen as the high-dose level in the 3-month study. Care should be taken that the low dose remains without any adverse effect to allow the determination of the NOAEL. In the test protocol of a 3-month toxicology study, a rationale should always be provided supporting the selection of the dose range. The results of the 3-month study allow for the design of the 6-month study in the rat and the 9-month study in the dog. In all the repeated-dose toxicology studies, satellite groups are included with rodents for toxicokinetic analysis. A summary of the critical elements of the test protocols for subchronic and chronic toxicology studies is given in Table 4.5.

4.3.3.5   Reproductive toxicology

All the tests covering all phases of the reproductive cycle, i.e. fertility → pre-natal development → post-natal development, are comprised in reproductive toxicology testing. In this chapter an overview is given of fertility tests in male and female animals, embryo–fetal development toxicity tests, pre- and post-natal development toxicity tests and juvenile toxicity tests.

Fertility

These tests are performed on male and female animals using the route of administration that is most relevant for the therapeutic application of the drug. Normally, 3 dose groups and 1 control group are used. The selection of the dose range is based on the experience gained from subacute toxicology studies. Approximately 24 animals per sex and per dose group are considered in fertility studies. A satellite group with fewer animals can be included for toxicokinetic analysis. The administration of the drug candidate is initiated 2 weeks prior to pairing for females and 4 weeks prior to pairing for males. Pairing is allowed for a maximum of 10 days and, if not successful the female is allowed to pair with a second male. When mating has taken place dosing continues until 1 week post-coitum for the females and until confirmation of fertility in the males. Females are sacrificed 1 week after cessation of dosing at day 14 of presumed pregnancy and males are sacrificed when fertility is confirmed in the females. The observations that are made in a male/female fertility study are summarised in Table 4.6.

The NOAEL of a fertility study is based on the statistically and biologically significant change towards controls of any of the parameters listed in Table 4.6. There may be different fertility NOAELs for male and female animals.

Embryo–fetal development

An embryo–fetal development test investigates the possible effect of the drug candidate on the development of the conceptus during the period of organogenesis. Normally, 3 dose groups and 1 control group are used. The selection of the dose range is based on the experience gained from subacute toxicology studies and the female fertility study. In the case of rabbits and mice for which not sufficient toxicology data exist, a dose range finding study with non-pregnant and later with pregnant animals is carried out to establish the dose range for the embryo–fetal development toxicology study. Female and male animals are paired and the females with a sperm positive vaginal smear are selected to become part of the main study. About 24 pregnant females are used for the main study. A satellite group with fewer animals is included for toxicokinetic analysis to evaluate possible transuterine transfer of the drug or one of its metabolites. The animals are dosed during the period of organogenesis and are sacrificed just before parturition. The uterus is excised and the fetuses isolated for examination. The observations that are made in an embryo–fetal development toxicology study are summarised in Table 4.7.

The structural changes of the fetuses are subdivided in birth abnormalities that are rare and most of the time lethal (e.g. excencephaly, spina bifida), minor abnormalities which are minor deviations from normal and that are

Table 4.6 Parameters of a male/female fertility study in the rat.

Parameters	Males	Females
General toxicity	Mortality Clinical signs Body weight Food consumption	Mortality Clinical signs Body weight Food consumption
Reproductive toxicity		Oestrous cycling (monitoring of vaginal smears) Confirmation of mating (sperm, copulation plugs) Copulation index Fertility index Pre-implantation loss Post-implantation loss
	Sperm motility Sperm count Sperm morphology	
Gross pathology		Weight of the gravid uterus Number of corpora lutea Number of implantation sites Number of resorptions Number of live embryos Number of dead embryos
	Weight of testes Weight of epididymides	
Microscopic pathology		Ovaries Uteri
	Testes Epididymides Prostate Seminal vesicles Coagulation gland	

Table 4.7 Parameters of the embryo–fetal development toxicology study in the rat.

General maternal toxicity	Mortality Clinical signs Body weight Food consumption
Gross pathology of the dams	Weight of the gravid uterus Number of corpora lutea Number/position of live and dead foetuses Number/position of resorptions Ovaries
Gross pathology of the foetuses	Body weight of the live foetuses Sex ratio of the live foetuses External abnormalities of the live foetuses Skeletal abnormalities of $\frac{1}{2}$ of the live foetuses Visceral abnormalities of $\frac{1}{2}$ of the live foetuses

found relatively frequently and deviations that are frequently found in control groups and are more frequent in the case of retardation of fetal development (e.g. extra pair of ribs, bent ribs, fused sternebrae). Two NOAELs can be derived from this study (one for maternal toxicity and one for embryo–fetal toxicity) and are based on the statistically and biologically significant change towards controls of any of the parameters listed in Table 4.7.

Pre- and post-natal development

A pre- and post-natal development study investigates the effects of the drug under development on pregnant and lactating female animals and on the development of the fetus and offspring following exposure of the female from implantation through weaning, i.e. from day 6 of pregnancy until day 21 of lactation for the rat. Three dose groups and 1 control group including each about 25 pregnant females are used. A satellite group with fewer animals is included for toxicokinetic analysis to evaluate the possible transfer of the drug or one of its metabolites to the offspring and excretion in milk during lactation. The dose range of this study is based on all the experience gathered with the repeated-dose toxicology studies up to 3 months, the fertility study in the female rat and the embryo-fetal toxicology studies in the rat and a second animal species. The route of administration that is most relevant for the therapeutic application of the drug candidate is selected. The pre- and post-natal development toxicology study is just only one of the many types of reproductive toxicology studies that are currently in use (e.g. 1-generation, 2-generations, 3-generations, continuous breeding, development neurotoxicity and extended 1-generation studies) but is the study that is most frequently used in drug development. The observations that are made in a pre- and post-natal development study are summarised in Table 4.8.

The number and type of observations listed are not exhaustive and can be extended with any other endpoint that is important for the toxicological and reproductive characterisation of the drug. One NOAEL can be derived from this study and is based on the statistically and biologically significant change towards controls of any of the parameters listed in Table 4.8.

Juvenile development

A juvenile development toxicology study is carried out to investigate the possible effect of the drug under development on the development of juvenile animals from weaning to sexual maturity. Many different study protocols are possible for juvenile toxicology studies. They may be tailored towards target organ systems undergoing significant growth and development or they may be more general with a dosing window that covers the development of all organ systems. An example is given in Table 4.9. One NOAEL can be derived from this study and is based on the statistically and biologically significant change towards controls of any of the parameters listed in Table 4.9.

Table 4.8   Parameters of a pre- and post-natal development study in the rat.

General maternal toxicity	Mortality
	Clinical signs
	Body weight
	Food consumption
Reproductive maternal toxicity	Parturition
	Litter size
	Implantations
	Gestation length
	Rearing behaviour
	Lactation
Gross pathology of maternal animals	Weight of major organs
	Weight of reproductive tissues
Microscopic pathology of maternal animals	Major organs with gross lesions
	Reproductive tissues
General pup toxicity	Survival
	Clinical signs
	Sex ratio
	Body weight
Developmental pup toxicity	Pre-weaning landmarks of development
	Reflexes
	Motor activity
	Learning and memory

4.3.3.6   Carcinogenicity

A carcinogenicity study is conducted when the drug under development is intended to be taken for a long period of time (>6 months) and there are indications that lesions found in the subchronic and chronic toxicology studies may develop into tumours. These tests are carried out in rats and mice that are normally treated via the oral route by gavage for a period of 24 months. In most instances 3 dose groups and 1 control group are used, but additional dose groups may be considered if the extrapolation of the dose range from 3-month studies is uncertain. The experimental conditions of a typical carcinogenicity study in rodents are summarised in Table 4.10.

One NOAEL can be derived from this study and is based on the statistically and biologically significant change towards controls of any of the parameters listed in Table 4.10. Important in the carcinogenicity study is the interpretation of the tumours in terms of their dose–response relationships and their relevance to man.

4.3.3.7   Immunotoxicology

In general, the design of a subacute toxicology study in the mouse or the rat using 3 dose groups, 1 control group and a toxicokinetic satellite group is taken

Table 4.9 General toxicity screening study design in juvenile rats.

Period	Dosing		Arm 1	Arm 2	Arm3
PND 0-5		PND1		Fostering of litters to 5/sex/litter	
		PND4		Culling to 4/sex/litter	
PND5-PNW9	X	PND21		Weaning	
	X	PND21-PNW8		Sexual maturation landmarks	
	X	PNW8		Serum biochemistry	
	X	PNW8-9		Ophthalmology	
	X	PNW9	Blood sampling for TK, sacrifice and organ weights, gross and microscopic pathology (10/sex)		
PNW9-14		PNW9-12		Neurobehavioural testing (10/sex)	
		PNW12			Reproductive assessment (20/sex)
		PNW14		Terminal sacrifice, hematology, serum biochemistry, organ weights, gross and microscopic pathology (10/sex)	

PND: post-natal day; PNW: post-natal week

as a basis for the conduct of a tailored immunotoxicology study. On top of the usual endpoints of a toxicology test, additional immunotoxicity parameters are added such as lymphocyte subset analysis to detect alterations in leucocyte populations (e.g. total T cells, total B cells, T helper cells), the determination of immunoglobulins (e.g. IgE, IgM), the determination of cytokines regulating innate immunity (e.g. tumour necrosis factor, chemokines) and cytokines regulating adaptive immunity (e.g. interleukins, interferon-γ). More extensive histopathological analysis can be performed on mesenteric, mandibular and popliteal lymph nodes, thymus, spleen and Peyer's patches in animals from all test groups. T-cell dependent anti-body response can be evaluated in the plaque-forming cell (PFC) assay at the termination of the immunotoxicology study. This test is based on the production of IgM anti-bodies by the B-cells of the spleen against sheep red blood cells and is a good indicator of the possible

Table 4.10   Critical test protocol elements of carcinogenicity studies in rodents.

Species	Mouse and rat
Test article formulation	Solution, emulsion, suspension, diet
Number groups	3–4 dose groups and 1 control group
Number of animals/sex/group	Minimum 50 + toxicokinetic satellite groups
Mode of administration	Gavage, diet
Duration of administration	Maximum 24 months
Observations	Mortality
	Clinical signs
	Body weight
	Body weight gain
	Food consumption
	Water consumption
	Hematology (at 12 m, 18 m and at end of study)
	Organ weights, all animals
	Gross pathology, all animals with specific attention to tumours
	Histopathology, all animals with gross pathology and tumours, specific attention to tumours
Toxicokinetics	Blood samples taken up to 6 months from animals at all dose levels
Toxicological parameters	Detailed description of all tumours with their incidences before and at termination of the study
	NOAELs for carcinogenicity and toxicity
Toxicokinetic parameters	t_{max}, C_{max}, AUC (0–24 h, last day), $t_{1/2}$ (0–24 h, last day)

influence of the drug molecule on immune response. Before sacrifice, the animals are injected with sheep red blood cells. At necropsy the spleen is excised and a suspension of spleen cells is prepared and incubated together with sheep red blood cells in culture. A so-called plaque (light zone) is formed around an IgM producing B-cell due to the lysis of the sheep red blood cells.

4.3.3.8   Neurotoxicology

To perform a neurotoxicology test the design of subacute or subchronic toxicology studies can be used with the addition of a number of specific endpoints. These, amongst many others, can be the measurement of acetyl and butyl cholinesterase activity in plasma, red blood cells and the brain, and a detailed neuropathological examination of the brain, the spine and peripheral nervous tissue in animals that have been perfused to that effect after sacrifice. Also, staining techniques (e.g. copper–silver stain) specific for neural tissue can be applied for histopathological examination. Additional neurobehavioural observational tests can be included such as water maze performance and passive avoidance performance tests.

4.4 Clinical development

In this section, a selection of methods and techniques is presented that are commonly used in clinical drug development, such as pharmacometric tools (e.g. PK/PD analysis, modelling techniques, and population kinetics), biomarkers, medical imaging techniques, human electrocardiography, and clinical trial methodology. Some of these methods and techniques are also used in nonclinical drug development (e.g. PK/PD, biomarkers, imaging techniques).

4.4.1 Pharmacometrics

Pharmacometrics is the emerging science of quantitative pharmacology. It is 'concerned with mathematical models of biology, physiology, pharmacology and disease used to describe and quantify interactions between xenobiotics and patients' [37]. It is the science of quantifying disease, drug and trial characteristics – in particular through modelling and simulation – that helps to increase the efficiency of the discovery, development and clinical use of new drugs. It is the basis of a new paradigm in innovative drug development known as model-based drug development, whereby disease, drug and trial models are used in concert to steer drug development, regulatory decision making and rational use of new drugs in clinical practice.

4.4.1.1 Drug models

Modelling and simulation have long been used to characterise, understand and predict exposure–response relationships of drugs, including various types of pharmacokinetic (PK), pharmacodynamic (PD), and PK/PD modelling techniques.

Individual PK analysis and *physiologically-based PK modelling* (PBPK) that have already been discussed in the nonclinical section of this chapter (Section 4.3.1.6), are equally useful in clinical pharmacokinetics and clinical drug development.

Population pharmacokinetic analysis and modelling aims at identifying and understanding the variability in clinical PK data amongst individuals from drug target populations. It thus helps to explain variability in drug efficacy and safety in various patient population groups and to define the optimum dosing strategy for new drugs. These 2 commonly used models estimate the fixed-effect (mean) and variability in the patient (sub)population, either by multiple measurements on each patient (the 2-stage approach using a rich data set), or either by sparse data collection on a limited number of patients at various time points (the nonlinear mixed-effect approach that is more appropriate in late clinical development).

PK/PD analysis and modelling links and integrates information from dose-systemic exposure relationships (PK) with information from systemic exposure-effect/response relationships (PD) allowing the characterisation and prediction of the time course of the intensity of the pharmacological effect in response to the administration of a given dose of the drug. It is particularly useful in early drug development to predict (desirable as well as undesirable) drug effects in humans from nonclinical data. Over the years, PK/PD modelling has developed from a purely descriptive approach to a mechanism-based and more recently to a systems-based approach, resulting in ever more accurate predictions. It is considered an important tool in the rational approach to individualised drug therapy.

4.4.1.2 Disease models

With the advent of systems biology, having its roots in the modelling of enzyme kinetics and signaling pathways, models of normal and pathophysiological states became available. Human disease models try to predict the natural progression of a disease, the influence of placebo and the normal or pathological course of biomarkers and clinical outcome measures. Recently, a whole-cell computation model was able to predict the phenotype from the genotype of a human pathogen, underlining the importance of the array of 'omics' (genomics, transcriptomics, metabolomics, proteomics, etc.) as well as bioinformatics in boosting the recent progress in this field.

4.4.1.3 Trial models

Modelling and simulation can be applied to the design of clinical trials (e.g. to predict the best suitable patient population to be studied) and the analysis of clinical data (e.g. use of population-based PK and PK/PD models). Currently, models of comparative efficacy, effectiveness and cost-effectiveness are being developed, as well as model-based meta-analyses. New techniques in the analysis of the vast amount of available data from clinical (drug) trials, like data mining, linkage analysis and intelligent big data analyses, were instrumental in the development and use of these models.

Pharmacometrics, by definition a multidisciplinary science, tries to integrate all these techniques in the model-based drug discovery and development approach, with the ultimate goal to increase the efficiency of pharmaceutical innovation. In particular, the FDA, in its Critical Path Initiative (CPI) White paper of 2004 and in its Guidance on End of phase 2a meetings of 2009, advocates the use of pharmacometrics to which drug developers have responded positively [38]. Pharmacometric tools have already proven their value and potential for optimal dosing recommendations, for the targeting of patients who will benefit most from the new drug, and for paediatric marketing authorisation applications.

4.4.2 Biomarkers

A biomarker is an indicator of (the activity of) a biological state. There are many biomarkers used in biomedical research in general and in drug development in particular. They can be classified in different ways according to:

- their nature: gene (profile), protein/drug target, metabolites of xenobiotics, endogenous metabolites, signalling pathway, cell, imaging, viral particles, bacteria, etc.;
- the biological state they are related to: physiologic or pathologic;
- their objective: diagnostic, pharmacologic, physiologic, toxicologic, therapeutic;
- their use: (early) diagnosis, progression or prognosis of disease, outcome of treatment.

They can be measured by a variety of methods, including physical examination, laboratory tests or imaging techniques.

Biomarkers can be used as a prognostic tool (if the underlying biological state/disease changes, the biomarker changes accordingly), or as a predictive tool (the biomarker changes are predictive of the final clinical outcome of an intervention, either drug or other type of treatment).

In order to be really useful in clinical research and clinical practice, biomarkers should be validated on the basis of pre-specified criteria, a process that can be complex and time consuming. A validated biomarker should be clinically relevant, sensitive and specific to the treatment effects (either desired efficacy or unwanted side effects), reliable, practical and simple in use.

Fully validated prognostic or predictive biomarkers can be used as surrogate markers in clinical trials with drugs, respectively as a substitute for disease activity (progression/regression, remission/relapse) or as a substitute for a primary clinical outcome measure (surrogate endpoint for efficacy, resistance or safety).

In early drug development, biomarkers are instrumental in enabling better and faster decisions in a number of areas such as drug candidate selection, early studies demonstrating the mechanism of action and the activity of the drug candidate in man, dose ranging, patient stratification, and drug safety management.

In late drug development, biomarkers are most useful as surrogate endpoints in clinical trials. If validated and accepted by regulatory authorities, their use can lead to smaller sample sizes, shorter duration of studies and reduced costs of clinical drug development. Well-known examples are the use of blood pressure as a surrogate for hard clinical cardiovascular events (stroke, myocardial infarction) or bone mineral density as a surrogate for bone fractures. These biomarkers react fairly quickly to treatment and can be frequently measured, whereas the corresponding clinical endpoints are rather rare and need considerably more time to reliably demonstrate treatment effects. Although many biomarkers exist and are tested, very few are validated and accepted as surrogate endpoints for clinical drug trials.

In some medical disciplines and therapeutic areas biomarkers are widely available and used on a regular basis (e.g. cardiovascular, virology, oncology), while in others they are very difficult to develop and to validate (e.g. central nervous system). An example of various types of biomarkers [39] is given in Table 4.11.

Table 4.11 Examples of biomarkers used in drug development.

Type	Biomarker	Method	Use
Exposure	Drug metabolite	LC-MS/MS	Bio-equivalence testing
Surrogate	Blood pressure	Sphygmomanometer	Cardiovascular events in clinical trials
Effect	Target-ligand interaction	PET imaging	Tissue distribution of target engagement of a drug
Efficacy	Plasma HIV-1 concentration	qRT-PCR	Monitoring of viral load in AIDS patients
Mechanism	Lamellar lysosomal bodies	Electron microscopy	Monitoring of development of phospholipidosis
Translational	Urinary metabolic profile	Metabonomics	Comparison of endogenous metabolism across species
Toxicity	Alanine aminotransferase	Enzymatic assay	Monitoring of toxic liver injury

qRT-PCR: quantitative reverse transcriptase polymerase chain reaction

4.4.3   Imaging techniques

Medical imaging technologies are defined as non-(or minimally) invasive means of visualising anatomical structures and physiological processes in living humans (and animals). They are a subset of imaging techniques in general. They were initially developed as diagnostic aids in clinical practice, but soon also became important tools in biomedical research including drug development. Molecular or targeted imaging is specifically interested in the dynamics of disease- or treatment (drug)-specific molecular changes *in vivo*. Some of these techniques have been specifically adapted for applications in small laboratory animals in toxicology (e.g. MRI, PET, micro-CT, SPECT, ultrasonography).

Medical imaging techniques are usually divided into 2 categories, i.e. those that provide primarily:

-   structural information, such as computed tomography (CT), magnetic resonance imaging (MRI), and ultrasound (US); or
-   functional or molecular information, such as positron emission tomography (PET), single-photon emission computed tomography (SPECT), functional MRI (fMRI), dual-energy X-ray absorptiometry (DEXA or DXA) and optical imaging.

Often, different imaging modalities are combined or merged in a multimodal approach (e.g. PET-CT scan) offering structural as well as functional information in a complementary way.

A summary of the working principle of these techniques and their use in (clinical) drug development is given below. More details can be found in the specialised literature.

4.4.3.1 Computed tomography (CT)

Conventional radiography uses external ionising electromagnetic radiation, such as X-rays, as energy wave source to produce images of (parts of) the inside of the human body. Computed tomography uses computer-processed X-ray projections from different directions to produce cross-sectional or tomographic 2D images of specific areas in the body. These slices can be stacked to form 3D images. The machine used is called a CT scanner and the image generated is a CT scan.

CT can generate accurate spatial anatomical information, but is not suitable in itself for molecular imaging. It is widely used to help in the diagnosis of multiple diseases in different organ systems (e.g. skeletal injuries, tumours, atherosclerosis). It should be kept in mind that exposure to ionising radiation like X-rays has the potential to increase the risk of cancer.

In clinical drug development, CT can be used as a diagnostic tool, but also as an imaging biomarker for the follow-up of the progression of the disease and its response to drug treatment. It is commonly used in combination with functional imaging techniques such as PET in the assessment of malignant tumours. This combination allows a more complete picture of the tumour's location, its growth and metabolism, and thus of the impact of targeted drug therapy on these variables.

4.4.3.2 Magnetic resonance imaging (MRI)

The generation of an MRI scan is based on proton nuclear magnetic resonance (NMR). The principle on which proton NMR is based is explained in Section 4.2.3.1.

Hydrogen has a high magnetic moment and is for almost 100% abundant in the human body. This is why only proton NMR is used in clinical imaging. The varying molecular structures and the different amounts of hydrogen in various tissues affect the behaviour (transitioning from a lower energy state to a higher energy state) of the hydrogen nuclei (protons) in the strong external magnetic field when irradiated with radio-frequency photons. Tissues with a high water content (e.g. blood) become magnetised to a higher degree than tissues with a lower water content (e.g. fat tissue) which makes it possible to produce an image. The computer converts the NMR signal mathematically into an image, by recovering spatial information using Fourier analysis. MRI can create 2D images or 3D volumes with very good contrast, although MRI contrast agents can be used for further image improvement. Proton NMR produces better images than X-ray CT, especially from soft tissues (heart, blood vessels, tumours, brain), so that it is particularly useful for the generation of structural information from these tissues. MRI is considered less risky than CT as it doesn't produce ionising radiation.

Apart from conventional MRI, several other MRI modalities have been developed, including functional MRI (fMRI) and magnetic resonance spectroscopy (MRS), which are used in drug development.

Functional MRI is able to measure brain hemodynamics, such as cerebral blood flow and brain tumour angiogenesis, as well as brain activity (where blood flow is supposed to be higher). This technique has for instance been used to evaluate the effects of anti-angiogenic anti-cancer drugs and candidate drugs to treat Alzheimer's Disease, stroke and seizures.

Magnetic Resonance Spectroscopy (MRS) is an associated technique able to study targeted metabolites in brain or tumour tissue. Apart from ^{1}H nuclei it can also detect ^{31}P nuclei as present in phospholipid metabolites such as phosphocholine (PC). It is used to evaluate brain tumours, epilepsy, and neurodegenerative disorders. ^{31}P-MRS turned out to be particularly useful to grade brain tumours and to distinguish tumour recurrence from radiation necrosis. In clinical drug development, this technique showed promising results as a pharmacodynamic marker for assessing tumour response to novel anti-cancer drugs.

4.4.3.3   Positron emission tomography (PET) and single-photon emission computed tomography (SPECT)

PET is a nuclear medical imaging technique that uses injected tracers (radio-pharmaceuticals) labelled with positron-emitting radioisotopes (e.g. ^{11}C and ^{18}F), whereas SPECT uses tracer probes labelled with gamma-emitting radioisotopes (e.g. ^{123}I, ^{99m}Tc). Both techniques allow the generation of 3D images of primarily functional processes in the body.

The most widespread used PET tracer is ^{18}F-FDG (fluorodeoxyglucose) that allows the study of the metabolic activity of normal versus malignant tissue (where it is strongly increased). In clinical practice, it is extensively used to detect and stage metabolically active tumours and metastases. It can also be used to predict the outcome of anti-cancer (drug) therapy, even earlier than other response criteria.

Tumour protein synthesis can be traced by PET (e.g. by using amino acid probes such as ^{11}C-methionine) or SPECT (e.g. by using ^{123}I-iodomethyl-tyrosine), as well as tumour DNA metabolism (e.g. with several PET tracers). These tracers are therefore useful tools for the evaluation of early tumour responses to cytostatic chemotherapy.

Another example of the potential of PET imaging in drug development is demonstrated by its use in the study of receptor occupancy. When new drugs with novel mechanisms of action are first tested in humans, one of the key questions is whether the compound interacts with its intended pharmacological target in man. Receptor occupancy or target engagement can be adequately studied if a valid PET-tracer of the receptor or other target is available early in clinical development. In this case, the PET probe of the receptor is displaced from the receptor by the new drug only if the new drug binds to a sufficient extent to the receptor. Such a study was used for the development of aprepitant, a novel neurokinin 1 (NK-1) receptor antagonist as an anti-emetic drug, with positive outcome and subsequent receptor occupancy guided choice of doses in early clinical trials [40].

PET/SPECT scans are often combined with CT or MRI, either with 2 machines or all-in-one (PET-CT), giving both functional and structural information superimposed. Because PET and CT both use ionising radiation, this application cannot be repeated too often.

4.4.3.4 Dual-energy X-ray absorptiometry (DEXA, DXA)
DEXA is the preferred imaging technique to study bone mineral density (BMD) noninvasively in humans. It is easy and quick to perform with minimal risk of radiation exposure. A DEXA machine produces 2 X-ray beams, one with high and one with low energy. For each beam, the amount of X-rays that passes through bone is measured. From the difference between the two, bone mineral density can be calculated. It is the method of choice for the diagnosis of osteoporosis and the monitoring of its treatment by anti-osteoporotic drugs.

4.4.3.5 Ultrasonography (US)
Ultrasonography provides the visualisation of deep structures in the body by recording reflections of echoes of pulses of ultrasonic waves directed to the tissues of interest. The frequencies used range from 1.6 to 10 MHz. The lower frequencies have a greater depth of penetration and are used for the examination of deep body structures such as thoracic or abdominal organs. The high-frequency waves are used for superficial structures such as skin and eyes.

Ultrasonography is widely use in medicine, with many diagnostic and therapeutic applications, whereby several modes of ultrasound are used, such as 2D, motion (M), and various Doppler modes. It is also an important imaging tool in clinical drug development. This can be illustrated with two selected examples:

- intravascular ultrasound (IVUS) to assess atheroma burden within the arterial vessel wall (anti-atherosclerotic drugs);
- echocardiography (2D mode for morphology, M mode for heart function and pulsed Doppler for blood flow) to assess the cardiac safety of many drugs, both in nonclinical toxicology and safety pharmacology, as well as in clinical trials in humans.

4.4.4   Human electrocardiography

Electrocardiography is a noninvasive transthoracic recording of the electrical impulses produced at every heart beat over a certain period of time. In humans, several thin skin surface wires (electrodes) are attached to the body, that conduct the electrical activity in pairs (leads) to a small device (electrocardiograph), that measures them and produces a read-out (electrocardiogram or ECG). The number of leads can vary from 3–4 (for continuous monitoring) to 12 (standard for research and cardiac safety aspects).

The ECG represents the sum of the individual action potentials of billions of cardiomyocytes (see Section 4.3.2.1, Figure 4.13). The electrical discharge of the heart at each heart beat is generated in the pacemaker cells of the sino-atrial (SA) node. At first, the atria depolarise and contract, then the ventricles. The electrical signal spreads through the atrio-ventricular (AV) node, over the bundle of His, to the right and left bundle branches ending in a dense network of Purkinje fibres (the so-called conduction system).

A typical ECG tracing during a normal heart beat at rest is shown in Figure 4.14. It is composed of a P wave (the result of atrial depolarisation), the QRS complex (formed by the depolarisation of the endocardial and epicardial cardiomyocytes) and a T wave (representing ventricular repolarisation). An additional U wave (of unknown origin) is usually hidden behind it.

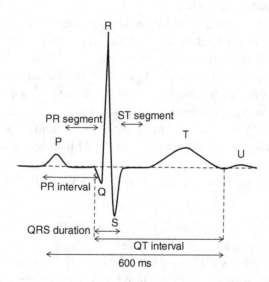

Figure 4.14   Normal human ECG tracing at rest.

The standard 12-lead ECG uses 10 skin electrodes attached to specific parts of the human body:

- 4 limb electrodes: on the left arm (LA), the right arm (RA), the left foot (F) and the right foot (N);
- and 6 precordial chest electrodes: V1 to V6 (each at a precise position).

Each lead traces the voltage difference between 2 of the electrodes and has a specific name, for example lead I records the voltage difference between the LA and RA electrodes. As each of the 12 leads records the electrical activity of the heart from a different angle, their combined use gives a fairly complete picture of the functional status of (the different anatomical areas of) the human heart.

ECG recordings have long been used in clinical practice as a diagnostic tool for several types of heart disease (e.g. myocardial ischemia and infarction, arrhythmias, left ventricular hypertrophy, pulmonary embolism). They also play an important role in the assessment of cardiac safety during the entire clinical development of every new drug. Some calculated variables, like ST segment depression (a biomarker for ischemic heart disease) and QT interval prolongation (a biomarker for a typical arrhythmia Torsade(s) de Pointes) are important outcome variables for the evaluation of either the efficacy of anti-anginal drugs or the safety of torsadogenic drugs.

For diagnostic and research purposes, the ECG can also be recorded during a *cardiac stress test*, usually an exercise tolerance test (on a treadmill or bicycle) or a pharmacological challenge test (e.g. by giving dobutamine) performed in a monitored clinical environment. During the entire stress test, the ECG is recorded and blood pressure is measured at regular intervals. The test may be accompanied by echocardiography (an ultrasound imaging technique) or myocardial perfusion imaging (using a specific radiotracer emitting gamma rays), thus generating sufficient information to gain a fairly good idea of the heart's capacity to respond to stress-induced ischemia.

Ambulatory electrocardiography or *Holter monitoring* allows continuous monitoring of the electrical activity of the heart for at least 24 h, and often 72 h or even a week. It is used to identify patients with certain types of arrhythmias and to monitor their subsequent response to drug treatment.

4.4.5 Clinical trial methodology

Clinical trials (structured investigations in humans) and clinical drug trials (studying the effects of drugs in humans) are the building blocks of the clinical development of a candidate drug. Therefore, it is important to have some prior understanding of the different methodological approaches available when studying the effects of drugs in humans in the early as well as in the late development phase. Most of the aspects discussed in this section are valid for all clinical trials, whether drug trials or not. Whenever useful, explanations or examples are given with drugs.

4.4.5.1 Types of clinical trials

Interventional or non-interventional clinical trials
In interventional (or experimental) clinical trials, the investigator intervenes in the behaviour or the exposure of the study participants (e.g. by administering a drug) with the intention to study the effects of this intervention on the subjects. In non-interventional (or observational) clinical trials the investigator collects (health) data from study participants by means of observation only, without interfering (i.e. without intervention by the investigator).

Controlled or uncontrolled clinical trials
Controlled clinical trials are trials in which different groups of subjects are differently exposed to a treatment and the results are compared between them, e.g. the control group receives nothing or a placebo, another group receives the test drug, and a third group might receive a comparator drug. They are also known as comparative trials. Uncontrolled clinical trials are trials in which only one single group of participants receives the test drug, without comparison with a control group. By definition this is an open (-label) trial, whereby participants as well as investigators know exactly which treatment is received.

Prospective or retrospective clinical trials
Prospective clinical trials are trials in which study participants are identified, eventually treated (by a drug) and then followed forward in time. Retrospective clinical trials are trials in which (drug-related) events or (drug) exposures that occurred in the past are studied by questioning the study subjects or by investigating existing data in (medical) files or databases.

Longitudinal or cross-sectional clinical trials
Longitudinal clinical trials are trials during which events are studied in the same subjects over a (long) period of time, allowing the measurement of an incidence (number of new cases within a specified period of time over the number of subjects studied, e.g. x new cases per 1000 persons per year). Cross-sectional clinical trials are trials in which events or (drug) exposures are observed at one particular point in time, allowing the measurement of a prevalence (proportion of the study population presenting a certain event or exposure, e.g. x cases per 1000 persons).

Clinical trials can be combined in different ways. For example, one clinical trial can be observational, retrospective and cross-sectional, while another clinical trial can be interventional, prospective and longitudinal.

The 4 common types of observational trials are cohort studies, case-control studies, cross-sectional surveys, and case (series) reports. The most common type of interventional trial is the randomised controlled trial (RCT), the 'gold standard' of interventional clinical studies.

The data and/or results of similar single trials can be combined in 'systematic reviews' and 'meta-analyses', which constitute a critical analysis of all the clinical trial data that are publicly available, thus frequently leading to a more balanced conclusion. This means that there is a hierarchy of evidence in clinical trials, starting with case reports carrying the lowest level of evidence, over cohort studies and single randomised clinical trials, up to meta-analyses of several randomised clinical trials carrying the highest level of evidence, as represented in Figure 4.15.

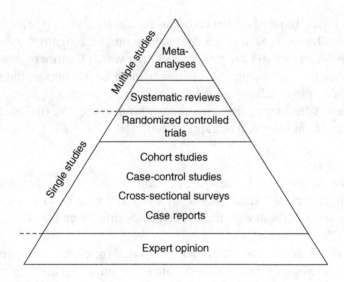

Figure 4.15 Pyramid with hierarchy of evidence from clinical trials.

4.4.5.2 The randomised controlled trial
The 'gold standard' of clinical trials is the randomised controlled trial (RCT) in which study participants are randomised to receive either the experimental intervention or treatment (for example, a new drug candidate) or another treatment as control or comparison.

Types of control
The control groups can be concurrent (i.e. drawn from the same study population) or external (either historical or current controls from another study). They can receive no treatment, a placebo, different doses of the same experimental drug, or an active (positive) control or comparator.

Randomisation

Allocation of treatment is done at random, thereby minimising systematic differences between groups. The process of randomisation is either simple (like tossing a coin, 1:1 randomisation), unequal (1:x:y randomisation), restricted in blocks of 4 or 6 subjects (for small or multicentre trials), or stratified (e.g. according to prognostic factors). For example, stratification can be done based on age or sex. Treatment allocation should be adequately concealed to the investigator team, either by a central randomisation procedure or by keeping the randomisation code in individual opaque sealed envelopes. The randomisation code can only be broken in exceptional circumstances, such as for serious safety reasons.

Blinding

A RCT may be blinded or masked. This means that some or all of the stakeholders involved in the study (i.e. the participants, investigators, outcome evaluators and statisticians) are unable to know which treatment was received. Unlike allocation concealment, blinding can be nearly impossible to achieve (e.g. when a bradycardic agent is tested). When both investigators and participants know which treatments are being administered, the trial is called open or open-label (but can still be randomised).

Study designs

There are several study designs possible to compare the intervention/ treatment groups or 'arms'. Some of the most widely used are described hereafter, each of them with their specific advantages and disadvantages.

Parallel group design   In a parallel group design, each study participant is randomised to one of two or more treatment groups that are followed in parallel. The comparative treatment period can be preceded by a run-in phase (in which all participants receive no treatment or placebo, either to randomise only stable participants or to exclude placebo responders) and/or followed by an extension period (e.g. all participants on the experimental drug) or a (placebo) wash-out (e.g. to study withdrawal effects). An example of a clinical trial with a parallel group design is schematically represented in Figure 4.16.
  The advantages of this design are that:

–   it allows informative comparison of several interventions/treatments (e.g. different doses of the candidate drug, placebo, and standard treatment);
–   it is less prone to bias (systematic tendency due to associated factors deviating the observed drug effect from its true value) (see also below);
–   it is the ideal design to demonstrate efficacy and safety, for dose finding and in late phase development (large and long-term studies).

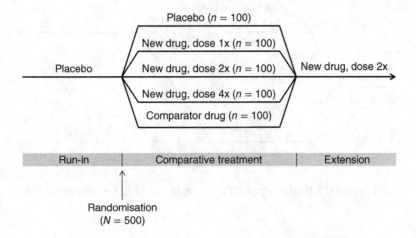

Figure 4.16 Parallel group design.

However, its disadvantage is that it usually needs larger sample sizes (between-subject comparison) and is more expensive.

Crossover design In a crossover design, the same group of study participants is given both or all treatments of interest in sequence, thus allowing within-subject comparison. The classic design is the 2 × 2 crossover design, where 2 treatments (A and B) are given over 2 periods (I and II) to 2 groups of study participants in 2 different sequences (AB and BA). After period I where participants receive either treatment A or B, they are switched or 'crossed over' to receive either treatment B or A in period II. If more interventions/treatments are to be compared, the designs become more complex (extra periods and extra sequences) and are known as higher-order crossover designs (including the Latin square design). A crossover design is presented in Figure 4.17 and a standard Latin square design in Figure 4.18.

The advantage of this approach is that smaller sample sizes are needed (each participant is its own control). It is most useful for bioequivalence studies and in early drug development for studies with single-dose administrations or short treatment durations. A major disadvantage is that it is less usable than parallel group designs because it is very demanding on sound methodology. The main problem is the carry-over of treatment effect from one period to the next. Therefore, a sufficiently long (placebo) wash-out interval has to be introduced between the different treatment periods to avoid that the following period(s) has (have) to be discarded. With the increasing length of each period and the increasing number of periods, the risk of drop-outs may be problematic. Only non-curable and rather stable diseases within the treatment or study period can be studied. Finally, attention should be paid to systematic differences between the treatment periods, e.g. participants may get used to

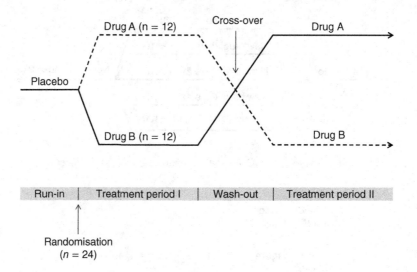

Figure 4.17   Crossover design. Full line: treatment arm BA; dashed line: group AB

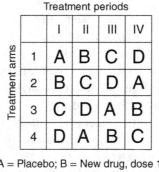

A = Placebo; B = New drug, dose 1×;
C = New drug, dose 2×; D = Comparator drug;
(n = 12 in each group)

Figure 4.18   Standard Latin square design.

a measurement or become more sensitive to the intended drug effect or a side effect.

Adaptive designs   In adaptive designs the initially planned design can be changed during the course of the study in accordance with the data generated during the trial. Because of the built-in flexibility, they are also called 'flexible designs'. Adaptive designs are a subset of flexible designs that allow only modifications that were planned or pre-specified in the study protocol, so that the redesign of the study does not undermine its scientific validity.

Possible adaptations are changes in sample size, dose (escalation) or randomisation schedule, dropping or adding a treatment arm, dropping or enriching subpopulations ('drop-the-losers' or 'enrichment' designs that target patients that can benefit the most), stop early (for efficacy, safety or futility reasons), and countless other variations.

The advantages of adaptive trial designs are that they may increase the efficiency of clinical drug development (reduction in size, time and costs of studies), and that fewer participants are assigned to inferior interventions/treatments. Major disadvantages are the increased complexity (deviating from the original question or the original patient population), the introduction of bias, and the fact that they are more difficult to replicate (limiting their reproducibility and generalisability).

Types of comparison

In comparative clinical trials, essentially 3 types of comparison are possible: superiority (A superior to B), equivalence (A equivalent to B), and non-inferiority (A not clinically inferior to B). Clinical trials can either be designed to show one of these or a combination (e.g. superiority to placebo and non-inferiority to comparator).

In new drug development:

1°/ *Superiority trials* intend to demonstrate that the response to the drug candidate is superior to that of the placebo and the active control. They are thus most convincing to demonstrate efficacy and are frequently used in phase 2 and phase 3 trials.

2°/ *Equivalence trials* allow the demonstration of therapeutic equivalence, i.e. the response to 2 or more drugs differs to an extent that is therapeutically unimportant. The (two-sided) equivalence margin (between lower and upper acceptable differences) should be pre-specified and justified in the study protocol. In clinical equivalence (CE) trials the demonstration of therapeutic equivalence is based on clinical outcome variables (e.g. blood-pressure reduction of the fixed association of 2 anti-hypertensive drugs versus the combination of the 2 single drugs), while in bioequivalence (BE) trials it is based on pharmacokinetic variables (a number of plasma versus concentration time curve descriptors). Examples of bioequivalence trials are the comparison between new formulations and the initial formulation (either during drug development or once the drug is on the market) and between generic products and the innovator drug.

3°/ *Non-inferiority trials* are designed to assess whether the drug candidate is not unacceptably worse, i.e. is as good as or better than current standard therapy or best available care. The new drug should not be clinically inferior by more than a pre-specified (one-sided) non-inferiority margin, i.e. the largest reduction in efficacy that is considered clinically irrelevant.

This design is often used in phase 3 studies when efficacious treatments already exist (and it is unethical to include a placebo arm) and the candidate drug is considered at least as good with some other advantages such as a better safety profile, patient convenience or cost effectiveness.

Although non-inferiority trials have gained popularity in drug development, their methodology and interpretation of results are not always well understood. For example, if in a non-inferiority trial the results show superiority of the new treatment over the standard, then superiority can be concluded. If on the contrary, non-inferiority is not demonstrated, this does not necessarily imply that the new treatment is inferior (Figure 4.19).

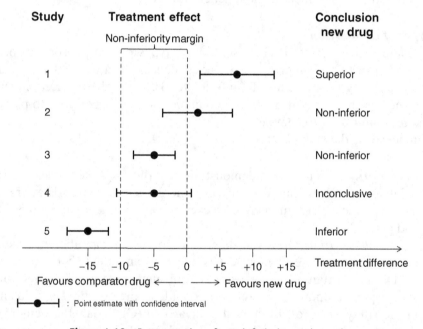

Figure 4.19   Interpretation of non-inferiority study results.

The choice of the non-inferiority margin is crucial in order not to introduce bias. If this margin is not sufficiently rigorously predefined, then an inferior drug could be accepted as non-inferior and become the standard in future drug trials, a phenomenon known as 'biocreep' leading to erosion of the quality of care.

4.4.5.3   Observational studies
In non-interventional or observational studies, study participants receiving a particular treatment (such as one or more drugs) are observed rather than being assigned to it (at random) by the investigator. This type of methodology is intensively used in clinical (pharmaco-) epidemiology research.

In the EU Clinical Trial Directive [41], a non-interventional drug trial is defined as follows: 'A study where the medicinal product(s) is (are) prescribed in the usual manner in accordance with the terms of the marketing authorisation. The assignment of the patient to a particular therapeutic strategy is not decided in advance by a trial protocol but falls within current practice and the prescription of the medicine is clearly separated from the decision to include the patient in the study. No additional diagnostic or monitoring procedures shall be applied to the patients and epidemiological methods shall be used for the analysis of collected data'. There are essentially 4 types of observational studies:

Case reports and case series

A case report is a simple description of clinical or other data observed in a single patient, such as a suspected side effect of a drug. A case series concerns a number of similar individual observations.

This type of observational study is widely used for routine pharmacovigilance once the drug is on the market (in the post-authorisation phase of drug development), where individual notifications of suspected drug side effects (through a yellow-card system or an electronic equivalent) are collected and analysed by Regulatory Agencies or the WHO Drug Monitoring Centre (Uppsala, Sweden). Although these studies are only descriptive in nature, they can play an important role in the detection of new safety signals that can be explored further. The advantages of these studies are that they are simple, easy and inexpensive, and that they are useful as an alert and for hypothesis generation. Disadvantages of case report studies include that they gather only anecdotal evidence, (exposure can only be roughly estimated) and that they are difficult to generalise.

Cross-sectional study

Cross-sectional studies collect data at one specific point in time. They allow a prevalence estimation, i.e. the number of persons with a certain characteristic (drug side effect) as a percentage of the persons at risk (exposed to the drug in the study), and are therefore also known as prevalence surveys. They are most suitable to study common diseases/side effects. Also, a wide variety of exposures and outcomes can be studied simultaneously and they are relatively inexpensive. However, they are only descriptive and hypothesis generating, and are unsuitable for rare diseases/side effects, prone to selection bias (selective choice of individuals to take part in the study) and provide only a snapshot with no information over the evolution over time.

Case-control study

In a case-control study, subjects with a certain disease or suspected drug side effect (the cases) are compared with subjects that do not present the disease of interest or side effect but are otherwise similar (the controls). The objective is to look back in time (retrospective) and identify the factor(s) or exposure(s) that may have caused the disease or side effect, for example, the suspected drug (class). A schematic representation is given in Figure 4.20.

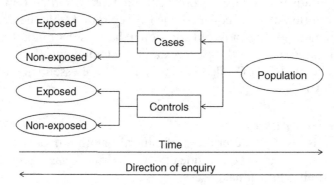

1) Select groups of diseased (cases) and non-diseased participants (controls)
2) Compare prior exposures between groups (no prevalence nor incidence estimation possible)

Figure 4.20   Case-control study.

The advantage of this approach is that it is the only practical way to study the aetiology of rare diseases/side effects. To demonstrate an association with the same statistical power, a case-control study would need to include only hundreds of patients, whereas a cohort study or RCT would have to include several (tens of) thousands of patients. Also, multiple side effects can be studied simultaneously, as well as side effects with a very long latency period. However, a case-control study provides no estimate of prevalence (artificially set at 50% by design, i.e. the same number of cases and controls) or incidence rate (proportion of new cases over time) and it is prone to different types of bias, mostly selection bias (whereby persons who decide to participate in the study are different from those who do not) and recall bias (cases tend to do more their best to remember the exposures that might have caused their disease than the controls).

Cohort study
A cohort or panel study is a study in which one or several groups of people with common characteristics (cohort) are followed over time (longitudinally), in order to make observations about the association between a particular exposure or risk factor and the subsequent development of disease or (side) effects. A schematic representation is given in Figure 4.21.

In clinical drug development, this design is often used in the post-authorisation phase to compare the effectiveness and safety of the new drug with standard therapy in real-life clinical practice. The longitudinal follow-up can be prospective (exposure is defined today and outcomes accrue in the

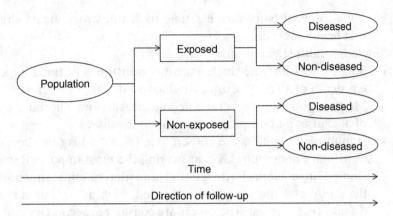

1) Selected groups of participants exposed to a new drug and non-exposed ones
2) Compare incidence of diseased between groups

Figure 4.21   Cohort study.

future) or historical (exposure was defined in the past and outcomes are collected today).

An advantage of cohort studies is that cases are incident (rather than prevalent) and thus more informative. They are also less subject to bias, and offer the only practical way to study a rare exposure (e.g. orphan drug). On the other hand, large study populations are needed that make cohort studies more expensive, and often long study durations make this study type sensitive to drop-outs.

A nested case-control study is a case-control study in a cohort study. Cases that occur in a cohort are matched with controls from the same cohort that did not (yet) develop the disease or side effect of interest. It allows considerable reduction of costs and efforts without much loss of statistical efficiency.

4.4.5.4   Study endpoints

An important consideration when designing a clinical (drug) trial is the choice of outcome variables or study endpoints, defined as a clear outcome measure associated with an individual study participant. There is an enormous variety of study endpoints and they can be categorised in many different ways:

- According to the type of variable:
  - Quantitative (continuous, numerical), representing a specific measure or count (e.g. cell count, systolic blood pressure).
  - Qualitative (categorical): characterising a certain quality, either binary/dichotomous (only 2 possibilities, e.g. death, gender), unordered or nominal (many equal possibilities, e.g. race), or ordered (several possibilities with different value, e.g. disease severity).

- • Time-to-event (survival): e.g. time to death, stroke, heart attack, or first hospitalisation.
- – Single or multiple endpoints:
  - • Single endpoint: one single outcome measure is deemed important, e.g. death of all causes, or death due to a disease of interest.
  - • Multiple endpoints: several outcome measures are chosen, e.g. death of all causes *and* hospitalisation due to the disease.
  - • If multiple endpoints are chosen, one (or more) is (are) considered as primary endpoint(s), i.e. answering the most important question studied in a clinical (drug) trial and determining the power of the study and the sample size needed, such as overall survival or disease-free survival. The others are considered secondary endpoints that answer other relevant but less important questions, such as reduction of the number of disease-related hospitalisations.
- – Hard and soft endpoints:
  - • Hard endpoints are non-ambiguous, such as death, myocardial infarction (MI) and bone fracture.
  - • Softer endpoints are blood pressure, serum cholesterol, quality of life (QoL) measures.
- – Clinical and nonclinical endpoints:
  - • Clinical endpoints are direct outcome measures of a clinical effect or benefit, such as reduction in (fatal) stroke or (fatal) MI.
  - • Nonclinical endpoints can be biochemical in nature (e.g. blood glucose), pharmacokinetic (AUC) or socioeconomic (QoL or quality-adjusted life years, QALYs).

Composite endpoints are combinations of 2 or more single endpoints. They have become particularly fashionable in cardiovascular drug development in order to increase the current low number of event rates in cardiovascular clinical trials (because patients are already well treated with a combination of several effective drugs). When single-event rates are low, the number of study participants needed to demonstrate a meaningful difference becomes very high and makes the trial very costly. For example, the primary endpoint can be a combination of cardiovascular death, stroke or nonfatal MI, whereby only one event can be counted for each patient (whatever comes first or with rules for hierarchy between endpoints). Although they increase the efficiency of clinical (drug) trials, composite endpoints can give results that are difficult to interpret [42]. As an example, in the secondary prevention of cardiovascular (CV) diseases, aspirin produces an 18% reduction in a CV composite endpoint (MI, stroke or CV death). However, a closer look at the separate endpoints reveals a 44% reduction in MI, a 22% reduction in stroke and no effect on CV death, making it particularly difficult to come to a unanimous interpretation of the results.

Surrogate endpoints are relatively simple laboratory or clinical measurements used as a substitute or marker for a clinically harder and more meaningful endpoint. They can be distinguished from simple biomarkers and intermediate endpoints in that they are better validated in reflecting and predicting hard clinical endpoints. They are particularly useful in early clinical drug development.

4.4.5.5 Statistical analysis issues

As biostatistics is a scientific discipline in itself, only a few issues that merit special attention in the context of the clinical drug development process are described.

First, it is very important that the statistical analysis plan of any clinical (drug) trial is thoroughly discussed with a (group of) biostatistician(s) before the start of the study. As much as possible, all planned statistical analyses should be pre-specified in the study protocol. Some intermediate analyses and modifications to the initial plan can be justified during the course of the trial, and even between database lock and the start of the analyses (*ad hoc* analyses). However, *post hoc* analyses, added after the completion of the planned analyses, can only be hypothesis generating and their results will have to be hypothesis tested in a new study.

Different sets of study participants can be analysed for different purposes:

- The 'intention-to-treat' (ITT) set includes all the study participants, regardless of whether they did or did not fully comply with the protocol (they are analysed in the group they were randomised in, even when they switched inadvertently to another treatment group; and also if their data are incomplete because of treatment withdrawal or protocol violations). This is the most conservative analysis (not prone to bias) and it is more pragmatic (closer to real life).
- The 'full analysis set' (FAS) includes all participants that received at least one dose of the intended treatment/drug. This is widely used to analyse drug safety.
- The 'per protocol' (PP) set includes only participants that were fully compliant with the study protocol. This analysis focuses rather on efficacy and is more explanatory.

The statistical plan can also include a number of subgroup analyses. These subgroups can be based on patient characteristics (age, disease severity), risk factors (blood pressure as a predictor of cardiovascular complications) or a specific trial outcome (myocardial infarction, stroke). They can be useful to identify subgroups of patients that are better responders, they can test whether randomisation worked properly, and they can be hypothesis generating for future studies. Common pitfalls are that the subgroups are often (too) small, that too many subgroups are analysed, and that they are performed *post hoc*, with increased risk of false-positive results. This phenomenon is known as 'data dredging' or 'data torturing' and can lead to overinterpretation of poor results as real evidence.

4.4.5.6   Study validity

The validity of the conclusions of a clinical (drug) trial is highly dependent on the use of a sound scientific methodology. The *internal validity* of a clinical study reflects whether the experimental or observed effects are a valid estimate of the true effects, and are not biased or confounded by systematic inequalities in other components (in other words, is the study properly done?). The *external validity* of a clinical study reflects whether the study sample is representative of a clinically relevant patient population, in other words, are the results generalisable to routine clinical practice? This is primarily determined by the inclusion and exclusion criteria for the study participants. The *assay sensitivity* of a clinical study reflects its ability to distinguish an effective treatment from a less effective or ineffective one, in other words, is the study design and conduct capable of demonstrating a difference?

The internal validity of a trial can be disturbed by many forms of bias (systematic errors in methodology) or confounding (influenced by a confounder that is both associated with exposure and outcome). Examples are selection bias (selective allocation of subjects to different study groups), observer bias (especially when judging subjective outcomes as in psychiatric studies), attrition bias (excluding participants from analysis for protocol deviations or loss of follow-up), publication bias (selective reporting of studies with positive results only), and confounding by indication (the indication for treatment with a drug may also be related to the outcome measure, leading to an imbalance between study groups).

In general, bias and confounding have to be controlled by a good study design, but confounding can also be controlled for by adjusting the statistical analysis.

The strict use of inclusion and exclusion criteria for participants in clinical trials in the pre-authorisation phase of clinical drug development (focusing on efficacy) limits their external validity and generalisability to routine clinical practice (interested in effectiveness). Hence, the importance of also performing *pragmatic clinical trials* with fewer restrictions on the included patient population and a special interest in outcome variables that are more meaningful to day-to-day health care.

4.4.5.7   Combining clinical evidence

During the clinical development of a drug, there are many instances when results of different clinical trials are to be combined to get an overall view of the drug's therapeutic potential (e.g. at different milestones, before marketing authorisation application, and once the drug is on the market).

Meta-analysis

Meta-analysis is a statistical method for combining evidence of multiple studies using a strict methodology in order to prevent bias. In its simplest form, it combines the effect sizes of a set of similar studies (aggregated data), weighted for heterogeneity between trials according to a specific model (the fixed-effect or the random-effects model).

The strength of the conclusions relies heavily on the (public) availability of the results of all the studies that have been performed (with good, bad or inconclusive results). As it is well known that drug trials suffer from publication bias (skewed versus positive trials), meta-analyses of drug trials tend to overestimate the real therapeutic benefits of drugs. In order to counter this problem, the following measures were taken at an international level:

– Most clinical trials with drugs have to be registered in a publicly available database before the start of the inclusion of participants (e.g. www.clinicaltrials.gov, www.controlled-trials.com, www.clinicaltrials register.eu). This recommendation is now also part of the Declaration of Helsinki, and thus of the Good Clinical Practice guideline.

– In particular, in Europe, there is great public pressure to make all results of clinical drug trials publicly available and the European Medicines Agency intends to proactively release clinical trial data of drugs with a marketing authorisation (www.ema.europa.eu > home > special topics > releasing clinical-trial data).

A more promising type of meta-analysis is based on individual participant/patient data (IPD), where investigators of several studies are contacted to share the individual patient data in order to pool them in one database for statistical analysis.

A network meta-analysis allows the comparison of multiple treatments (drugs) even when they have not been compared directly in the individual trials. For example, when drug A was shown superior to B in trial 1, while drug B was shown superior to drug C in a similar trial 2, a proper network meta-analysis would be able to conclude that drug A is superior to drug C although they have not been compared head-to-head.

It is even possible to combine evidence from interventional trials and observational studies. This is particularly important because observational studies are only able to demonstrate an association between exposure and outcome, but do not allow direct causal inference between the two. They are dependent on circumferential evidence that supports causality (e.g. replication of results, the strength and consistency of the association), as well as on confirmation of the results from randomised controlled trials.

Evidence-based medicine (EBM)

Evidence-based medicine is defined as 'the conscientious, explicit and judicious use of current best evidence in making decisions about the care of individual patients' [43]. It carefully assesses all the available evidence on the benefits and risks of (new) treatments (also drugs), helping clinicians in decision making for their patients. Its practice on an individual patient level has now evolved to evidence-based health care (EBHC), where EBM principles are used on a strategic level by health care policy makers and health technology assessment (HTA) organisations (for reimbursement of drugs), and on an operational level by health care institutions and professional organisations (for establishing clinical practice guidelines, care paths, prescription formularies, and pharmaceutical care).

The Cochrane collaboration is a worldwide independent organisation 'internationally recognised as the benchmark for high-quality information about the effectiveness of health care' (www.cochrane.org). They publish online, as part of the Cochrane Library, the largest collection of RCTs and the Cochrane Database of Systematic Reviews. Some national Cochrane centres are very active in performing independent meta-analyses of clinical trials and observational studies performed with new drugs.

4.4.5.8   Reporting of results

The interpretation of the statistical results of a clinical (drug) trial assumes extensive crosstalk between statisticians and clinicians. Statistical significance is not the same as clinical relevance.

The format in which the results are presented also merits attention. Usually, clinical trial reports give estimates of treatment effects, confidence intervals and p values. Some prefer to report effect size in relative terms (e.g. new drug N versus comparator or placebo C), either as

- Relative risk or risk ratio (RR): the risk of the outcome in group N divided by the risk in group C. If is greater than 1, than the new drug carries more risk than C.
- Odds ratio (OR): a surrogate and complex measure for relative risk, particularly useful in case-control studies when the drug effect under study is rare (a rare side effect) and the OR nearly equals the RR (which cannot be calculated itself).
- Hazard ratio (HR): used in survival analysis for time-to-event measures. The rate of dying (or reaching another event) in group N divided by the rate of dying (or other event) in group C. If it is greater than 1, than the new drug carries more risk than C.

While clinicians, health technology assessment (HTA) organisations and health care policy makers prefer it in absolute measures:

- Absolute risk reduction (ARR) or risk difference (RD): the risk of the outcome in group N minus the risk in group C. The relative risk reduction can be substantial, but the absolute one minor.

- Number needed to treat (NNT): 1/ARR, the number of patients to be treated with N in order to induce 1 extra therapeutic event (by reaching it when it is favourable or by preventing it when it is unfavourable) in comparison with C in the time course of the trial. The lower the number, the more effective the new drug.
- Number needed to harm (NNH): 1/ARR, the number of patients to be treated with N to induce 1 extra side effect in comparison with C in the time course of the trial. The higher the number the better.

There is also a plethora of summary tables, schemes and figures that are used in clinical trial reports and publications, most of them in relation to the methodology used (the study design scheme, the study participant flow diagram), and the trial results (survival curve, plasma concentration versus time curve, waterfall plot, Forest plot, funnel plot).

Several guidance documents are available to help investigators in reporting and publishing clinical (drug) trials, such as the CONSORT statement for RCTs (CONsolidated Standards Of Reporting Trials), the PRISMA statement (Preferred Reporting Items for Systematic reviews and Meta-Analyses), and the STROBE statement (Strengthening The Reporting of Observational studies in Epidemiology) (www.consort-statement.org; www.prisma-statement.org; www.strobe-statement.org).

4.4.6 Organisational challenges in clinical drug trials

The organisation of a clinical drug trial is a challenge, as well for a small open pilot study in one centre as for a large international randomised controlled phase 3 trial (tens of thousands of patients, hundreds of centres, ten countries). Many stakeholders are involved and the trial has to be performed under fairly high pressure to deliver optimal quality, within strict timelines and within the allocated budget. A number of *practical* operational issues need to be tackled before, during and at the end of a clinical drug study.

4.4.6.1 Before the start of the study

All activities have to be meticulously planned well in advance (several months for a small study up to a year for large-scale studies) so that the trial can start on time:

- a risk analysis should be performed and a risk management plan should be drafted;
- all necessary study documents should be prepared: study synopsis (for preliminary discussions with advisers and investigators), product file (IMPD, IND), investigator brochure, detailed study protocol, (electronic or paper) case report file (CRF) to collect all the participant's study

data, information and consent form for study participants, clinical trial application (CTA), contracts between all parties involved;

– the participating countries and centres should be selected, generally based on a number of criteria checked during preliminary country and centre feasibility studies;

– depending on the study, a number of independent committees can be set up, such as a:

- Data Monitoring Committee (DMC) or Data and Safety Monitoring Board (DSMB), responsible for the follow-up of study (safety) data, intermediate statistical analyses, and stopping rules;
- Executive and/or Steering Committee, a multidisciplinary group of medical and scientific experts that manage the study independent of the sponsor;
- Adjudication or Critical Events Review Committee, a small group of experts that adjudicate primary endpoints and safety endpoints;

– the study database should be set up and everything that is needed to collect, check, review and clean-up the sometimes massive amount of incoming data;

– the manufacturing (or purchase or renting) and the entire logistics of all study material should be organised, e.g. all study drugs (new candidate, placebo, comparator), biological samples material, same equipment for all centres (bone densitometer, treadmill for exercise tolerance test);

– all necessary agreements from all competent authorities and ethics committees involved should be obtained as quickly as possible;

– appropriate training for the investigator teams should be organised as needed, e.g. on GCP, pharmacovigilance, study outcome criteria (in particular, when subjective in nature as in psychiatry); and

– finally, all participating centres should be set up so that they are ready to include the first participant (first participant first visit, FPFV).

4.4.6.2 During the study

Once the trial has started, the focus changes to the recruitment of study participants, the risk-based monitoring of the study, the safety follow-up and the progress reporting of the study:

– during the recruitment period (from FPFV till last participant in, LPI), the inclusion of participants is closely monitored, both quantitatively and qualitatively, so that appropriate measures can be taken quickly (open new centres, retrain investigators, modify the study protocol by substantial or non-substantial amendment);

– regular monitoring activities are scheduled in order to control the quality of the data collected, either by on-site monitoring (a clinical research associate or CRA visiting the centre), remote monitoring (a CRA using phone, e-mail, videoconference, or monitoring eCRFs from his desk), or central (statistical) monitoring (performed by data managers or statisticians using algorithms to look for aberrant trends or outliers);

– medical review of collected data is performed by trained physicians, to check whether these data are medically valid, complete and coherent. Similarly, all safety data are thoroughly reviewed (pharmacovigilance) and reported to (other) investigators, competent authorities, and ethics committees within set tough timelines for immediate reporting (death within 7 days, and serious adverse events within 15 days);

– regular blind data reviews are organised in order to clean the database in real time, without waiting till the end of the study;

– annual study progress reports and safety reports are to be prepared and sent out to participating investigators, ethics committees and competent authorities;

– regular meetings of the DMC/DSMB are scheduled to have an independent intermediate look at the accumulated data, to decide whether the study can continue as planned, or whether the protocol should be amended, or whether the study should be stopped prematurely for either exceptional efficacy in one group, inacceptable safety reasons, or for futility (useless to proceed as the chance to confirm the initial hypothesis has become negligibly small).

4.4.6.3 At the end of the study

After the last participant last visit (LPLV), a range of activities take place to assess the results as quickly as possible:

– a final blind review of the database is planned, before final clean-up and database lock;

– the frozen database is transferred to the statisticians (as much as possible, independent of the sponsor) for full statistical analysis before decoding;

– the results are interpreted by a panel of clinical experts (e.g. the Executive or Steering Committee), as much as possible independent of the sponsor;

– the participating centres are closed (return unused study medication, verify the completeness of the investigator study file, make arrangements for archiving);

– the end of the study is notified to the competent authorities and ethics committees;

– investigators and participants are informed of the results of the study, the study synopsis is made public, and the full study report is written.

Finally, the communication of the results in public is planned: when and where will they be presented in congresses, when and where will they be made public (in a public database, on a corporate website), and when and where will they be published in a scientific or medical journal. This is sometimes problematic, as there might be a conflict between the drug company's wish for provisional confidentiality and the society's call for full access to clinical trial data.

References

[1] Li P, Zhao L. (2007) Developing early formulations: Practice and perspective. *International Journal of Pharmaceutics* **341**, 1–19.

[2] Hansen SH, Peterson-Bjergaard S, Rasmussen KE. (2011) *Introduction to Pharmaceutical Chemical Analysis*. Wiley, Chichester.

[3] Brittain HG. (2009) *Polymorphism in Pharmaceutical Solids*, Informa Healthcare, New York.

[4] Banker GS, Rhodes CT. (2006) *Modern Pharmaceutics*, 4th edn. Marcel-Dekker, New York.

[5] Yan Z, Caldwell GW (eds.). (2004) *Methods in Pharmacology and Toxicology Optimization in Drug Discovery – in vitro Methods*. Humana Press, Totowa, New Jersey, USA.

[6] Tozer TN, Rowland M. (2006) *Introduction to Pharmacokinetics and Pharmaco-Dynamics: The Quantitative Basis of Drug Therapy*. Lippincott Williams and Wilkins, Baltimore.

[7] Shargel L, Yu A, Wu-Pong S. (2012) *Applied Biopharmaceutics and Pharmacokinetics*, 6th edn. McGraw Hill Medical, New York.

[8] Rowland M, Tozer TN. (1995) *Clinical Pharmacokinetics Concepts and Applications*. Lippincott Williams and Wilkins, Baltimore.

[9] Gibson GG, Skett P. (2001) *Introduction to Drug Metabolism*, 3rd edn. Nelson Thornes Publishers, Cheltenham.

[10] Hsieh Y, Chen J, Korfmacher WA. (2007) Mapping pharmaceuticals in tissues using MALDI imaging mass spectrometry. *Journal of Pharmacological and Toxicological Methods* **55**(2), 193–200.

[11] OECD SERIES ON PRINCIPLES OF GOOD LABORATORY PRACTICE AND COMPLIANCE MONITORING (1998), Number 1, OECD Principles on Good Laboratory Practice (as revised in 1997), ENV/MC/CHEM(98)17, OECD, Paris.

[12] ICH safety guidelines http://www.ich.org/products/guidelines/safety/article/safety-guidelines.html

[13] Gad SC. (2012) *Safety Pharmacology in Pharmaceutical Development: Approval and Post Marketing Surveillance*, 2nd edn, CRC Press, Taylor & Francis Group LLC, Boca Raton, Florida.

[14] Leishman DJ, Beck TW, Dybdal N *et al.* (2011) Best practice in the conduct of key nonclinical cardiovascular assessments in drug development: current recommendations from the Safety Pharmacology Society. *Journal of Pharmacological and Toxicological Methods* **65**, 93–101.

[15] Morganroth J, Gussak I. (2005) *Cardiac Safety of Noncardiac Drugs. Practical Guidelines for Clinical Research and Drug Development*. eds. Humana Press Inc., Totowa, New Jersey.

[16] Lu HR, Vlaminckx E, Van de Water A *et al.* (2006) In-vitro experimental models for the risk assessment of antibiotic-induced QT prolongation. *European Journal of Pharmacology* **553**, 229–239.

[17] Hamill OP, Marty A, Neher E *et al.* (1981) Improved patch-clamp techniques for high-resolution current recording from cells and cell-free membrane patches. *Pflügers Archiv* **391**, 85–100.

[18] Dubin AE, Nasser N, Rohrbacher J *et al.* (2005) Identifying modulators of hERG channel activity using the PatchXpress planar patch clamp. *Journal of Biomolecular Screening* **10**, 168–181.

[19] Aubert M, Osterwalder R, Wagner B *et al.* (2006) Evaluation of the rabbit Purkinje fibre assay as an in vitro tool for assessing the risk of drug-induced torsades de pointes in humans. *Drug Safety* **29**, 237–254.

[20] Roche M, Renauleaud C, Ballet V *et al.* (2010) The isolated rabbit heart and Purkinje fibers as models for identifying proarrhythmic liability. *Journal Pharmacological and Toxicological Methods* **61**, 238–250.

[21] De Clerck F, Van de Water A, D'Aubioul J *et al.* (2002) In vivo measurement of QT prolongation, dispersion and arrhythmogenesis: application to the preclinical cardiovascular safety pharmacology of a new chemical entity. *Blackwell Science Fundamental & Clinical Pharmacology* **16**, 125–140.

[22] Hondeghem LM, Lu HR, van Rossem K *et al.* (2003) Detection of proarrhythmia in the female rabbit heart: blinded validation. *Journal of Cardiovascular Electrophysiology*, **14**, 287–294.

[23] Valentin JP, Hoffman P, De Clerck F *et al.* (2004) Review of the predictive value of the Langendorff heart model Screenit system in assessing the proarrhythmic potential of drugs. *Journal of Pharmacological and Toxicological Methods* **49**, 171–181.

[24] Gelzer AR, Ball HA. (1997) Validation of a telemetry system for the measurement of blood pressure, electrocardiogram and locomotor activity in Beagle dogs. *Clinical Experimental Hypertension* **19**, 1135–1160.

[25] Murphy DJ. (1994) Safety Pharmacology of the respiratory system: Techniques and study design. *Drug Development Research* **32**, 237–246.

[26] Irwin S. (1968) Comprehensive observational assessment: 1a. A systematic quantitative procedure for assessing the behavioural and physiologic state of the mouse. *Psychopharmacologia (Berl.)* **13**, 222–257.

[27] Mattsson JL, Spencer PJ, Albee RR. (1996) A performance standard for clinical and functional observational battery examinations of rats. *Journal American College Toxicology* **15**, 239.

[28] OECD Guidelines for the testing of Chemicals, OECD publications, Paris, 2006 http://www.oecd.org/env/ehs/testing/oecdguidelinesforthetestingofchemicals.htm.

[29] Hayes AW, Kruger CL. (2014) *Principles and Methods of Toxicology*, 6th edn. CRC Press, Taylor and Francis Group.

[30] Gad SC. (2006) *Animal Models in Toxicology*, 2nd edn. Taylor and Francis.

[31] Shayne CG. (2009) *Drug Safety Evaluation*, 2nd edn. Wiley-Interscience.

[32] Jacobson-Kram D, Keller KA (eds). (2006) *Toxicological Testing Handbook Principles, Applications and Data Interpretation*, 2nd edn., Informa Healthcare USA Inc., New York.

[33] Hodgson E (ed.). (2010) *A textbook of Modern Toxicology*, 4th edn. John Wiley & Sons Publications.

[34] Faqi AS (ed.). (2013) *A Comprehensive Guide to Toxicology in Preclinical Drug Development*, Elsevier-Academic Press.

[35] Moore MM, Honma M, Clements J *et al.* (2007) Mouse lymphoma thymidine kinase gene mutation assay: Meeting of the international workshop on genotoxicity testing, San Francisco, 2005. *Mutation Research* **627**, 36–40.

[36] ICCVAM Test method Evaluation report, Appendix G: ICCVAM recommended HET-CAM test method protocol, November 2006.

[37] Barrett JS, Fossier MJ, Cadieu KD *et al.* (2008) Pharmacometrics: a multidisciplinary field to facilitate critical thinking in drug development and translational research settings. *Journal of Clinical Pharmacology* **48**, 632–649.

[38] Marier JF. (2011) Paving the way with pharmacometrics. *Drug Discovery and Development*, www.dddmag.com/articles/2011/04/paving-way-pharmacometrics.

[39] Wang F. (2008) *Biomarker Methods in Drug Discovery and Development. In series Methods in Pharmacology and Toxicology.* Humana Press, New York.

[40] Hargraves RJ. (2008) The role of molecular imaging in drug discovery and development. *Clinical Pharmacology and Therapeutics* **83**(2), 349–353.

[41] Directive 2001/20/EC of the European Parliament and of the Council of 4 April 2001 on the approximation of the laws, regulations and administrative provisions of the Member States relating to the implementation of good clinical practice in the conduct of clinical trials on medicinal products for human use. *Official Journal of the European Communities* 1.5.2001, L 121/34–44.

[42] Montori VN, Permanyer-Miralda G, Ferreira-Gonzalez I *et al.* (2005) Validity of composite end points in clinical trials. *British Medical Journal* **330,** 594–596.

[43] Sackett DL, Rosenberg WM, Gray JA *et al.* (1996) Evidence based medicine: what it is and what it isn't. *British Medical Journal*, **312** (7023), 71–72.

5
The Early Development of a New Drug

5.1   Introduction

Once a drug molecule has been selected as a 'lead molecule' in drug discovery because it shows promise to be developed into a human medicine, it transitions from the largely non-regulated and highly flexible discovery environment to a highly regulated development environment. This is a significant step in the drug life cycle. Because a drug molecule is developed in a step-wise fashion, its potential as a real drug candidate is explored in what is called 'early drug development'. The objectives of early drug development are to:

-   provide sufficient pre-clinical evidence on the quality, safety and efficacy of the drug candidate, so that it can be tested in humans;
-   demonstrate that it can be safely used in humans, both in healthy volunteers and in patients, and that its human pharmacokinetic profile is compatible with further development; and
-   provide clinical evidence that the drug candidate shows sufficiently convincing initial signs of a relevant therapeutic effect in the intended patient population to allow it to be taken forward into late development.

Early drug development is generally subdivided into two major parts.

The first part precedes the First-in-Human (FIH) clinical trial and is referred to in this book as the 'pre-clinical phase'. This is a critical step in early development because it will provide the data that are necessary to conclude whether the new drug molecule is sufficiently bioavailable and safe to be tested in man for the first time. This is the part of early development

Global New Drug Development: An Introduction, First Edition.
Jan A. Rosier, Mark A. Martens and Josse R. Thomas.
© 2014 John Wiley & Sons, Ltd. Published 2014 by John Wiley & Sons, Ltd.

where most contributions come from the chemical/pharmaceutical and nonclinical development streams. Also, limited exploratory clinical trials can be conducted during this phase without an extensive nonclinical safety dataset. In such case very low subtherapeutic doses of the drug molecule are used to explore some critical characteristics (e.g. pharmacokinetics) in man to accelerate development or to support the selection of a drug molecule for development.

The second part of early development is the 'clinical phase' where the drug candidate is typically first administered as a single ascending dose to human volunteers (phase 1a), followed by repeated ascending dosing in human volunteers (phase 1b), and finally administered in different doses and dose regimens to relatively small numbers of carefully selected patients (phase 2a). Also, chemical/pharmaceutical and nonclinical development continues by upscaling chemical manufacturing and further improving pharmaceutical formulations and by providing further nonclinical safety data to support future clinical development.

At the end of early development when the results from the clinical phase 2a trials ('Proof-of-Concept' or 'Proof-of-Confidence' trial and others) are available chemical/pharmaceutical, nonclinical and clinical data are integrated and evaluated and a 'go/no go' decision is made relating to the transfer of the drug candidate to late development.

Therefore, this chapter consists of a section on the pre-clinical phase and a section on the clinical phase of early development. Each of these sections is organised according to the contributions made by the three main drug development streams, i.e. chemical/pharmaceutical, nonclinical and clinical, followed by a discussion of data integration and decision making.

5.2   Pre-clinical phase

5.2.1   Chemical and pharmaceutical development

5.2.1.1   Development of a new synthesis method

When the new drug molecule is transferred from medicinal chemistry in discovery to chemical development, its synthesis will undergo a number of changes. The chemical synthesis of a new drug molecule is explored for the first time by medicinal chemistry and the quantities produced at laboratory scale are just sufficient to characterise it for its structural, chemical, physico-chemical, pharmacological, and to some extent its pharmacokinetic and toxicological properties. Chemical development, on the other hand, focuses on the development of a synthesis process that is capable of supplying the new drug in sufficient amounts for use in extended nonclinical experiments, clinical trials and finally for the market. This calls for a reassessment of the original synthesis process and takes into consideration aspects such as quality, cost of goods, yield, upscaling, good manufacturing practices, occupational safety and health and environmental safety. The objective of chemical development at this stage in early development is to make sure that sufficient drug material is available for the start of GLP-compliant nonclinical testing and for the development and production of clinical phase 1 formulations. The unit in the chemical development department that is responsible for the elaboration of the first chemical synthesis procedures in early development is known as the 'kilolab' because its objective is to provide sufficient amounts of drug substance (up to 1 kg) of a sufficiently high quality. As further upscaling is required during drug development, the manufacturing process will gradually be upgraded and introduced into a 'pilot plant' where chemical reactors are available to produce larger amounts of drug material.

5.2.1.2 Formulation development

Pre-formulation and formulation research

When a new drug molecule leaves the medicinal chemistry laboratories as part of the formal transfer of knowledge from discovery to (early) development, one of the very first questions to be answered is how to introduce this new drug molecule into a (dosage) form that is suitable for administration to experimental animals and to human volunteers and patients via the intended route of administration. This early development work is referred to as 'pre-formulation work' or 'pre-formulation research'. The objective of pre-formulation research is to investigate the physicochemical characteristics of the new active ingredient that are important for the development of an effective pharmaceutical formulation. These characteristics are, for example, solubility in water and other pharmaceutically acceptable solvents, pKa, $\log P_{ow}$, vapour pressure, surface characteristics, kinetic pH profiles, light and heat sensitivity, stability in acid or alkaline media and polymorphic modifications. These data provide insight in the bioavailability, bioaccumulation and stability of the active ingredient and offer guidance on the selection of the techniques to be used for the development of the most suitable form for administration. For example, if a drug is very poorly soluble in water, a simple pharmaceutical form such as a syrup is not the best choice because the active ingredient will not completely dissolve in the aqueous medium with a very poor bioavailability as a result.

For decades, the drugs that were developed by pharmaceutical R&D companies were characterised by a relatively good water solubility. Good solubility in water has two major advantages:

– good absorption from the gastrointestinal tract after oral administration;
– only simple pharmaceutical technologies are required for the incorporation of the active ingredient into dosage forms such as tablets and capsules.

However, through the application of highly sophisticated approaches in drug discovery such as molecular design, many recently discovered drug molecules have a low to a very low aqueous solubility (e.g. <0.01 g/L). In molecular design the molecular structures of candidate molecules are generated 'in silico' with the objective to obtain an optimal fit with the binding site of the macromolecular pharmacological target. A disadvantage of this approach is that structural fine tuning may have a negative impact on the solubility characteristics of the new drug molecule. Many – if not all – drug development organisations searching for highly active drugs are now faced with the challenge to find the right pharmaceutical formulation and dosage form to overcome problems of drug disposition due to their low water solubility. Often, if no pharmaceutical technology is available that is capable to ensure sufficient bioavailability of a poorly water soluble drug molecule it may be withdrawn from development even when it is pharmacologically very active.

In support of pre-formulation and formulation research for the development of oral formulations, a classification system was developed that allows for the classification of drug molecules according to their water solubility and permeability through biological membranes [1]. This biopharmaceutical classification system (BCS) allows the classification of drug candidates into 4 major classes:

- Class 1: High solubility, high permeability and rapid dissolution;
- Class 2: Low solubility and high permeability;
- Class 3: High solubility and low permeability;
- Class 4: Low solubility and low permeability.

High solubility means that the highest dose strength is soluble in 250 mL or less in aqueous media over a pH range of 1–7.5 at 37 °C, rapid dissolution requires more than 85% of the drug substance to dissolve within 30 min at 0.1N HCl, pH 4.5 and pH 6.8 and high permeability means that the extent of oral absorption is more than 90% of the administered dose. In the absence of any in vivo drug disposition data permeability is measured by means of the Caco-2 in vitro test system (Section 4.3.1.1). A number of examples of BCS classification are given in Table 5.1.

Drugs with a high permeability and very poor water solubility (BCS class 2) may pose a challenge in pharmaceutical development. These problems can be overcome by the application of pharmaceutical formulation technologies such as solid dispersions and nanosized suspensions. These formulation approaches, however, are much more complicated to develop and to introduce into a pharmaceutical manufacturing plant for later supply to clinical development and the market.

Table 5.1 Example of classification of drugs in the BCS system [1].

	High solubility	Low solubility
High permeability	**BCS class 1:** Acetaminophen Propranolol Metoprolol Valproic acid	**BCS class 2:** Carbamazepine Cyclosporine Digoxin Ketoconazole Tacrolimus
Low permeability	**BCS class 3:** Cimetidine Ranitidine	**BCS class 4:** Chlorthiazide Furosemide Methotrexate

Excipients

Although the active ingredient is the most important constituent of the drug product, the inactive ingredients or excipients constitute the major part of the formulation and – combined with the selected formulation technology – constitute the basis for the performance (e.g. bioavailability), the stability and the manufacturability of the drug product. The objective of including excipients in a formulation is to allow the drug product to establish its integrity (e.g. filling agents in tablets) or to make use of their intended properties such as anti-oxidation, penetration enhancement, disintegration and control of release. Notwithstanding the fact that excipients are selected based on their low chemical reactivity, it is not excluded that they can still interact with each other and with the active ingredient. The phenomenon whereby excipients react with each other or with the active ingredient is called 'excipient incompatibility' and may lead to the reduction of the stability of the drug product. Sometimes, excipients are used to assist in the manufacturing process and are then referred to as 'processing aids', but may/do not appear in the drug product. Some excipients are 'generally regarded as safe' and are known as 'GRAS' excipients, while others may have some chemical and biological activity and show toxicity (e.g. cyclodextrines). An overview of different types of excipients [2] with some examples is given in Table 5.2. For each of the excipients used, their presence in the formulation must be justified. The use of excipients is justified if their quantity in the drug product ranges between a preset minimum and a maximum value. When excipients are used, for example, as diluents to reconstitute a drug product, it is necessary to investigate any incompatibilities between the original formulation and the diluted formulation such as potential for precipitation, chemical

Table 5.2 Types of excipients with examples [2].

Type of excipient	Examples
Adsorbent	Aluminium hydroxide, calcium silicate, microcrystalline cellulose, magnesium aluminium silicate
Emollient	Aluminium monostearate, coconut oil, glyceryl monostearate, lecithin, myristyl alcohol
Emulsion stabiliser	Aluminium monostearate, carrageenan, carboxymethyl cellulose, glyceryl monostearate, magnesium aluminium silicate, myristyl alcohol, polyvinyl alcohol, xanthan gum
Gelling agent	Aluminium monostearate, carrageenan, xanthan gum
Dispersing agent	Aluminium oxide, carboxymethyl cellulose, microcrystalline cellulose, phospholipids, polyoxyethylene sorbitan fatty acid esters (Tweens), vitamin E polyethylene glycol succinate
Antioxidant	Ascorbic acid, vitamin E polyethylene glycol succinate
Anti-microbial agents	Benzalkonium chloride, boric acid, chlorhexidine, cetylpyridinium chloride, ethyl and methyl paraben, thiomersal
Tablet and capsule filler	Calcium silicate, dextrin, microcrystalline cellulose, corn starch, fructose, lactose, magnesium oxide, mannitol
Tablet and capsule lubricant	Calcium stearate, glyceryl monostearate, lauric acid, magnesium stearate, polyethylene glycol, stearic acid, polyvinyl alcohol, sodium lauryl sulfate, zinc stearate
Tablet and capsule desintegrant	Carboxymethyl cellulose, corn starch, guar gum, magnesium aluminium silicate, microcrystalline cellulose
Coating agent	Carboxymethyl cellulose, cetyl alcohol, hydroxypropyl cellulose, sucrose, titanium dioxide, polyvinyl alcohol
Emulsifying agent	Cetyl alcohol, glyceryl monostearate, hydroxypropyl cellulose, lanolin, lecithin, myristyl alcohol, poloxamer, polyoxyethylene castor oil derivatives, vitamin E polyethylene glycol succinate, polyoxyethylene sorbitan fatty acid esters (Tweens), polyoxyethylene stearates, sodium lauryl sulfate
Tablet binding agent	Corn starch, dextrin, guar gum, hydroxypropyl cellulose, lactose monohydrate, magnesium aluminium silicate, sucrose, vitamin E polyethylene glycol succinate
Chelating agent	Disodium edentate, hydroxypropyl-β–cyclodextrin, sulfobutylether-β -cyclodextrin
Ointment base	Coconut oil, lanolin, paraffin, polyethylene glycol, vitamin E polyethylene glycol succinate, cetyl alcohol, glycerine
Dissolution enhancer	Hydroxypropyl-β-cyclodextrin, sulfobutylether-β-cyclodextrin, polyethylene glycol, pyrrolidone
Anti-caking agent	Calcium silicate, magnesium silicate, magnesium oxide
Glidant	Magnesium silicate, magnesium oxide
Skin penetrant	Oleic acid, palmitic acid, pyrrolidone
Wetting agent	Poloxamer, polyoxyethylene castor oil derivatives, polyoxyethylene sorbitan fatty acid esters (Tweens), polyoxyethylene stearates, sodium lauryl sulfate, sorbitol
Thickening agent	Carboxymethyl cellulose, guar gum, hydroxypropyl cellulose, magnesium aluminium silicate, myristyl alcohol, potassium alginate, xanthan gum

reaction and, hence, overall change in stability. These incompatibilities need to be identified early in development.

Tox formulations

One of the earliest formulation activities in drug development is the selection of a formulation for the new drug molecule allowing the best possible bioavailability in experimental animals. To be able to demonstrate any toxicity it is essential that there is sufficient systemic exposure to the drug and that the formulation is well tolerated by test animals. The first pharmaceutical formulations that are developed for *in vivo* toxicology and safety pharmacology studies are commonly referred to as 'tox formulations'. Numerous approaches have been used to develop tox formulations for poorly water soluble drug candidates. Examples of excipients that can be used in the preparation of tox formulations for oral administration are hydroxypropyl-β-cyclodextrin, polyethylene glycol (PEG) with neutralisation of alkaline molecules with citric acid or acid molecules with NaOH and nonionic surfactants such as polysorbates (e.g. Tween 80). Care should be taken that the excipients are well tolerated by the experimental animals. Dogs, for example, do not tolerate polysorbates as formulation components for oral formulations. In the development of intravenous formulations care should be taken that excipients do not contribute to or exacerbate the intravenous intolerance of certain drugs.

Development of a formulation for clinical phase 1

The formulation approaches used for pre-clinical toxicology testing can – in principle – also be used for FIH clinical trials when nonclinical pharmacokinetics have demonstrated their good bioavailability and that the excipients used have been shown to be well tolerated.

While the first liquid formulations are used in *in vivo* toxicology experiments in pre-clinical development, formulation research is continued to further improve bioavailability and tolerability with the objective to obtain the most suitable formulation for clinical phase 1 studies. This involves the testing of numerous excipients and combinations thereof. Once the new formulation shows promising results in *in vitro* release tests, its performance is further tested *in vivo* in a limited number of dogs. The improved formulation then replaces the original tox formulation for all further nonclinical and clinical development. The search for the right formulation for phase 1 clinical development can sometimes be very demanding. For example, a company that recently developed a new drug against HIV, had to evaluate approximately 120 different formulation approaches including micronisation, nanonisation, solid dispersions, lipid mixtures and combinations thereof before a suitable formulation was found to be successfully introduced into phase 1 clinical development. Formulations for clinical phase 1 trials should in general remain stable for the duration of the trials that generally cover weeks or months.

The formulation of a drug candidate that is used for the first time in patients must also comply with the quality requirements that have to be met by every drug, i.e. the formulation must be of high quality, be manufactured under Good Manufacturing Practices (GMP) and be released on the basis of clearly described quality parameters tested by methods that are sufficiently validated for the phase of development. There is considerable debate about these quality requirements, because the final analytical methods and quality specifications are not yet available at this early stage of development. The analytical methods are not yet validated to the level that is required for a marketed drug because the methods are still under development. The composition, the manufacturing process, and the quality specifications of a phase 1 formulation are described in the CMC section of the IND application (USA) or in the IMPD section of the CTA (EU). Regulatory authorities review the IND and IMPD data and decide whether a phase 1 clinical trial can proceed on the basis of chemical/pharmaceutical and nonclinical data.

Degradation

Degradation products are formed as a result of the influence of light, temperature, pH or water or due to a reaction of the active ingredient with an excipient and/or with the packaging material. Organic impurities may appear during the production of an active ingredient but they can also appear during its storage. The impurities that appear during storage are more appropriately called 'degradants' because they result from degradation processes of the active ingredient. It is possible that the active ingredient in the drug product degrades during storage and it is therefore important to put forward limits to the potential level of degradation in the drug product. The degradation of the active ingredient may already start at the moment when the active ingredient is introduced into the manufacturing process, resulting in an amount of degradation product at the moment of the final QC release. If this is the case, the level of degradation should be measured and reported in the regulatory dossier. If this is not the case, the stability studies will need to address degradation by means of appropriate stability indicating analytical methods and determine the maximum level of degradation that occurs up to the shelf life of the drug product by means of accelerated and long-term stability studies.

5.2.1.3   Analytical development

An important activity in drug development is analytical development. There is not one single activity – clinical, nonclinical, chemical, pharmaceutical, production or supply chain – that does not rely on or can proceed without the support of the analytical development laboratories. The major objective of analytical development is four-fold:

- the development of quality specifications for the release of active ingredient, excipients, drug product, starting materials, reagents, solvents, catalysts and intermediate products in the manufacture of the active ingredient and the drug product;
- the development and validation of analytical methods to test the quality specifications of in-process controls during manufacture and of stability indicating analytical methods;
- the conduct of stability studies to establish shelf-life specifications and re-test dates of the active ingredient, the intermediates in chemical and pharmaceutical manufacture and of the drug product and of any material for which stability data are required;
- the development of pharmaceutical analytical methods required for the conduct of special studies during drug development such as the investigation of the interaction between the active ingredient and excipients in the drug product.

The most advanced industrial analytical laboratories are equipped with state-of-the-art apparatus to conduct assays such as impurity profiling, chiral separations, stability screens and long-term stability studies. Analytical development already starts during the discovery and continues throughout development. During early development the focus is on method development and on the application and fine tuning of the analytical method to be used to test the active ingredient and the drug product (or any other material) for quality and stability. The analytical methods developed for quality assessment and stability assessment are known as 'release methods' and 'stability indicating analytical methods', respectively.

5.2.1.4 Development of early quality specifications

During the early development of a new drug, the active ingredient and drug product are assigned quality specifications that are fine-tuned as more manufacturing experience is obtained and drug development proceeds. During the later stages of development (i.e. in clinical phases 2b and 3) these quality specifications are further refined and fixed into final quality specifications for the active ingredient and drug product as they will be used on the market. The approach followed for the development of the 'final' quality characteristics that have to be submitted to the regulatory health authorities is presented in Section 6.2.1.3.

It is important that the choice of a specification is justified both during development and when the new drug is registered. Questions such as 'why were these specifications proposed?', 'why is this analytical method preferred over an alternative one to test the parameter?', 'why are these limits set and can they be narrowed?' are raised by analytical chemists in anticipation to the questions raised by reviewers of regulatory authorities. It should be emphasised that the specifications assigned to the active ingredient and to the drug product at this stage of early development are preliminary in nature and change during the course of development until they become the final specifications in late development.

Quality specifications for the active ingredient
A quality specification is assigned to a material or a process that defines the quality of the material or the efficiency of a process. A specification is a combination of:

– a parameter that describes a specific characteristic;
– an acceptance criterion or limit that determines the value of the parameter that should be reached; and
– an analytical method to test the parameter to inquire whether the parameter complies with the acceptance criterion.

Such a parameter can be the particle size of an active ingredient, the pH of a solution during a manufacturing process, the impurity level in the active ingredient or the degradant level in the drug product. In order to test the parameter an analytical method is developed to determine whether a predetermined value (a limit value or a range of values) is reached and the quality can be assessed. A quality specification is therefore used to release material for use in a clinical trial or for further treatment during manufacture.

An active ingredient should comply with a number of quality specifications that can be categorised as 'general' and 'specific' quality specifications. General quality specifications are described in or derived from an official pharmacopoeia (USP or Ph. Eur. or another official monograph) and tested by methods described in these pharmacopoeias. Specific quality specifications may or may not refer to parameters described in or derived from an official pharmacopoeia but they differ from general quality specifications in that they are specific for the active ingredient. At the beginning of the development of a new drug, the parameters and limits that are assigned to a material (such as the active ingredient) are relatively broad because not much data and knowledge is available and provisional limits are assigned to these parameters for quality control. Near the end of development, these parameters and limits are tightened or relaxed based on the experience accumulated during development allowing their fine tuning. For example, while the assay limits for the active ingredient may be 95–105% during early development, they may be tightened to 98–102% later during development because knowledge on the reproducibility of the manufacturing process resulted in the narrowing of the in-process controls of the production.

The general tests that apply to an active ingredient are:

-   visual characteristics (e.g. colour of a powder);
-   identity (e.g. UV spectrum, IR spectrum, NMR spectrum, mass spectrum, melting point, LC retention time), assay (level of purity, preferably measured by means of LC);
-   impurities (organic and inorganic impurities and residual solvents by means of LC, GC, atomic absorption).

Other tests are:

-   pH of a solution of the active ingredient;
-   refraction index;
-   melting point;
-   particle size (expressed as a particle-size distribution);
-   polymorphic modification;
-   chirality in the case of stereochemical substances;
-   water content;
-   impurity tests for inorganic impurities (e.g. sulfates, chlorides, calcium);
-   microbial purity.

These quality specifications are reviewed by the regulatory authorities in view of a clinical trial or a marketing authorisation. From the specifications listed above, some are selected at the start of development, while others may be added or even removed near the end of early development or the beginning of late development, if justified. Alternatively, other specifications can be added to obtain a better control of the quality of the active ingredient. The limit assigned to a specification has an important impact on the reproducibility of the manufacturing process. Because experience with the large-scale production of an active ingredient is limited at the time of registration of a new drug, the limits assigned to specifications have to be sufficiently narrow to guarantee the quality of the materials, but not so tight that the manufacturing of the product is jeopardised. In other words, there needs to be a balance between the quality that can be reached and the manufacturability of the product.

Quality specifications for the drug product
The quality parameters assigned to a drug product in early development include a description of the dosage form (e.g., size, thickness, and diameter of a tablet), an identification test, an assay test and a test for impurities and degradation. The identity test should be specific and capable of differentiating between active ingredients with a closely related molecular structure. This requires a combination of two independent tests based on different physical principles (e.g. NMR and IR) or the same test using different experimental

conditions such as a combination of the determination of a LC retention time with two different eluents. When LC is combined with tandem MS (MS/MS) detection, then specificity is high enough for one test to be conducted. The quantitative determination of impurities should be conducted by means of a stability-indicating LC method. Because the level of synthesis impurities is quantified in the active ingredient, it is not required to test these again at the level of the drug product unless the synthesis impurity is also a degradation product of the active ingredient. The test for degradation of the active ingredient in the drug product can possibly be removed from the specifications if it can be shown that no degradation occurs under the specific storage conditions of the drug product. The quality parameters can be expanded with additional dosage specific parameters as presented in Table 5.3. The specification setting for specific attributes may be applicable to drug products containing polymorphic and/or chiral active ingredients or active ingredients that degrade (rapidly) and to *in vitro* dissolution characteristics and microbial purity of drug products. It goes beyond the scope of this book to discuss these parameters in detail and further reference is made to the applicable ICH guideline Q6. In Section 6.2.1.3 on the late development of the drug product, the way in which final quality specifications are set is discussed in more detail. Table 5.3 presents an overview of traditional finished drug product specifications [3] that provide guidance in defining quality specifications for the formulations used in early development.

A quality specification – in short 'specification' – should not only be used at the moment of release of the drug product, it can also be used as a 'shelf-life' specification, i.e. a specification that applies at the end of a storage period of a product and that represents the quality that the product should have at the end of its shelf life. A limit can have a fixed numerical value or a range of values, or non-quantifiable criteria that are assigned to raw materials and finished products such as an organoleptic property. The analytical procedure can be an official pharmacopoeial monograph or a method developed for that purpose to test the parameter. The statement 'compliant with the specification' means that the parameter is tested by means of a validated analytical method and the measured result lies within the limits of the quality criterion.

5.2.2   Nonclinical development

5.2.2.1   Pharmacokinetics

In drug discovery it is not only important to characterise the pharmacological activity of a new drug molecule but also to make sure that the drug candidate or its active metabolite reaches the target site in sufficiently high concentrations to exert the intended effect. Pharmacokinetics is therefore an important factor in the decision-making process of the release of a drug candidate into early drug development.

Table 5.3 Example of possible drug product specification.

	Solid oral dosage form (coated and uncoated)	Oral liquids	Parenteral solution
General tests	i. description of the dosage form (e.g., size, thickness, and diameter of a tablet) ii. identification test, by means of two independent tests iii. assay, preferably a stability-indicating and impurity detection HPLC method iv. impurity test to measure the level of degradation and residual solvents if applicable		
Specific tests	i. *in vitro* dissolution ii. disintegration iii. hardness iv. friability v. uniformity of dosage units vi. water content vii. microbial limits	i. uniformity of dosage units ii. pH iii. microbial limits iv. anti-microbial preservative content v. anti-oxidant preservative content vi. extractables vii. alcohol content viii. dissolution ix. particle size distribution x. re-dispersability xi. rheological properties xii. re-constitution time xiii. water content	i. uniformity of dosage units ii. pH iii. sterility iv. endotoxins/pyrogens v. particulate matter vi. water content vii. anti-microbial preservative content viii. anti-oxidant preservative content ix. extractables x. functionality testing of the delivery system xi. osmolarity xii. particle size distribution xiii. re-dispersability xiv. re-constitution time

(Source: ICH Guideline Q6A [3]. Reproduced with permission of ICH.)

The first screening tests that are normally carried out in drug discovery are *in vitro* absorption (e.g. PAMPA, Caco-2 test), *in vitro* interaction with transport peptides (e.g. P-gp in Caco-2 cells), *in vitro* plasma protein binding, comparative *in vitro* metabolism profiling using liver post-mitochondrial (S9) fractions or microsomes from various animal species and *in vitro* identification and inhibition of metabolising enzymes. Liver microsomes are derived from subcellular fractions of liver cells (hepatocytes) and carry key drug-metabolising enzymes such as cytochrome P450 enzymes and glucuronyl transferases. Apart from subcellular fractions intact hepatocytes in culture are also used for the study of drug metabolism *in vitro*. Typical *in vivo* studies performed in drug discovery are single-dose pharmacokinetics in one or two species (e.g. rat and dog) via the relevant routes of administration to characterise the absorption and elimination rates of the new drug molecule.

Based on the pharmacokinetic data generated in discovery a more detailed and advanced kinetics and metabolism study package is designed in the pre-clinical phase of early development to better understand species differences in kinetics and drug metabolism. The main objective of this approach is to obtain data that allow the estimation of the systemic exposure of humans to the drug candidate necessary to exert the intended therapeutic effect. The results of these studies are important for the determination of the recommended safe starting dose of a FIH clinical trial.

Following single-dose pharmacokinetic studies via the oral and parenteral routes (e.g. intravenous, intramuscular) of administration, multiple-dose studies are carried out to characterise phenomena such as drug accumulation or liver enzyme induction. Also, the influence of food intake and various early pharmaceutical formulations on the pharmacokinetic behaviour of the candidate drug are studied at this stage in different animal species (e.g. mouse, rat, dog, and monkey). Data from all these *in vivo* studies are used to optimise the blood sampling schedule of repeated dose toxicokinetic studies. A toxicokinetic study allows for the determination of the systemic exposure to the drug candidate and/or its metabolites in toxicology and safety pharmacology studies and the study of AUC or C_{max} versus toxicity relationships. When single-dose intravenous pharmacokinetic studies are available for different animal species allometric scaling of some important pharmacokinetic parameters such as the volume of distribution (V_d) or total body clearance (Cl_{tot}) to man becomes possible and allows for the simulation of plasma concentration versus time curves in man for different levels of absorption of the drug candidate from the gastrointestinal tract.

The pharmacokinetic characterisation and the conduct of toxicokinetic studies are not possible without the development a reliable and validated bioanalytical method. Currently, LC with MS/MS detection is the most commonly used analytical technique for the determination of the concentration of drug molecules and their metabolites in biological fluids and tissues.

To enhance the understanding of the availability of the absorbed drug molecule to target tissues, a detailed comparison of the binding to plasma proteins between various experimental animal species and man is needed. The repartition of the drug candidate between plasma and red blood cells can also be important in pharmacokinetic modelling, certainly for those drug molecules that bind to constituents of red blood cells (e.g. hemoglobin).

A more detailed comparative *in vitro* metabolic profiling with identification of the molecular structures of the metabolites is performed in pre-clinical development. To this effect non-labelled (cold) as well as radio-labelled (^{3}H, ^{14}C) drug molecules are used. Hepatocytes, liver S9 fraction and/or microsomes from various experimental animals (e.g. mouse, rat, rabbit, dog, monkey) and man are used to discover pertinent differences in liver metabolism. This provides useful information for the extrapolation of toxicological and pharmacological effects between animal species and from animals to man. The identification of the metabolising enzymes such as cytochrome P450 isoforms involved in the biotransformation of the drug molecule and the study of their interaction (inhibition, induction) are also done in this phase of drug development.

Since experience has shown that the metabolic profiles obtained *in vitro* are not always fully predictive of the *in vivo* situation, a first metabolic screen in plasma and excreta (urine, faeces) can be performed during this phase of development. A mass-balance study using a radio-labelled drug molecule can be performed to study the distribution of the excretion of radioactivity over the various routes of excretion (urine, faeces, exhalation). Radio-labelled material also allows for the study of the tissue distribution of the molecule and its metabolites using whole-body autoradiography (WBA). This technique is useful to explain toxic effects in organs or tissues where the drug or one of its metabolites is accumulated. The whole-body autoradiographs obtained at different time points also provide information on the rate of elimination of the radioactivity from the tissues concerned.

5.2.2.2 Safety pharmacology

Primary pharmacodynamic, secondary pharmacodynamic and safety pharmacology studies are all pharmacology studies used in drug research and development. The first category of studies investigates the effects and the mode of action of new drug molecules in relation to their desired therapeutic use. The second category addresses more the safety aspects of a drug candidate and investigates effects on pharmacological targets that are different from the desired pharmacological target. Safety pharmacology studies investigate adverse effects of a candidate drug on essential physiological functions within the therapeutic dose range and above.

The main three physiological systems investigated in safety pharmacology in early drug development are the cardiovascular, the respiratory and the central nervous systems. Effects on the functioning of the gastrointestinal system such as gastric emptying and intestinal transfer are also addressed in many instances. The study of effects on liver and renal function is normally integrated in toxicology studies.

Cardiovascular safety tests have as the main objective to assess the effects of the candidate drug on ventricular re-polarisation and pro-arrhythmic risk. The QT interval (Figure 4.10) is a measure of the duration of the ventricular action potential.

When ventricular re-polarisation is delayed, the QT interval is prolonged and that is indicative of an increased risk of ventricular tacharrthythmia leading to Torsade(s) de Pointes and cardiac arrest. Ventricular depolarisation and re-polarisation is a complicated series of changes of ion currents through ion channels of the cardiomyocyte membrane (Figure 5.1).

Five phases can be distinguished in the action potential:

– Phase 0: Depolarisation (from −90 mV to +20 mV) by a rapid transient influx of Na^+ (I_{Na}) through Na^+ channels.
– Phase 1: Initial rapid re-polarisation by inactivation of the Na^+ channels and transient efflux of K^+ (I_{to}) through K^+ channels.
– Phase 2: Plateau phase through a balance between the influx of Ca^{++} (I_{Ca}) through L-type Ca^{++} channels and outward re-polarising K^+ currents.
– Phase 3: Late rapid re-polarisation by efflux of K^+ (I_{Kr} and I_{Ks}) through delayed rectifier K^+ channels.
– Phase 4: Resting membrane potential (−90 mV) maintained by the inward rectifier K^+ current.

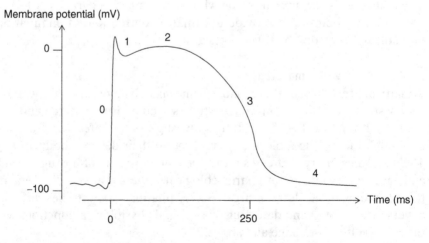

Figure 5.1   Phases of action potential.

The delay of ventricular re-polarisation can result from decreased inactivation of the Na^+ and Ca^{++} currents, increased activation of the Ca^{++} current or the inhibition of one or more K^+ currents. The rapidly and slowly activating components of the delayed rectifier K^+ current (I_{Kr} and I_{Ks}) seem to have the most influential role in determining the duration of the action potential and thus the QT interval. The human ether-à-go-go-related gene (hERG) encodes for the human K^+ channel that is responsible for the I_{Kr}. The inhibition of this channel is the most common mechanism of drug-induced QT interval prolongation.

During the selection process of a drug candidate in late discovery already some safety pharmacology screening tests are performed. These are in most cases rapid *in vitro/in vivo* secondary pharmacology screens and some *in vitro* cardiovascular safety screens. The secondary pharmacology screen generally consist of the study of the interaction of the drug candidate with a limited set of enzymes, receptors, transporter peptides and ion channels and of its activity in some *in vivo* pharmacology models.

It is important that new molecules are already tested for their effect on K^+ channels in the discovery phase using the *in vitro* hERG patch clamp assay. Also, the hERG ion channel binding assay is used as an initial screen for QT prolongation but its predictive value is considered as limited.

A positive outcome of the hERG patch clamp assay can already trigger more advanced multi-ion channel cardiovascular safety tests in the discovery phase of the drug candidate such as the Guinea pig right atrium assay (force and rate of contraction), the dog or rabbit heart Purkinje fibre test (action potential prolongation) or the isolated perfused rabbit (Langendorff) heart test (action potential prolongation, coronary artery flow). Even at the stage of late discovery an intravenous anesthetised dog cardiovascular safety test can be performed before deciding to release the drug candidate to early development.

In early development a more extensive secondary pharmacology screen is carried out using animal, tissue and cell-based systems and is aimed at detecting autonomic, CNS, cardiovascular, allergy, inflammation and gastrointestinal activity. The results of such a screen may also help to better understand the adverse effects observed in toxicology studies (e.g. decreased gastric emptying due to interaction with cholecystokinin). The safety pharmacology studies that are carried out in the pre-clinical phase consist in most instances of the cardiovascular and respiratory safety test in the conscious dog, the modified Irwin's test in the rat for central nervous systems effects and a gastrointestinal transit test in the rat. The effect of the drug candidate on the central nervous system is assessed in a single-dose neurobehavioural test in the rat at various dose levels. Assessment of hepatic and renal function is included in the toxicology studies in the rat and the dog. Depending on the toxicological characteristics of the drug candidate more specific secondary pharmacology tests can be added such as gastric emptying, inhibition of platelet aggregation or hemolysis.

A clearly positive outcome of any of the safety pharmacology tests triggers the conduct of more advanced/specific tests or can be a reason to discontinue development. Independent of the outcome of the pre-clinical safety pharmacology studies human volunteers participating in the FIH trial are closely monitored for cardiovascular function. In the event of any doubt on other safety pharmacology effects (e.g. neurobehavioural effects) specific monitoring for these effects is considered.

5.2.2.3   Toxicology

Toxicology studies in drug development have to be performed in accordance with internationally agreed test guidelines [4, 5] and good laboratory practices [6]. The tests that are conducted in the pre-clinical phase of early development can be subdivided into acute toxicity, repeated-dose toxicity, genotoxicity and local tolerance studies. The results from these studies are essential to the determination of the recommended safe starting dose in the FIH clinical trial.

Acute toxicity studies

During the late discovery phase, in an effort to select the most suitable molecule for early drug development, single-dose toxicity studies are carried out in several animal species. Some of these tests are repeated in early development using a more optimised dose range and in accordance with international guidelines. The animal species used for acute toxicity studies in this phase of development are usually mice and rats, while the routes of exposure are predominantly the oral and the intravenous routes.

Repeated-dose toxicity studies

When a drug candidate is introduced into early development, little or no information is available on repeated-dose toxicology. A repeated-dose toxicity test is pivotal in the pre-clinical phase since it is designed to provide the dose level from which a safe starting dose can be calculated and the safety parameters can be derived that need to be monitored in the FIH clinical trial.

At the start of the pre-clinical phase, the best possible pharmaceutical formulation for use in toxicology studies is developed. This formulation should be such that it is easy to produce, easy to handle, sufficiently stable, well tolerated by test animals for the projected routes of exposure and that it ensures the highest possible bioavailability of the drug candidate. Based on the late discovery acute toxicology data short (e.g. 5 days) dose range finding studies are conducted. The two animal species that are most used at this stage are the rat and the dog. Based on the effects observed in these studies, the best possible dose range can be estimated for a subacute toxicology study (2-week or 4-week studies). The conduct of a subacute toxicology study should be sufficient to provide a good point of departure for the calculation of a safe starting dose for the first human trial.

The selection of the dose levels for the subacute toxicology study is a delicate process that has to take toxicity as well as toxicokinetic aspects into consideration. Three dose levels are normally selected of which the highest dose should be able to demonstrate clear toxicity (e.g. significant changes in serum biochemistry, histopathological changes) but without influencing the survival of the animals. The lowest dose should remain without any effect. The mid-dose is situated in between. The dose levels usually differ by a factor 2 to 5. To assess the reversibility of the toxic effects observed, a high-dose satellite group can be included that is kept in the test for another time period (e.g. 1–2 weeks) without treatment.

To ensure the safety of the volunteers participating in a FIH clinical trial involving a single administration and then followed by a limited repeated dose clinical trial (e.g. 1 week) the conduct of a 2-week or a 4-week toxicology study in two animal species is generally sufficient. The minimal duration of toxicology studies to address the safety of clinical trials during drug development is shown in Table 5.4 [7].

Table 5.4 Minimum duration of toxicology studies to support the conduct of clinical trials.

Maximum duration of clinical trial	Minimum duration of a repeated dose toxicology study	
	Rodents	Non-rodents
Up to 2 weeks	2 weeks	2 weeks
Between 2 weeks and 6 months	Same as clinical trial	Same as clinical trial
More than 6 months	6 months	9 months

(Source: ICH Guideline M3(R2)[7]. Reproduced with permission of ICH.)

The highest dose level without an adverse effect (no-observed-adverse-effect-level, NOAEL) of the most sensitive and/or most relevant animal species is taken as the point of departure for the calculation of a safe starting dose. The NOAEL can be based on any of the toxicological endpoints of subacute toxicology studies. The adverse or toxic effect that constitutes the basis for the NOAEL should be statistically significantly different from control, should show a dose–response relationship and preferably be corroborated by another parameter indicating toxicity to the same target (e.g. increased serum transaminase levels combined with single-cell necrosis in the liver).

Genotoxicity studies
Genotoxicity testing in drug development is important for the identification of drug molecules that are capable of inducing genetic damage. This can be the

fixation of DNA damage after mitosis such as gene mutations (e.g. base-pair substitution, frame shifts), chromosomal damage and recombinations (chromosome aberrations) and numerical chromosome changes (aneuploidy). These changes can lead to carcinogenicity and heritable diseases.

Depending on the results from the screening tests performed in discovery, a battery of genotoxicity tests according to international test guidelines [4, 5] is devised to address gene mutations, chromosomal aberrations and aneuploidy. The minimal battery of tests to be conducted normally consists of two *in vitro* tests, i.e. a bacterial reverse gene mutation test (e.g. Ames test) and a mammalian cell forward gene mutation test (e.g. mouse lymphoma assay), and one *in vivo* chromosome aberration and aneuploidy test (e.g. mouse micronucleus test). The mouse lymphoma assay also permits the detection of chromosome aberrations when cell colony sizing is considered. Another option is to skip the *in vitro* mammalian cell tests and immediately conduct a micronucleus test after the Ames test. The *in vitro* assays are carried out in the absence and in the presence of an external metabolisation system (post-mitochondrial fraction (S9) supplemented with an NADPH regenerating system) derived from arochlor- or phenobarbital-induced rat livers to mimic rodent liver oxidative metabolism. Using S9 liver fraction in genotoxicity screening is very important since it has been established that many mutagens are formed through oxidative bioactivation of the parent compound. The mouse micronucleus test is an *in vivo* test and thus already includes factors such as bioavailability, metabolism and tissue distribution. To make sure that the *in vivo* test is sufficiently representative, pharmacokinetic evidence has to be delivered to demonstrate that the parent compound and its (active) metabolites have reached the tissue of investigation, i.e. bone marrow. An alternative way to make sure whether the drug candidate has reached the target tissue is to dose up to toxic levels (maximum tolerated dose) or in the event of low toxicity to dose up to the limit dose of 2000 mg/kg body weight for single dose exposure and 1000 mg/kg body weight for repeated-dose exposure. Normally, the micronucleus test is a single-dose genotoxicity test in the mouse but it can also be integrated in a subacute toxicity test in the rat.

In the event of borderline gene mutation results or test results that are not compliant with the quality criteria, the same test is performed again. For an equivocal gene mutation test result, normally a clearly negative mouse lymphoma test should provide sufficient comfort but in case of any doubt another mammalian cell gene mutation test can be considered (e.g. HPRT test in CHO cells). If results are still equivocal additional genotoxicity tests can be carried out *in vivo* such as the UDS assay (DNA repair), the COMET assay (DNA damage), molecular characterisation of genetic changes and assays with transgenic rodent systems (e.g. mutamouse test).

In the event of borderline chromosomal aberration results (e.g. the mouse lymphoma assay or the micronucleus assay) the conduct of an *in vitro* chromosomal aberration assay using human peripheral lymphocytes can be used. This test permits the full analysis of chromosomal aberrations in human cells in metaphase. *In vivo* confirmation can be done in the in rat cytogenetic assay where chromosomal aberrations are scored in bone marrow cells in metaphase. Also in this *in vivo* test, evidence should be delivered that the parent compound and metabolites have reached the bone marrow or that dosing was done up to the maximum feasible dose.

If the results of the minimal testing battery are clearly negative no further genotoxicity testing is required in drug development. In certain cases additional testing is performed if the molecular structure shows genotoxic structural alerts. If the results are clearly positive and confirmed in additional testing then the drug candidate is withdrawn from development. Often, in the case of a very promising pharmacological activity, the relationship between certain molecular moieties and genotoxicity is investigated and structural changes may be suggested to remove the effect.

Genotoxicity testing of a drug candidate is normally limited to the hit-to-lead and early and late lead optimisation phases in discovery and the pre-clinical phase in drug development. Later in development and as a result of the upscaling and optimisation of chemical synthesis impurities may arise in the drug under development that will need genotoxicity evaluation if potential mutagenic moieties are present. In the event that the drug under development has been shown to produce tumours in rodent systems and no non-genotoxic mechanism of action can be demonstrated, additional genotoxicity testing can be considered on a case-by-case basis.

Local tolerance studies
Depending on the projected clinical use of the drug candidate local tolerance studies are initiated in pre-clinical development. This is the case for drugs that will be brought into contact with mucous membranes (e.g. eye, conjunctivae, respiratory tract, rectum, vagina) or will be applied via the parenteral route (e.g. subcutaneous, intramuscular, intravenous, intraperitoneal). In the first instance *in vitro* assays are conducted to get a first idea of the irritation potential of the drug candidate such as the bovine corneal opacity and permeability assay (BCOP) and the hen chorio-allantoic membrane assay (HET-CAM). These tests are most of the time applied in the discovery phase to select late lead molecules before they are released to early development. In the case of candidate drugs for oral administration these local tolerance *in vitro* screening tests are also carried out in early development for occupational safety purposes. Since there is a significant increase of product use in early development the risk becomes greater for laboratory personnel to come into contact with substances that can irritate the eyes and the respiratory passages.

Even when parenteral drug candidates have been cleared for their potential to irritate mucous membranes using *in vitro* assays, still more representative test models are necessary before allowing the drug candidate to be used in a FIH clinical trial. For the development of parenteral drugs further testing is needed *in vivo* to rule out any possible intolerance towards the active ingredient and formulation components. *In vivo* parenteral tolerance models may include intramuscular injections in the rabbit, subcutaneous injections in the rat tail or intravenous injections in the dog with subsequent clinical observations and histopathological examination of the site of injection. Experience has shown that these *in vivo* models are much more predictive for local intolerance in humans than *in vitro* models because a living vascular system is necessary to mimic inflammatory processes as a result of chemical action.

5.2.3   Clinical development

In the pre-clinical phase of early drug development the main focus of clinical development is on the preparation of the clinical phase when the data produced by nonclinical development provide sufficient evidence that the drug candidate can be safely administered to man. The planning and preparation for the clinical phase consists of the participation in the risk assessment of the drug candidate based on the nonclinical database, the preparation of a clinical development plan and the preparation of the protocol for the First-In-Human (FIH) study. Another activity of clinical development in this early phase is to help in the selection of the best possible lead drug molecule in late discovery and to obtain early information on the pharmacokinetic behaviour of a drug candidate in man. This activity is referred to as phase 0, microdose or exploratory pharmacology studies in man.

5.2.3.1   Phase 0, microdose or exploratory studies

The inclusion of this type of preliminary studies in humans in the pre-clinical phase of early drug development is a matter of debate. Some consider all drug studies in humans by definition as belonging to the 'clinical' phase of drug development, hence the use of the term 'phase 0' studies. Others are of the opinion that this type of early exploratory studies in man allow for a better preparation of the first full-scale in human (FIH) study, and still others regard them as an additional tool in the selection process of the best possible lead molecule for transfer from discovery to development. They are in fact conducted in the transition zone between late discovery and early clinical development.

Phase 0, microdose or exploratory clinical studies are preliminary small-scale studies in humans, with one or a small number of different candidate drugs, as part of the selection procedure of the drug candidate to be taken forward to the more formal FIH clinical trial. Exploratory clinical studies have a very flexible design and can already be initiated in the late phases of drug discovery to make choices that are based on human data rather than only on data from nonclinical animal models. In many cases there are differences in pharmacokinetic behaviour of drug candidates between animals and man, as well as between profiles of drug metabolism *in vitro* (with human microsomes or hepatocytes) and in humans. The suboptimal knowledge of the pharmacokinetics of drug candidates in man in early development is an important factor in drug failures. Too low concentrations and too short exposure times at the target site can be the reason for lack of efficacy, whereas too high concentrations for too long at non-target sites can be the reason for toxicity.

There are many approaches possible in exploratory clinical studies [8–11]. They can be subdivided into dosing strategies in the microgram dose range (microdose studies) and at subtherapeutic and therapeutic dose levels. For each of these approaches a minimal nonclinical data package is required (Table 5.5) before starting exploratory clinical studies.

Subpharmacological trace doses (maximum 100 µg/administration) that are well below the toxicity threshold are sufficient to determine basic pharmacokinetic parameters in humans such as:

- plasma elimination half-life ($t^1/_2$);
- total body clearance (Cl_{tot});
- volume of distribution (V_d); and
- tissue distribution (e.g. CNS penetration and receptor occupancy).

This type of study requires the least nonclinical safety information (Table 5.5).

To make it possible to measure plasma drug concentrations after dosing of only microgram quantities ultrasensitive techniques are used requiring drug molecules labelled with radionuclides. Drug molecules labelled with ^{14}C are

Table 5.5 Phase 0 approaches with purpose and minimal nonclinical dataset.

Dose	Dosing frequency	Purpose	Nonclinical data
≤100 µg 1/100th of NOAEL 1/100th of MABEL	Single	Target receptor binding (PET); tissue distribution (PET); plasma PK (AMS)	Extended single-dose toxicology study in one rodent species
Max. 500 µg total, ≤100 µg/admin. 1/100th of MABEL	Multiple	Target receptor binding (PET); tissue distribution (PET); plasma PK (AMS)	7-day toxicology study in one rodent species; SAR for genotoxicity
Up to ½ NOAEL, therapeutic range	Single	Plasma PK with non-labelled test substance	Extended single-dose toxicology study in one rodent and one non-rodent species; Ames test; safety pharmacology core battery

NOAEL: no-observed-adverse-effect level; MABEL: minimum anticipated biological effect level; SAR: structure-activity relationship used for the application of accelerator mass spectrometry (AMS) [12] and with ^{11}C or ^{18}F for positron emission tomography (PET) (Section 4.4.3.3). A great advantage of the use of these radionuclides is that their incorporation in the drug molecule does not change its physicochemical, pharmacokinetic and biological characteristics. AMS is used for the determination of traces of drug molecules and their metabolites in body fluids. The radioactive dose to which a volunteer is exposed when receiving a microdose of a ^{14}C-labelled drug molecule for AMS tracing is only a fraction of the natural radiation levels, so that even children can be included in exploratory clinical studies. Only 20 μL of a plasma sample is already sufficient to study the pharmacokinetics of a drug candidate. The study of the pharmacokinetics of a drug candidate is much less obvious with PET because of the very short half-life of the ^{11}C positron emitting radionuclide (20 min). PET is applied for real-time noninvasive tomographic imaging of the tissue distribution of drug–receptor complexes by means of sets of tomographic images (PET camera) with a very high resolution and sensitivity. Whereas the drug candidate can be administered via the oral route with AMS, the intravenous route is preferred for PET applications.

Microdosing can be applied for the selection of drug candidates with a similar pharmacodynamic potency on the basis of their pharmacokinetic properties in man. The candidate with the best profile (e.g. high bioavailability, long plasma half-life) can then be selected for more extensive nonclinical testing in preparation for a FIH clinical trial. Another approach of selection is sequential, which means that the best possible lead drug molecule can first be tested for its pharmacokinetic behaviour in man. If the result is satisfactory the molecule can be selected for transfer to early development. If not, it may be modified chemically and tested again until an optimal result is obtained. Microdosing can also be used to confirm metabolic pathways in man that have been previously identified in *in vitro* human metabolising systems. Experience has shown that the metabolic profile of a drug obtained *in vitro* with human microsomes or hepatocytes is not always the same as that obtained in man.

An important limitation of microdosing used in the context of the early determination of pharmacokinetic parameters is that it supposes that the pharmacokinetics of the drug candidate is linear from the microdose range up to the therapeutic range. This is not always the case because of possible saturation of metabolic enzymes and/or transporter systems that can only be determined with classic bioanalytical methods at therapeutic dose levels. In any case, since microdosing allows for the selection of drug candidates directly in man, the results obtained have a high predictive value and the more frequent application of these approaches can accelerate drug development and reduce the use of experimental animals in nonclinical development.

5.2.3.2 Planning and preparation of the clinical phase

Risk assessment of the drug candidate on the basis of pre-clinical data
The clinical development team participates in the overall risk assessment preceding the decision to proceed or not with the drug candidate to clinical studies in humans. It is important to evaluate whether the safety issues observed during pre-clinical development (preliminary toxicology and safety pharmacology) could pose any (serious) problem during clinical development.

Depending on the nature and severity of the observed safety issues, they will either:

– Preclude further development of the drug candidate in man.
– Need no specific follow-up during early clinical development, apart from the usual attentive monitoring of safety and tolerability in these studies.
– Need special attention during the first clinical studies in man. Some of the safety issues (e.g. QT interval prolongation) might be considered manageable provided strict monitoring of this safety variable is possible in study participants (e.g. regular ECG testing post-dose).

In the latter case, clear instructions should be given to clinical investigators (under 'Guidance for the investigator' in the investigator's brochure (IB) and more detailed in the study protocol) to mitigate any risk.

Preparation of the clinical development plan
The clinical development plan of a new drug describes the planned clinical studies to obtain a market authorisation for one or several indications, as well as the post-authorisation studies during the first years that the drug will be on the market.

For each individual study, the type of study (phase 1 to 4), objective, study participants (healthy volunteers, type of patients, number), single centre or multicentre (if multinational, world regions to participate), and start and end dates are determined.

Some of the clinical studies are fairly typical as their nature and objective are common for nearly all new drug candidates, for example the single ascending dose (SAD) study to test the safety and tolerability in human volunteers, the ADME study (absorption, distribution, metabolism and excretion of the drug in humans), the POC (Proof-of-Concept) study in patients, the dose-response study in patients, the pivotal phase 3 study and the Post-Authorisation Safety Study (PASS). They are part of all clinical development plans of new drugs but need to be adapted to the specificities of the guidelines on clinical drug development for the targeted disease and for the drug class under study.

Other studies are more specific for the therapeutic domain and/or the drug under study. For most therapeutic domains and for several drug classes, specific guidelines (from EMA, FDA and expert groups) recommend which type of clinical studies should be conducted to bring a drug candidate successfully to the market.

The timing of the different studies and their interdependence is extremely important. Some of the studies need to be performed consecutively (because the next one is dependent on the results of the previous one), while others can be planned in parallel. As a result, a number of key dates (stage gates, milestones) are planned: go/no go for early clinical development, go/no go for late clinical development, marketing authorisation file submission date (first and subsequent indications), with the patent expiry date as reference.

Even at this early stage, the drug development team must have the final goal in mind, i.e. a successful marketing authorisation for the new drug. The clinical drug development plan must reflect the intended strategy to bring an innovative drug to the market with a positive benefit/risk ratio and with at least one or more competitive advantages.

Once the Clinical Development Team has prepared the final draft of the plan, it is discussed and fine tuned internally in the Project Team in consensus with the views of all other departments being represented. At this stage, the plan is often discussed with external experts in the field of interest, either individually or gathered in an Advisory Board, and adapted as needed. Also, scientific advice can be asked to regulatory agencies, be it the EMA or the FDA or other national authorities.

Finally, the clinical development plan is integrated in the overall development plan as one of the essential elements of the total package of information allowing top management to decide on a go/no go for the clinical phase of early development (Section 5.2.4).

Preparation of the First-in-Human (FIH) study

The First-in-Human study, formally also known as First-in-Man (FIM) study, is the very first full study of the candidate drug in humans, usually healthy volunteers, with the objective to test the bioavailability, safety and tolerability of single ascending dose administrations.

The planning of this study needs careful preparation taking into account all the data that have been produced in the pre-clinical phase. Therefore, the clinical development team sits together with the chemical/pharmaceutical and nonclinical development teams to perform a structured risk analysis and to develop a strategy to mitigate these risks in the clinic.

General guidance for early clinical studies with drugs in humans has been already available since 1983 [13] and served as a basis for subsequent and current regulations. For many years, and especially for the development of small molecules, these guidelines were deemed satisfactory.

Since the TeGenero incident in 2006 in the UK [14], whereby the first single administration of a CD28 superagonistic humanised monoclonal anti-body (TGN1412) created a cytokine storm in 6 healthy volunteers with consequent systemic organ failure and the need for emergency intensive care till recovery, more specific guidelines have been issued to help sponsors and investigators in the planning, the design and the conduct of FIH studies.

The EMA/CHMP 'Guideline on strategies to identify and mitigate risks for FIH clinical trials with investigational medicinal products' of 2007 [15], describes issues for consideration on a case-by-case basis when planning a FIH study.

They propose that prior to the start of any FIH study:

- A risk assessment should be done, considering especially the mode of action of the drug candidate, the nature of the drug target, specific chemical and pharmaceutical issues (strength and potency determination of the drug, qualification of the material used, reliability of very small doses), and specific nonclinical aspects (the relevance of animal species and models used, and availability of non-standard PK-PD/toxicology/ safety pharmacology data).
- A strategy should be available to mitigate and manage these identified risks, including the careful estimation of the first dose to be used in humans, paying special attention to a number of aspects of the study protocol and the trial conduct (choice of study participants, route and rate of administration of the first dose, sequence and interval between dosing of participants within the same dose cohort, transition to the next dose cohort, dose escalation increments, stopping rules and decision making, monitoring and communication of adverse events/reactions), and performing the trial only in phase 1 centres with experience in FIH studies.

Risk analysis These guidelines are particularly suitable for so-called 'higher risk' drug candidates, e.g. drugs acting on multiple signalling pathways or via a cascade system with amplification of effects, but are also very useful for any new substance to be first tested in humans, as already proposed by Kenter and Cohen [16] soon after the TeGenero case in 2006.

Kenter and Cohen proposed a set of 8 'issues of concern' to be considered in a rational risk analysis before starting any FIH study, for example the level of knowledge about the mechanism of action of the drug candidate, previous exposure of human beings to products with a similar biological mechanism, induction of primary or secondary mechanisms in animals or in human cell material, selectivity of the mechanism to target tissue in animals, analysis of potential effects, pharmacokinetic considerations, predictability of the effect(s), and can effects be managed in the clinic?

Since July 2012, this 'structured risk analysis' (complemented with 2 additional issues of concern: study population, interaction with other products) is part of the 'template research protocol' proposed by the Dutch Central

Committee on Research involving Human Subjects (CCMO) for any interventional clinical trial.

Risk management According to the results of the risk assessment, a strategy should be developed to manage the identified risks during the FIH trial. The following aspects need special consideration:

– Careful determination of a safe starting dose and potential adverse reactions as identified in nonclinical safety studies. A specific plan for monitoring these likely reactions should be available so that clinical investigators can identify them in time and treat them as necessary. This includes the availability of adequate medical staff and examinations, antidotes when they exist, access to emergency care as well as long-term follow-up.
– Choice of study population, increasing the dose, administration of doses, stopping rules and decision making, is described in more detail in Section 5.3.3.1 dealing with the conduct of FIH studies.
– Choice of an appropriate study centre with adequate facilities and well-trained investigators and staff, and sufficient experience in the conduct of FIH studies.

A lot of information on best practices in planning and performing FIH studies can be found in guidance documents such as the EMA/CHMP guideline of 2007 [15], the FDA guidance 'Estimating the safe starting dose for healthy volunteers' (2005) [17], the ABPI (Association of the British Pharmaceutical Industry) document 'First in Human Studies: Points to Consider in Study Placement, Design and Conduct' (2011) [18], and the more general 'Guidelines for phase 1 clinical trials' from the ABPI (2012 edition) [19].

Performing such a structured risk analysis and developing a risk-mitigation strategy on a case-by-case basis helps sponsors and investigators to plan the FIH study, Expert Advice Groups to comment on the draft protocol, as well as Ethics Committees to conclude whether the intended FIH study is finally acceptable.

5.2.4 Integration and decision making

By the end of the pre-clinical phase of early development a clear understanding is obtained of the complexities of the chemical synthesis process and how to proceed with the upscaling of manufacturing. Because the chemical, physicochemical and biopharmaceutical characteristics of the active ingredient are quite well understood the development of a suitable formulation and dosage form for clinical phase 1 and potentially also for clinical phase 2 can start.

In addition, impurity profiles are well characterised to allow nonclinical development to assess the full safety profile of the active ingredient.

All data on the quality, chemical synthesis, pharmaceutical formulation, physicochemistry, pharmacokinetics, metabolism, toxicology and safety pharmacology of the drug candidate are evaluated to ascertain that it:

- can be synthesised with high purity and formulated into a drug product for the FIH trial;
- is sufficiently systemically available to be able to exert its pharmacological activity;
- is free of unacceptable toxicological effects;
- has been demonstrated to have a no-observed-adverse-effect-level (NOAEL) in several animal species allowing the derivation of a maximum recommended safe starting dose (MRSD) in humans;
- has been sufficiently characterised from a toxicological and safety pharmacological point of view to allow careful monitoring of the health status of human volunteers in the clinic.

In addition, before deciding to administer a drug candidate to man it is essential to ascertain that the drug candidate is not genotoxic. In case of doubt, additional studies have to be conducted to make sure that it doesn't cause any damage to genetic material. If it is not possible to unequivocally demonstrate that the drug candidate is not genotoxic, it cannot be administered to healthy volunteers and is usually withdrawn from development. In exceptional cases, however, these compounds can be administered to patients when the intended pharmacological effect is based on a genotoxic mechanism of action, as is the case with some cytotoxic drugs in oncology.

From a safety pharmacology point of view the drug candidate should not impair normal cardiovascular function *in vivo* (e.g. anesthetised dog model, conscious dog model) at exposure levels that are well beyond the maximum level of optimal pharmacological activity. In case of doubt, confirmatory *in vivo* testing may be required as well as mechanistic studies to better understand the underlying cause of the effect and its significance to man. Minor effects on respiratory function or on the central nervous system can be accepted if they appear at dose levels well beyond the NOAEL value from which the MRSD will be derived and if they can be easily monitored and kept under control in the clinic.

The repeated-dose toxicology studies in pre-clinical development provide important information on the pharmacokinetics (toxicokinetics) and the safety of the drug candidate. They should be able to demonstrate sufficient safety at the systemic exposure levels that are necessary to obtain the desired pharmacological effect. The outcome of the repeated dose (14-day or 28-day) toxicology study is not only important for the calculation of the MRSD but also for the identification of possible toxic effects in man. The awareness of these effects will allow the clinician to detect and monitor any possible early signs of toxicity during the clinical trial. Examples are a change in serum transaminases (e.g. ALT, AST) and blood coagulation parameters in the case of liver toxicity or a change in hematological parameters in the case of toxicity to the bone marrow.

From the NOAEL, a Human Equivalent Dose (HED) is derived by applying an allometric scaling factor to extrapolate this dose from the experimental animal to man. Allometric scaling among experimental species is based on body surface rather than on body weight and is a widespread practice in the determination of the HED for FIH trials. It is based on the assumption that toxic endpoints such as the maximum tolerated dose (MTD) scale well across species when doses are normalised to body surface area [20, 21]. Scaling based on body surface takes account of the lower (oxidative) metabolism rate of larger species whereby less parent compound is eliminated through hepatic metabolism. As a result of this the parent compound is present in higher systemic concentrations with higher toxicity as a possible consequence. This approach assumes that toxicity is only produced by the parent and not by metabolites formed through oxidative metabolism, which is not always the case. If there is information available indicating that toxicity seen in experimental animals is due to a metabolite rather than to the parent compound and that this metabolite might also be present in man another approach can be considered.

To derive the HED, the NOAEL of each animal species is multiplied by a conversion factor that is the ratio of the animal K_m to the human K_m. K_m is the ratio of body weight to body surface for each animal species and expressed as kg/m^2. This conversion factor is a unitless number that converts the NOAEL of each animal species (expressed in mg/kg body weight) to the corresponding human dose (expressed in mg/kg body weight), which is equivalent to the animal's NOAEL on a mg/m^2 basis.

$$HED\ (mg/kg) = NOAEL\ (mg/kg) \times (Animal\ K_m/Human\ K_m)$$

The animal species that generates the lowest HED is the most sensitive species. Correcting for body surface area increases safety in clinical trials because it results in a more conservative starting dose estimate. Deviations from the body surface area approach are possible but they should be justified, for example in the case where the NOAEL values are similar across species. The conversion of animal doses to the HED using standardised conversion factors is shown in Table 5.6 [22].

Table 5.6 Conversion of animal doses to HED based on body surface area [22].

Species	Weight (kg)	Body surface (m^2)	K_m (kg/m^2)
Human (adult)	60	1.6	37
Human (child)	20	0.8	25
Baboon	12	0.6	20
Dog	10	0.5	20
Monkey	3	0.24	12
Rabbit	1.8	0.15	12
Guinea pig	0.4	0.05	8
Rat	0.15	0.025	6
Hamster	0.08	0.02	5
Mouse	0.02	0.007	3

The MRSD is calculated from the most appropriate human equivalent dose (HED) by dividing it by a safety factor. The most appropriate HED is selected from the animal species that is most representative for the assessment of human safety. Important in the selection of a representative animal species are pharmacokinetic data from pharmacokinetic studies as well as from toxicology studies and data from *in vitro* comparative metabolism studies and explorative animal metabolism studies. The appropriateness of the animal toxicology model for the pharmacological effect in the event of exaggerated pharmacological effects may also play a role in the decision-making process. If there is no pharmacokinetic, metabolism or pharmacological reason to make a selection, the HED from the most sensitive species, i.e. the lowest HED, is chosen for the calculation of the MRSD.

To derive the MRSD from the HED, a safety factor is introduced to compensate for variability in extrapolating animal toxicity results to humans. The uncertainties that are compensated by such safety factors are, for example, a greater sensitivity of humans to the pharmacological activity of the drug candidate in comparison to the experimental animals used, difficulties in detecting certain toxic effects in animals that can be prominent in humans (e.g. pain, mental disturbances) or for which there is no appropriate animal model, differences in pharmacokinetics and metabolism across animal species and differences in sensitivity across the human population. Generally, a default safety factor of 10 is applied, but this can be increased as a function of the nature of the toxicity detected in animal experimentation. Examples are a very variable systemic exposure (often due to the very low bioavailability of the drug candidate), steep dose–response curves, irreversible effects and toxicities which are very difficult to monitor in the clinic with noninvasive techniques (e.g. histopathological changes). Also, unexplained mortality, which sometimes happens in dogs, may be a reason to increase this safety factor. Decreasing this safety factor is less evident but can sometimes be applied if the compound belongs to a pharmacological and molecular class for which there exists a lot of evidence that animal data are very predictive for human toxicity.

There are many other different approaches possible for the derivation of a MRSD for a FIH clinical trial. Allometric scaling of pharmacokinetic parameters across several experimental species (e.g. mouse, rat, rabbit, dog, monkey) can be used to extrapolate to PK parameters in humans and thereby simulate the pharmacokinetic profile of the drug candidate in man. This approach provides an estimate on the doses required to achieve pharmacologically active systemic levels of the drug candidate in man.

An approach to the calculation of a safe starting dose in FIH trials that is followed for biopharmaceuticals (e.g. monoclonal anti-bodies, not addressed in this book) but that can also be applied for 'small molecules' is the "Minimal Anticipated Biological Effects Level" (MABEL). The calculation of the MABEL utilises *in vitro* and *in vivo* pharmacokinetic/ pharmacodynamic (PK-PD) data such as the binding of the drug molecule to the target (e.g. membrane receptor), the degree of occupancy of the target, concentration–response relationships *in vitro* in target cells from humans and relevant animal species and dose–response relationships *in vivo* in the relevant animal species. When the NOAEL and the MABEL are different then preference is given to the lowest value for the calculation of a safe starting dose. To further limit the potential of adverse effects in humans safety factors may be applied to calculate the safe human dose from the MABEL. Criteria that are considered in selecting a safety factor are the novelty of the drug molecule, biological potency, mode of action, species specificity and the shape of the dose–response curve.

5.3   Clinical phase

The second part of early development is the 'clinical phase' where the drug candidate is typically first administered as a single ascending dose to human volunteers (phase 1a), followed by repeated ascending dosing in human volunteers (phase 1b), and finally administered in different doses and dose regimens to relatively small numbers of carefully selected patients (phase 2a). A lot of flexibility is allowed at this stage and often a number of trials in early clinical development are combined in one single clinical trial protocol. In specific cases, such as the development of anti-cancer drugs, the drug candidate can be directly administered to patients. During the clinical phase of early development, chemical/pharmaceutical and nonclinical development continues by upscaling chemical manufacturing and further improving pharmaceutical formulations and by providing further nonclinical safety data to support future clinical development.

5.3.1   Chemical and pharmaceutical development

During the pre-clinical phase of early development, chemical and pharmaceutical development focuses on the development of a new synthesis method to prepare for the increasing demands for active ingredient for nonclinical testing. Once nonclinical testing has demonstrated that the drug candidate is sufficiently bioavailable and safe and the decision is taken to conduct a phase 1 clinical trial, chemical and pharmaceutical development engages in a programme to reach the following long-term objectives for the active ingredient and the drug product:

- a suitable manufacturing process;
- a thorough understanding of the physicochemical characteristics;
- the development of preliminary quality specifications ('specs');
- analytical methods to test these specifications;
- pharmaceutical drug formulations for use in 1a/b and 2a phase clinical trials;
- manufacturing processes for these formulations;
- (preliminary) quality specifications of these formulations;
- analytical methods to test these specifications;
- a stability profile of the active ingredient;
- the determination of a projected – preliminary – shelf life for the drug product.

In order to achieve these objectives, a chemical and pharmaceutical development plan is prepared that incorporates the individual steps that have to be followed to develop the new drug product. The development plan also includes the relationships between the individual steps. For example, the plan indicates when the first batch of active ingredient is to be manufactured in the chemical pilot plant and when the preliminary specifications should be ready for both the active ingredient and the pharmaceutical formulation.

It should be emphasised that during these early phases in development it is still far from clear whether the drug candidate will make it to the end of the development programme. Nevertheless, already at this stage in development it should be considered whether there is a need for the construction of a new manufacturing unit or a pharmaceutical plant to be able to ensure sufficient supply of the market once marketing authorisation is obtained.

During these early phases, the focus is on the generation of knowledge about the active ingredient and the drug product necessary for the development of a final manufacturing process, analytical methods, quality parameters and storage conditions. The data that are collected during these early phases are still preliminary and subject to continuous change. These changes are carefully managed and recorded to keep track of the development status of the active ingredient and the drug product and to create a chain of knowledge from the start to the end of development. For example, during early development, the active ingredient is assigned a quality parameter such as a maximum allowed level of impurity of 0.3% (w/w). This parameter will change during development because new conditions and parameters are introduced in the manufacturing process that increase the purity of the active ingredient and reduce the maximum allowed level of impurity to 0.1% (w/w). In other words, the 'impurity profile' of the active ingredient improves as development progresses. Figure 5.2 presents a scheme in which three manufacturing processes for an active ingredient are developed. During the earlier phases of development, manufacturing process version B is used as opposed to the process A used in medicinal chemistry. As a result of the changes introduced to increase yield and quality of the active ingredient, a new synthesis process version C is developed in which intermediate C is replaced by intermediate E. This leads to an impurity profile of the active ingredient identified as impurity profile C. The decision is then taken to use this material in further clinical studies such as a therapeutic exploratory study. Finally, further changes to the process lead to process version D that will be used for the final therapeutic confirmatory clinical trials in late development and leads to an impurity profile D.

These changes are carefully controlled and managed and it is important to introduce them during the early phases of drug development because late drug development requires active ingredient and drug product both manufactured

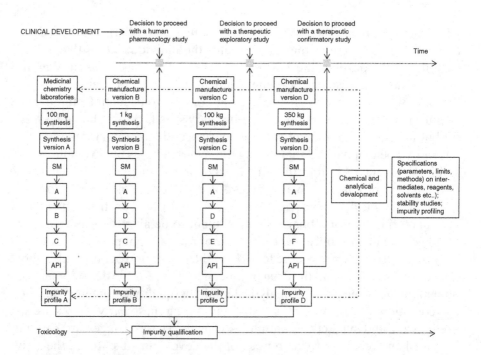

Figure 5.2   The development of a new chemical synthesis process for the active ingredient.

by means of processes that are very similar to the ones that will be used to supply the market if and when the drug is approved. Therefore, while early development focuses on the generation of knowledge and the improvement of processes and parameters, late development concentrates on the 'freezing' of this knowledge into final quality specifications, parameters, manufacturing processes, in-process controls, procedures, shelf lives, etc. (Section 6.2.1.3).

5.3.1.1   Early development of a manufacturing process

As discussed above, the chemical development of a new drug starts with the physicochemical characterisation of the active ingredient. This is initiated during late discovery. These studies are continued and assist process chemists and pharmaceutical scientists in their search for a manufacturing process. For example, when different polymorphic forms of the drug candidate are identified, process chemists conduct an exhaustive study on the manufacturability of these polymorphs and their stability while pharmaceutical scientists evaluate the impact of these polymorphs on bioavailability. The main objective of chemical development at this stage of development is to produce a high-purity active ingredient at a small scale for clinical development and at a large scale for the market. Because the synthesis process of the active ingredient developed originally by medicinal chemistry produces only small quantities of compound (milligrams to grams) it needs to be scaled up to volumes that can vary from a few hundred kilograms to ton quantities. Simultaneously, efforts are made to reduce cost and increase quality and yield. This means that changes are continuously being made during the development of an active ingredient that impact on its quality, impurity profile and on the performance of the drug product. For example, a change in particle size as a result of the introduction of a milling step, may have an impact on the bioavailability of the active ingredient. When the drug development organisation is not in the position to manufacture the active ingredient itself it has to select a reliable chemical manufacturer that is capable of manufacturing batches of active ingredient of increasing size under GMP conditions. Starting materials, solvents, reagents and catalysts have to be characterised and quality specifications (parameters, limits, methods) assigned to each of them. The intermediates that are manufactured during the synthesis process and have to be transported from one production site to another have also to be tested for stability to be able to define appropriate transportation and storage conditions to prevent degradation. Appropriate storage conditions and – if required – a re-test date is assigned to the active ingredient. A crucial part of chemical and analytical development is the identification, quantification and qualification of impurities that appear at the different stages of the synthesis process. Figure 5.3 schematically presents a synthesis process and indicates the steps in the synthesis where impurities may be introduced and/or formed.

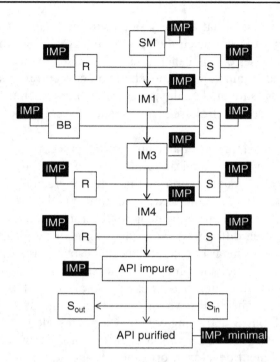

Figure 5.3 A synthesis process and the origin of impurities. IMP: impurity; SM: starting material; R: reagent; S: solvent; IM1, IM2 etc: Intermediate; BB: backbone structure of the molecule; API impure: crude unpurified API; Sin: solvent in; Sout: solvent out; IMP, minimal: API with minimal impurities.

An investigation is conducted to know which impurities are formed at what stage of the synthesis process and how they are introduced. Impurities can be generated as side products of chemical reactions in the synthesis process or can be introduced as impurities present in starting materials, solvents, catalysts and reagents. Impurities can also be formed through reactions (e.g. condensation reactions) between impurities. In addition, during the synthesis process degradants may be formed that appear as impurities in the final active ingredient. When impurities are shown to have biological activity with potential safety concerns, steps have to be taken to reduce their concentration or to eliminate them completely from the active ingredient. Impurities can be removed using different techniques such as drying (e.g. for volatile solvents), extraction (washing) with solvents, recrystallisation, precipitation and preparative chromatography. The concentration of impurities can be reduced drastically when these techniques are applied when they are present in the percent and pro mille range. However, the complete elimination of impurities (to concentrations at and below the ppm range (e.g. in the case of mutagens) is often impossible to accomplish. In such cases the source of the impurities has to be identified and removed from the synthesis process whenever this is possible.

Only recently, the International Conference on Harmonization (ICH) released a guideline that addresses the approaches that can be followed to develop a manufacturing process of an active ingredient [23]. It distinguishes between a traditional and an advanced approach in chemical development. A traditional chemical development project focuses on the following objectives:

– the development of a stable (semi-)synthetic manufacturing process;
– the process is controlled by operating conditions and in-process controls (temperature, stirring rates, pressure, etc.) that are either fixed (a given temperature and pressure) or constitute a range (e.g. a range between 45–60 °C);
– the process uses starting materials (SM) that are transformed into intermediates (IM) and comply with quality specifications and makes use of reagents, solvents, catalysts or other materials that comply with specific quality requirements;
– the process leads to an active ingredient that – after one or more purification steps – is tested against quality specifications.

The result of a traditional approach is a manufacturing process that leads to an active ingredient that complies with predetermined quality requirements. In order to achieve that objective, all steps in the synthesis are 'fixed' to assure that the output (yield, quality) is 'fixed' and consistent. The development of such a chemical manufacturing process is based on knowledge of organic chemistry and process engineering. There is a very narrow range within which changes may occur or be implemented during the execution of the process and operating outside these ranges may (or may not) impact the quality or yield. The problem with these 'fixed' processes is that it is not clear how a simultaneous change of process parameters impacts on the output because no experimental data are available that investigate the impact of these concomitant changes. These processes lead to products for which the quality is tested at the end and process success is guaranteed by assessing its outcome. Any change to this 'fixed' manufacturing process may result in changes in the quality and purity of the active ingredient that are difficult to predict because there is no experimental data that show a link between individual and potential changes (in operating conditions, in material attributes) and their impact (on quality, on yield). Also, a change to the process will need to be considered as a change requiring prior regulatory approval because the fixed process is described as such in a registration dossier and constitutes the 'manufacturing contract' between the marketing authorisation holder and the regulatory authorities. As any synthesis process submitted in an application for drug approval should be considered a commitment between the marketing authorisation holder and the regulatory authorities, any change to that fixed process requires prior approval putting a high administrative burden on the drug development organisation as well as on the regulatory authorities. If the operating conditions of a process would be presented by means of a cylinder whereby the cylinder's diameter would indicate the degree of variability that can be allowed in the process, a 'fixed' process could be presented as a very narrow cylinder (Figure 5.4), while the process in which the operating conditions are broad could be presented by means of a cylinder with a larger diameter (Figure 5.4). Broad operating conditions require a good understanding of the impact and feasibility of these operating conditions, the quality of the materials used and their impact on the next steps and on the final active ingredient. In contrast with the traditional approach of chemical development, the *advanced* approach in chemical development requires each step to be thoroughly investigated in order to identify the range of operating conditions (broad or tight) and the quality attributes of the materials (e.g. water content, impurity profile) used in the process. While the traditional approach assigns critical quality attributes (CQAs) to the active ingredient in view of its impact on the performance of the finished drug product, the advanced approach assigns CQAs to each material introduced into the process in view of their impact on the quality of the active ingredient. In other words, for each step in the process, experimental data show the impact of the (range of the) quality of incoming materials and of the operating conditions on the output of the process. These experiments are complex as different variables and parameters may be changed simultaneously and an experimental design approach is required. The end result of this experimental design in the advanced approach is the construction of a 'design space' in which material attributes and operating conditions may vary without impact on the yield and quality of the output and without the need for regulatory approval from the regulatory bodies. Obviously, the traditional approach and the advanced approach may be combined in a single manufacturing process development and some processes may be kept under tight control (either because experimental design data have shown that this is necessary or because experience and historical data have shown that the fixed approach leads to outputs shown to be acceptable) or may be conducted with a certain degree of freedom based upon the design space results. This is schematically presented in Figure 5.4.

5.3.1.2   Chiral active ingredients

Of all molecules that are in development or drugs that are on the market about 50% appear as chiral drugs, i.e. drugs with a stereochemical centre. During the early stages of development the attention to the chiral character of a molecule is critical and many efforts go into the elucidation and characterisation of chiral molecules. It is therefore appropriate to address the chemical development of these molecules. When a new active ingredient is a chiral molecule or contains stereochemical centres chemical development together

Traditional approach: process is 'fixed';
Manufacturing process is tightly controlled;
Qality is tested at API level

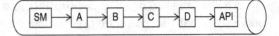

Traditional approach: manufacturing process is
not tightly controlled but the impact on the yield
and quality of API is guranteed

Advanced approach: the conditions of each step
are such that there is data to show that the operating
conditions and quality attributes of the materials
used are within the design space and assure good
quality output

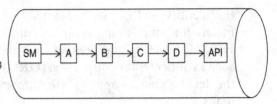

Combination of traditional and advanced approach:
The step SM to A and D to API is based upon
experimental design and design space approaches.
Steps B to C are either based on a traditional approach
or a design-based approach

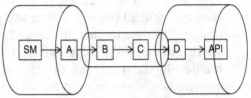

Figure 5.4 Traditional versus advanced development of a chemical manufacturing process.

with analytical development conduct studies to explore the chiral character of the active ingredient.

The development of stereochemical drugs poses formidable challenges to chemical and analytical scientists. The complexity of developing stereochemical drugs has increased considerably over the previous decades. It is difficult to obtain a pure chiral compound as the synthesis or separation of the preferred enantiomer may prove to be difficult and costly. Different resolution methods are available to the process chemist to separate the pure enantiomer from a reaction mixture such as diastereoisomer crystallisation, chemical or enzymatic kinetic resolution, preferential crystallisation or chromatographic resolution. The synthesis of a stereochemical drug focuses on the introduction of the stereogenic centre in the molecule and maintenance of the desired configuration. The introduction of the stereogenic centre is a crucial step in the chemical development of the new drug molecule and parameters such as reaction time, pressure, temperature, stirring speed as well as the quality of ingoing materials and reagents should be fully controlled and validated so as to assure a consistent yield and output of the relevant reaction step. This should be described in great detail in the regulatory dossier together with data (process parameters, quality control of intermediates, reagents, etc.) ensuring the reproducibility of the process. The maintenance of the desired configuration should be assured by the development of appropriate and justified in-process controls so as to guarantee consistent output over the full synthetic process and subsequent manufacturing campaigns.

It is a challenge to develop appropriate and validated analytical methods to make sure that the synthetic process can be steered and controlled in such a way that the output guarantees a pure enantiomer. The analytical methods for the quality control of stereochemical purity have to show unequivocally:

-   the identity and the stereoisomeric purity of the active ingredient by means of methods such as optical rotation, melting point determination, HPLC using chiral stationary phases and non-chromatographic methods such as optical rotary dispersion (ORD), circular dichroism (CD), NMR;
-   the development of appropriate stereochemical purity specifications and limits;
-   the development of in-process control methods, specifications and limits to assess the stereochemical process steps;
-   the development of quality (identity, purity) release methods, specifications and limits to assess the stereochemical purity for QC release of the starting material(s), intermediate(s), reagents and active ingredient;
-   the development and use of reference material that needs to be characterised over and beyond the analytical techniques used to assess the structure, configuration, purity and identity of the active ingredient;
-   the development of stability-indicating methods that are capable of showing any deviation from the original stereochemical purity of the drug from the moment of release and during storage;
-   the development of a method that assures the stability of the stereochemical purity of the active ingredient during introduction of the compound into the manufacturing process and the finished product;
-   the racemic character of the end-product of a synthesis, for example if it is not clear from the synthesis route.

In the description of the synthesis of the chiral active ingredient, it is important to show at which point in the synthesis and in which site in the molecule the stereochemical centre is introduced. Because this is an important step in the synthesis, all in-process controls, reagents and solvents that are critical for this step must be described in detail in the registration dossier. In addition, data must be made available that show that the reproducibility of the synthesis process is guaranteed.

The development of a stereochemical drug not only poses a number of chemical and analytical challenges, it will also impact the nonclinical and clinical development work. In some cases, the problem of developing enantiomers is simplified by the fact that both molecules have identical activities. For example, dobutamin-enantiomers are both positive inotropes, the enantiomers of ibuprofen act as anti-inflammatory agents, both enantiomers of warfarin and phenprocoumon are anti-coagulants and bupivicaine enantiomers act as local anesthetics. However, in other cases, one of the enantiomers is pharmacologically active, while the other is not. This is the case with propranolol where the l-enantiomer acts as a beta blocking agent, while the d-enantiomer does not, or in the case of sotalol where the d-enantiomer is a type-3 anti-arrhythmic, while the l-enantiomer is a beta-blocking agent.

5.3.1.3 Development of a formulation for clinical phase 2

To allow phase 2a clinical trials to be conducted, a formulation is developed that can be manufactured on a relatively larger scale and that is stable for the duration of the clinical trial. In some (rare) cases phase 2a formulations are identical to phase 2b/3 formulations. In most cases, however, phase 2a formulations still need to be optimised to improve organoleptic properties, increase bioavailability and to assure manufacturability on a larger scale for phase 3 trials and the market. Regulatory approval of a phase 2a finished drug product is based on the submission to and review by the authorities of an IND (USA) or IMPD (EU). Table 5.7 offers a comparative overview of the objectives and characteristics of both phase 1 and phase 2a formulations. During phase 1 and phase 2a – when the human pharmacology studies and the therapeutic exploration trials are conducted – the manufacturing process development is still in an early stage and the focus is primarily on creating manufacturing conditions for the product that sustain a continuous supply of clinical trial medication to the clinical trial site.

Once the results of the human exploratory trials have become available, the knowledge of the active ingredient and drug product has increased considerably. It is now known which quality parameters are useful to test the quality of the product and which methods are most suitable to test these parameters. It is also known which manufacturing processes are sufficiently robust and capable of generating a stable supply chain in the future. Also, for both

Table 5.7 Formulations during early development and their characteristics.

	Objectives of formulation	Characteristics of formulation	
Phase 1	Used for phase 1 trials to explore of the safety, PK and tolerability of the new active ingredient	i. ii. iii. iv.	Quality specifications are preliminary Manufactured on small scale Analysed by means of analytical methods that are not validated fully Stable for the duration of the phase 1 trial
Phase 2a	Used for phase 2a trials to explore an appropriate dosage strength	i. ii. iii. iv. v. vi.	Quality specifications are more advanced Offers an indication of the final formulation Manufactured on pilot scale but assures consistent output First supply chain Analysed by means of analytical methods that are validated sufficiently for the objective of a phase 2 trial Stable for the duration of the phase 2 trial

active ingredient and drug product, the stability characteristics are known as well as their shelf life and appropriate storage conditions. In summary, the active ingredient and drug product are ready for the final development phase in which this knowledge will be further extended and validated. Although processes, specifications and methods are still preliminary at this stage, the knowledge base has already reached a level that is sufficiently mature to initiate the final development activities in phase 3. During late development, the focus will be on consolidating all the knowledge on the final manufacturing process under full-scale conditions, the validation of these processes, the setting of final quality specifications of both active ingredient and drug product and on the validation of the analytical methods used to test both.

5.3.1.4   Development of a pharmaceutical manufacturing process

The development of the manufacturing process of the drug product is a key part of drug development. The objective is to develop a manufacturing process that is capable of producing a formulation that ensures a bioavailability of the active ingredient that is sufficiently high to obtain the desired therapeutic effect. The process should be stable, i.e. it should yield the same product consistently with the same high level of quality and should also be robust, i.e. it can be transferred to another site and still be capable of producing a drug product with the same quality characteristics. As the development of a product proceeds through different stages (clinical phases 1, 2 and 3) and the drug products used in clinical trials during each of these stages may differ, the pharmaceutical manufacturing processes are continuously modified during development.

5.3.1.5   Stability testing in early development

One of the main objectives of analytical development is to conduct stability investigations of the active ingredient and of the drug product with the objective to put forward a re-test date and shelf life respectively and to determine the quality specifications for the drug product. Both active ingredients and drug products are also subject to stability investigation under various storage conditions. When an active ingredient or intermediate(s) are transported between different continents or manufacturing sites, the transport must be simulated in the laboratory to assure that transport is not adversely affecting the quality of the material. From these studies, appropriate storage conditions and shelf lives for the transported materials can be derived. Stability studies are initiated at the interface between late discovery and early development and generally start with stress stability studies to explore potential degradation. As soon as the first batches of active ingredient and drug product are manufactured, they are introduced into formal stability studies. The introduction of batches of both active ingredient and drug product (or intermediates during manufacture) into stability studies, is continued during late development (Section 6.2.1.4).

Stress stability and screening stability

One of the first stability studies that is conducted with the active ingredient is stress testing. It is important to submit active ingredients to extreme conditions in order to detect potential or real degradation products that could form in less extreme storage conditions. Generally, stress stability studies are conducted on one lot of active ingredient that is subjected to temperatures that are increased by 10 °C at a time (e.g. to 50 °C, 60 °C) in conditions of extreme humidity but also under oxidative stress (H_2O_2) or light (photolysis). Sensitivity to hydrolysis (decomposition under the influence of water at different pH) is also a part of stress testing. These stress studies are conducted during early development because the knowledge gained is valuable for the development of stability-indicating analytical methods and is required before the initiation of the first stability studies of the active ingredient.

Stability testing of the active ingredient

One of the main objectives of analytical development is to conduct stability investigations of the active ingredient. During the conduct of the first clinical studies (clinical phases 1 and 2a), stability studies are initiated under conditions that are determined by regulatory guidelines. Stability studies must be conducted for active ingredients in the packaging that is used during the clinical studies (and later in the commercial packaging). The quality specifications that are assigned to the active ingredient are considered to be the test parameters at the start of and during the stability tests. The frequency of testing decreases with the duration of the stability study. Initially the frequency is high, i.e. at 1, 3, 6, 9, 12 months for the first year but then decreases to every 6 months for the second year (18 and 24 months) and thereafter annually. These batches are stored under 'ICH storage conditions', i.e. storage conditions that are put forward by ICH and defined in detail in ICH guidelines [24] (Table 5.8).

Table 5.8 ICH stability conditions (RH: Relative Humidity).

Intended storage conditions	Study	Storage conditions for study	Minimum period covered by data at submission
General	Long term	25 °C ±2 °C / 60% RH ±5% RH, or 30 °C ±2 °C / 65% RH ±5%RH	12 months
	Intermediary	30 °C ±2 °C / 65% RH ±5% RH	6 months
	Accelerated	40 °C ±2 °C / 75% RH ±5% RH	6 months
Refrigerator	Long term	5 °C ±3 °C	12 months
	Accelerated	25 °C ±2 °C / 60% RH ±5% RH	6 months
Freezer	Long term	−20 °C ±5 °C	12 months

(Source: ICH Guideline Q1A(R2)[24]. Reproduced with permission of ICH.)

In general, each batch of active ingredient manufactured during early development is tested for its stability. As a result, before the start of late development a considerable amount of stability data is collected from which appropriate storage conditions and a re-test date are derived. Each of these batches is kept on stability for 3 years. There are a number of conditions that need to be met if the stability study is to be of value to support clinical trials. At least three batches of active ingredient should be put on stability and the container/closure system of the stability batches is identical to the container/closure system of the batches used for clinical trials.

Stability testing of the drug product

Prior to and during the phase 1 and 2 clinical trials, a number of drug product batches are 'put on stability', i.e. they are introduced into an ICH stability study. This signifies that batches are stored for a specified duration under well-defined conditions of temperature and humidity and are tested at specific time points. During early development these batches are either experimental batches resulting from formulation or manufacturing process research or clinical batches that are used during the human pharmacology and therapeutic exploratory trials. These batches are also stored under 'ICH storage conditions'.

During these stability studies, the quality parameters assigned to the drug product are tested to investigate whether they change during storage. If, during development, new quality specifications are added, these will be subject of a stability inquiry in the batches to which these new quality specifications are assigned. For drugs that have to be stored at temperatures below $-20\,°C$, the storage conditions and shelf life are determined on a case-by-case basis. It is not uncommon that drug products (e.g. tablets, solutions) discolour under the influence of light. The sensitivity of a drug product to light is a common problem that is investigated by conducting a photostability study on a 'representative batch', e.g. a batch that is identical to the batches that will be used in a clinical trial. Oral dosage forms that contain a colourant are submitted to this stress test in order to detect potential discolouration during use. If the stress stability study shows that the active ingredient is photolabile, a photostability study should also be conducted on the finished product [25] and another colourant is to be added that does not discolour in the formulation matrix, or – alternatively – the colouring agent needs to be removed. Photographic pictures illustrating the discolouration generally accompany the stability study report.

The duration of the stability study of the drug product that is used in a clinical trial depends on the duration of the clinical trial. For example, when a phase 1 study is planned, the phase 1 formulation will be put on stability during 1–2 months because the duration of a phase 1 study is of the same order of magnitude. The same principles that apply for the stability testing of the active ingredient are used for the stability testing of the drug product: a number of conditions need to be met if the stability study is to be of value for regulatory purposes. These requirements are:

- at least three batches should be put on stability, two of these batches should be at least pilot batches and one batch can have a smaller size;
- the qualitative and quantitative composition of the stability batches is identical to the qualitative and quantitative composition of the batches for the clinical trial;
- the container/closure system of the stability batches is identical to the container/closure system of the batches for the clinical trial.

As argued by EMA, the use of an 'overage' to compensate for degradation that occurs during storage or to extend the shelf life of the product is not recommended. On the other hand, overages added to compensate for losses during to a production process are accepted but there should be a justification why this is done. Information must be given on the quantity of the overage added, the reason for the overage (stability or production loss), and the justification.

5.3.1.6 The container closure system

The container closure system of a drug product consists of the outer packing (bottle, carton box) and of the primary packaging that contains the individual units such as tablets, capsules or a solution or suspension. The pharmaceutical development project includes studies that show the suitability of the primary packaging for the drug product for storage and transportation. This consists of short-term or long-term stability studies that not only investigate the stability of the formulation when stored in the primary packaging but also the potential interaction between the primary packaging and the formulation such as leaching of chemicals (e.g. plasticisers) from a plastic bottle into a liquid formulation or adsorption or absorption (extraction) of the active ingredient onto/in the recipient material. The choice of the materials of the primary packaging (e.g. ACLAR^R for blisters, polypropylene, polyethylene or (coloured) glass for bottles) needs to be justified in view of their protective effect on the stability of the formulations. In addition, in many cases, the tablets, capsules or liquid formulations are shipped in bulk quantities and the compatibility between the recipient for bulk transport and the formulation need to be assessed. The choice of the materials of the primary packaging should be justified not only from a viewpoint of compatibility with the formulation constituents but also from a viewpoint of integrity (e.g. container-closure tightness). When the container/closure system includes dosing devices such as a dropper pipette, an injection device, a dry powder inhaler, a nose spray or eye drops, it is necessary to investigate whether these dosing systems function correctly and consistently deliver the correct dose to the patient.

For dosage forms that are sterile, the integrity of the container closure system with respect to its prevention of microbial contamination should be assessed.

5.3.1.7   Further development and quality by design

Different approaches may be followed in the development of a drug product for introduction into late development. These range from simple, straightforward development activities that are based on development experience with similar products or highly sophisticated pharmaceutical development processes using a 'design space' approach. Pharmaceutical development focuses on five objectives:

–   the clear definition of the objective of the development that is made explicit in a 'Quality Target Product Profile' (QTPP);
–   the identification of the critical quality attributes (CQAs) for the drug product;
–   the identification of the critical quality attributes of the constituents (active ingredient and excipients);
–   the selection of the manufacturing process; and
–   the selection of appropriate specifications (parameters, limits and methods) or 'control strategy' development.

The 'Quality Target Product Profile' or QTPP is a 'prospective summary of the quality characteristics of a drug product that ideally will be achieved to ensure the desired quality, taking into account safety and efficacy of the drug product' [26]. The intended clinical setting and therapeutic objective, the route of administration, the selected dosage form, the delivery systems, the dosage strength(s), the container closure systems and other characteristics of the finished product that affect its *in vivo* performance and their relation with the intended quality requirements (sterility, purity, stability and release) are part of the QTPP. The determination of the critical quality attributes or CQAs consists in identifying the physical, chemical, biological, microbiological properties or characteristics of a material (excipients) and of the drug product that ensure the desired product quality. The search for an appropriate manufacturing process and the development of a control strategy are the other main objectives of a QTPP. Pharmaceutical development scientists use a range of approaches to develop drug products from a 'minimalistic' approach to a 'Quality by Design' or QbD approach.

A quality by design approach is an 'enhanced' approach towards product development in that its focus is on determining not only the right parameters of the manufacturing process and in the specifications of the drug product but rather to conduct an in-depth investigation of each and every material introduced in a manufacturing step of the drug product. Quality by design is defined in ICH Q8 Annex as 'a systematic approach to development that begins with predefined objectives and emphasises product and process understanding and process control, based on sound science and quality risk management'. The result of a QbD approach is to obtain a clear picture of the impact of each material and parameter on the product's performance but also making available a 'space' within which these parameters can vary without affecting the product's performance. In other words, instead of reducing the knowledge about a drug product's performance to the setting of parameters either in production or in final specifications, QbD generates a complete picture of all the variables that may impact on the products performance, their relationship and the degrees of freedom in which these parameters can vary without affecting the product's performance. That is why QbD is also known as a 'holistic' approach to pharmaceutical product development.

The two concepts that are core to the QbD approach are the critical quality attribute (CQA) and the Critical Process Parameter (CPP). A critical quality attribute is a 'physical, chemical, biological or microbiological property or characteristic that should be within an appropriate limit, range, or distribution to ensure the desired product quality', while a critical process parameter is a 'process parameter whose variability has an impact on a critical quality attribute and therefore should be monitored or controlled to ensure the process produces the right quality'. Both definitions refer to a principle that is to build the quality of the product into the manufacturing process and into the constitutive materials that enter the manufacturing process, instead of testing the quality at the end of a (fixed) manufacturing process.

5.3.2 Nonclinical development

All nonclinical safety and exposure data that are required to conduct a FIH clinical trial have been produced during the pre-clinical phase of early development. Once clinical development has started, nonclinical development continues to develop pharmacokinetic and safety data to allow the drug candidate to be administered to man for longer periods of time and also to allow the inclusion of women of child-bearing age in clinical trials. All issues that were identified in previous nonclinical experiments and in clinical trials with volunteers are addressed in this phase of early development. During this phase there is a continuous improvement of the form and the impurity profile of the drug candidate and of the pharmaceutical formulation. The introduction of new formulations requires bioequivalence studies in animals before they are administered to humans. Once more evidence becomes available from clinical trials that the drug candidate is pharmacologically active at safe dose levels, drug–drug interactions can be investigated *in vitro* and *in vivo* in experimental animals before studies are initiated in humans. Depending on the intended treatment regime longer-term toxicology studies and reproductive toxicology studies are started towards the end of early development that continue into late development. For drugs that have to be taken for very long periods of time (lifetime), preliminary toxicology studies are also initiated to get prepared for the start of carcinogenicity studies in two animal species in late development.

5.3.2.1   Pharmacokinetics

Plasma kinetics

Normally, plasma kinetics and absolute bioavailabilty of the candidate drug should have been sufficiently characterised in the rat and the dog (or other appropriate species depending on the drug candidate) for single and repeated dosing in the pre-clinical phase of early drug development. In the clinical phase of early development many pharmacokinetic parameters are derived from toxicokinetic studies. These are toxicology studies combined with the determination of the concentration of the drug molecule and/or its metabolites in plasma at time points that best characterise their plasma kinetics. The simultaneous study of toxic effects and plasma kinetics increases the understanding of the relationship between toxicity (at different target sites) and the plasma concentration required to elicit toxicity. Most of the time, C_{max} is considered for acute effects and the AUC (for a defined time period) for chronic effects to study such relationships. Once a relationship is established between pharmacokinetic parameters and safety data in the clinic after single and repeated exposure it can be compared against those obtained in several animal species. This allows the selection of the most appropriate nonclinical animal species to continue toxicology testing. The selection of such animal species is also useful for the conduct of bioequivalence studies of new forms (e.g. salts, free acid, free base, spray-dried, micronised, nanosized) of the drug candidate and their corresponding pharmaceutical formulations. Bioequivalence studies are pharmacokinetic studies where the plasma kinetics of new drug forms or formulations are compared against the kinetics obtained with a drug form or formulation used thus far in the clinic. Such studies are necessary to demonstrate the superiority or equivalence of the new pharmaceutical formulation before allowing it to be tested in man.

Apart from a more detailed characterisation of the plasma kinetics of the drug candidate in a greater number of animal species (e.g. mouse, rabbit, minipig, monkey) after single exposure, the most important challenge in pharmacokinetics in this phase of development is to understand the kinetics of repeated dosing. Frequently asked questions are related to the linearity of plasma kinetics (linear relationship between the AUC and the dose), bioaccumulation, enzyme induction, the time at which the steady-state plasma concentration (C_{ss}) is reached and which is the most appropriate dosing regimen (once a day (qd), twice a day (bid), thrice a day (tid)) to attain a steady plasma concentration at therapeutic levels as quickly as possible after the start of dosing.

Beside the knowledge of plasma kinetics in adult animals at this stage of development the understanding of plasma kinetics of the parent drug in pregnant animals in embryo–fetal development and in pre- and post-natal development studies is also important for the interpretation of reproduction toxicology effects.

As more data become available on the metabolism of the drug candidate in several animal species and in humans new bioanalytical methods have to be developed and validated to be able to establish the plasma kinetics of major drug metabolites that could have an impact on the safety profile of the drug candidate in man.

Tissue distribution

The database on tissue distribution at the beginning of the clinical phase in early development may generally be limited to one or sometimes two animal species and is most of the time of a semi-quantitative nature. In this phase of development, the number of animal species is increased according to the needs of toxicity testing. Also, pigmented animals (e.g. rat) may be envisaged to specifically study the accumulation of the drug molecule or one of its metabolites in the eye and in the skin (melanin binding). To support the interpretation of embryo–fetal toxicology studies and to investigate species differences in embryo–fetal development effects, the transfer of the parent drug and/or its metabolites through the placenta is studied at different time points. Transfer of the drug molecule or one of its metabolites can also be assessed by the toxicokinetic analysis of foetuses and pups during reproduction toxicology studies. The quantitative determination of parent compound or metabolites in body fluids and tissues at various time points after single-dose or repeated-dose administration allows for the calculation of the tissue/blood ratio and the elimination kinetics from tissues after single dose and repeated-dose administration. Such data provide more insight into the relationship between the toxic effects in certain tissues and the presence of the drug molecule or one of its metabolites. If a metabolite producing tissue specific toxicity in animals would also be found in man, it is critical to understand the toxicity threshold of that metabolite in man to be able to adapt the dosing regimen in subsequent clinical trials.

The uptake and release of the drug molecule and its metabolites in tissues is greatly influenced by transporter proteins. P-glycoprotein (P-gp), for example, is localised in intestine, kidney, placenta and brain. P-gp can limit oral drug absorption by transporting the drug molecule back into the intestinal lumen and can limit the entry of substrate drugs into the central nervous system. Examples of transporter peptides operative in liver tissue are given in Table 5.9.

Table 5.9 Transporter peptides in the human hepatocyte.

Direction of transport	Transporter peptides
Blood → cell	OCT1, OATP1B1, OATP1B3
Cell → blood	MRP3
Cell ↔ blood	OATP2B1, NTCP
Cell →bile	BSEP, BCRP, MDR1, MRP2

Many transporter peptides are operative in transmembrane transport of endogenous substances. A typical example is the uptake of bilirubin glucuronide in hepatocytes and its excretion in the bile. If a drug molecule is a substrate to one of these transporter peptides the excretion of bilirubin in the bile can be decreased or inhibited with jaundice as a clinical consequence. Otherwise, drugs interfering with the normal function or biosynthesis of these transporter peptides can alter the availability of the drug candidate to the tissues where it is supposed to exert its pharmacological action.

Drug metabolism
Mass-balance studies can be conducted in preparation for the FIH clinical trial or thereafter. Mass balance data provide insight in the distribution of the drug molecule and its metabolites combined (in the case of radiolabelled studies) between urine, faeces, exhaled air and carcass over different time points until complete excretion. These data give an indication of the degree of absorption, excretion and accumulation as a function of time. Most of the time, these studies are combined with the isolation and identification of metabolites in blood, urine and faeces. For the study of the excretion of metabolites in bile and entero-hepatic circulation separate, more complicated, studies are required where the bile of one rat is cannulated and led into the intestine of a second rat.

In this phase of early drug development, the knowledge of the metabolic pathways of the drug candidate is refined and the number of species increased according to their need in pharmacological, safety pharmacological and toxicological models (e.g. minipig, Guinea pig, monkey, rabbit).

On the basis of the knowledge gathered on the metabolic pathways of the drug candidate in several animal species and how they relate to each other, a human metabolism study is designed. Human volunteers are given a single dose of the drug candidate and blood, urine and faeces samples are collected at different time points in accordance with the plasma kinetics obtained during the FIH clinical trial. The concentration of the most important metabolites identified in *in vitro* metabolism studies with human hepatocytes and various animal species is determined by bioanalytical methods developed for that purpose. These methods can also be applied for the determination of metabolites excreted in the milk of lactating animals in reproduction toxicology studies and the evolution of the concentration of these metabolites as a function of time in repeated-dose toxicology studies and in clinical trials.

The detailed knowledge of the metabolic pathways and the enzymes involved may provide inspiration for the design of prodrugs to improve the safety and efficacy of the drug molecule. A prodrug is a chemical structure that, for example, is better absorbed from the gastrointestinal tract and from which the active drug molecule is released through liver metabolism or the activity of plasma esterases. Prodrugs are often designed for parenteral applications to improve local tolerance and to regulate the release of the active drug from the injection site.

Liver enzyme induction
The investigation of liver enzyme induction *in vivo* is typically combined with the 3-month toxicology studies in the rat and the dog or any other species that is relevant to the development of the drug candidate. At the end of the 3-month treatment period the livers of the animals are isolated and microsomal fractions prepared to measure total protein, total cytochrome P450 content and the activity of a series of enzymes which were identified earlier *in vitro* to play a role in the metabolism of the candidate drug.

Besides the measurement of the activity of the metabolising enzymes the concentration of the enzyme protein and the extent of gene expression can also be determined in hepatocytes derived from repeated-dose toxicology studies. When drug molecules induce their own metabolism (autoinduction) a steady decrease of the plasma concentration of the unchanged drug becomes evident in repeated-dose pharmacokinetic or toxicokinetic studies.

As the drug candidate progresses through this phase of early development nonclinical assays are initiated to study possible drug–drug interactions with drugs that may be taken by the target patient population together with the drug candidate. Such studies are first done *in vitro* where the drug candidate is incubated with human liver fractions in the presence and absence of the drugs that are expected to be taken concomitantly. The determination of the parent drug and its metabolites provide information as to whether the metabolism of the drug candidate is modified by the other drugs. This may be a decrease as well as an increase of its metabolism. A typical example of drug-drug interactions is that of ritonavir and grape fruit juice that inhibit the activity of CYP3A4 and increase the plasma concentrations of many drugs. Some more examples are given in Table 5.10 (http://medicine.iupui.edu/clinpharm/ddis/table.aspx).

5.3.2.2 Toxicology

Repeated-dose toxicology
Based on the results from the subacute toxicology studies in the rat and the dog or any other appropriate animal species (e.g. minipig, monkey) a 90-day

Table 5.10   Some examples for substrates, inducers and inhibitors of the most commonly investigated cytochrome P450 isoforms.

CYP isoform	Substrate	Inhibitor	Inducer
1A2	amitryptiline	ciprofloxacin	omeprazole
2C9	diclofenac	fluconazole	rifampin
2C19	lansoprazole	omeprazole	prednisone
2D6	tamoxifen	fluoxetine	dexamethasone
3A4	ritonavir	ritonavir	rifabutin

toxicology study is designed. The 90-day toxicology study is a pivotal study in drug development since it provides reliable information on possible chronic toxicity and carcinogenicity and is used to estimate the best possible dose range for longer-term toxicology studies. The minimum number of animals per dose group and per sex is 10 for the rat and 3 for the dog. For the rat study, a satellite group of 3 animals per dose group and per sex is taken for toxicokinetic analysis. A satellite group is not necessary in the dog study since a sufficient volume of blood can be obtained from the animals of the main group for toxicokinetic analysis. The sampling scheme for toxicokinetics is based on the knowledge acquired from the pharmacokinetic and toxicokinetic data obtained in the pre-clinical phase. A minimum of three dose levels and one control should be considered.

Depending on the findings in the subacute toxicology studies and in the FIH clinical trial, the observational battery of the 90-day toxicology study can be extended on a case-by-case basis. For example, the hematology and serum biochemistry investigations can be further expanded to include a more detailed analysis of white blood cell morphology, hormonal or metabolic parameters or endpoints relating to immuno- or neurotoxicity. Apart from the addition of more tissues to be examined, a more detailed histopathological examination can be performed on tissues that have been formerly identified as target tissues using electron microscopy or more specific histological staining techniques. Other examples are the measurement of specific enzyme activities in target tissues and the use of imaging techniques such as DXA, MRI and ultrasonography (Section 4.4.3).

The results from the 3-month studies in rats and dogs provide a firm basis for the dose selection and the detailed analysis of the target organs in the chronic toxicology studies in rats (6 months) and dogs (9 months). These studies normally start towards the end of the clinical phase in early development and are finalised before the results of clinical phase 2b in late development become available. The data from the 3-month and chronic toxicology studies in the rat help in the design of the carcinogenicity studies in the rat. Normally, no carcinogenicity studies are performed in dogs and monkeys. Sometimes, hamsters are used but this is rather seldom. If the results of the clinical trials are promising for the drug candidate and there is a real chance that development will be continued, preparations can be made for the conduct of a carcinogenicity study in a second animal species. In most cases this is the mouse. Unless acute toxicity data have already been produced in the mouse in the last phases of drug discovery, a 5-day dose range finding study has to be conducted to be able to estimate an accurate dose range for a subacute toxicology study. Once toxicity has been characterised in subacute toxicology studies a well-designed 3-month study can be carried out to provide a sound rationale for the dose setting of a mouse carcinogenicity study. In parallel with the elaboration of an optimal dose range for longer-term mouse studies toxicokinetic data and metabolism data have to be produced. These data are important to identify and understand differences in toxicity between mouse, rat and man.

Genotoxicology

Additional genotoxicology studies can be performed to address uncertainties in some genotoxicity study results obtained in the pre-clinical phase or in the event of the identification of new impurities with mutagenic molecular alerts as a result of upscaling of chemical manufacturing.

When new impurities have been identified in new production batches at concentrations beyond the identification threshold (0.1% (w/w) for a daily dose of less than 2 g/day) they have to be investigated for the presence of genotoxicological structural alerts [27]. Such a structure–activity relation screen can be performed using empirical or rule-based systems (DEREK, ToxTree) and/or QSAR-based systems (MultiCASE, Leadscope). In the event structural alerts are detected that might indicate a possible mutagenic activity several actions can be taken. If it is not easy to remove this impurity from the active ingredient a simple gene mutation test (e.g. Ames test) can be performed on the isolated (or newly synthesised) impurity. In such a case a loading of minimum 250 μg/plate is recommended [28]. When it appears that the impurity is positive in the Ames test and it is very difficult to completely remove the impurity from the active ingredient further tests (including in vivo tests) can be performed to assess the genotoxicity of the impurity following a weight-of-evidence approach. If genotoxicity is confirmed, then the pragmatic approach of the Threshold of Toxicological Concern (TTC) can be taken [29–33]. The TTC is a daily dose of 1.5 μg/day and is associated with an acceptable cancer risk for pharmaceuticals of $1/10^5$ over a lifetime. The TTC is a very conservative approach since it is based on cancer data from the most sensitive animal species of which the dose with 50% tumour incidence has been extrapolated to an incidence of $1/10^6$. When impurities are found in the active ingredients that are positive in the Ames test deviations from the TTC are justified if:

– evidence is delivered that the impurity is not genotoxic in vivo (e.g. destruction of the impurity in the gastric content) or that the

mechanism of genotoxic action is threshold sensitive (which is very hard to demonstrate);
- exposure is shorter than one year (staged TTC approach [33, 34];
- a life-threatening condition has to be treated;
- the life expectancy of the patient is less than 5 years;
- exposure to the impurity through other sources (e.g. food) is much greater.

From the TTC and the estimated maximum daily intake the maximum concentration of the genotoxic impurity in the active ingredient can be calculated. Based on this figure chemical manufacturing has to investigate whether it is possible to produce batches with an impurity concentration that remains below the limit based on the TTC.

Local tolerance

Since larger quantities of drug candidate are manipulated by laboratory and manufacturing personnel and accidental dermal contact with the drug molecule is more likely to occur, the database for occupational safety is further completed with local tolerance data. For drug candidates that are not developed for dermal applications, testing for primary skin irritation and skin sensitisation can be carried out at the beginning of the clinical phase of early development.

Primary skin irritation is the inflammatory response of the skin to chemicals after a single contact of short duration and is assessed in the first place in *in vitro* skin toxicity models such as 3D skin irritation (e.g. reconstituted human epidermis (RHE) model). When *in vitro* skin irritation testing is negative a confirmatory test in a single rabbit can still be carried out to exclude any possibility of skin irritation.

Skin sensitisation is the allergic reaction of the skin to chemicals. During a first skin contact, the drug molecule can penetrate the skin and bind to proteins to form haptens that are recognised by the dendritic cells in the epidermis. These cells then migrate to the closest lymph nodes where the antigen is presented to T-lymphocytes causing the proliferation of a T-lymphocyte population that is sensitised against the drug molecule. The first skin contact with the drug molecule may occur without the production of any skin reaction. However, upon repeated skin contact later on skin reactions are produced such as redness and swelling. The test model that is currently most used is the local lymph node assay (LLNA) in the mouse.

If it appears that the drug molecule absorbs light in the 270–800 nm range, easily distributes to tissues that are sensitive to light (e.g. skin, eyes) and shows the tendency to produce reactive molecular species upon exposure to UV/visible light, the criteria are fulfilled for the conduct of a phototoxicity test. Phototoxicity testing can also be initiated when sensitivity to sunlight has been observed in the FIH clinical trial. The potential of the drug candidate to produce phototoxicity should be assessed in the first place by conducting *in vitro* assays. The assay that is most used to date is the *in vitro* neutral red uptake inhibition phototoxicity test. This does not necessarily mean that the drug candidate will cause phototoxicity in humans after systemic exposure but it is a strong indication for closer follow-up in the clinic or for further confirmation in other *in vitro* test systems such as the reconstituted human epidermis test and *in vivo* testing in pigmented and non-pigmented animal models.

Reproductive toxicology
Once the results of the FIH clinical trial are available and the results from the phase 1 clinical studies look promising the planning can start for the conduct of studies that investigate the possible effects of the drug candidate on the critical phases of the reproductive cycle (Figure 5.5).

Through the pathology examination of the reproductive tissues in the 4-week and 3-month toxicology studies already direct effects on reproductive function can be revealed. Examples are a decrease in testicular weight and depletion of sperm cells in the seminiferous tubules of the testicles as indicators of a decrease in male fertility. However, to obtain a complete picture on the possible effects of the candidate drug on reproductive performance and development more specific tests in experimental animals are required. These are fertility tests in male and female animals (Segment I), embryo–fetal development tests (Segment II), pre- and post-natal development tests (Segment III) and juvenile toxicology tests.

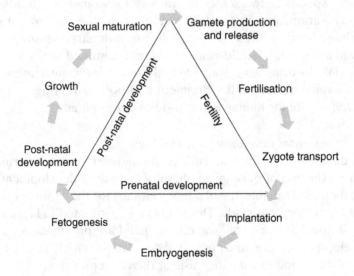

Figure 5.5 The reproductive cycle.

Fertility

Fertility tests are usually performed in the rat and cover a premating period, the mating period and a post-coital period so that any effects on the reproductive organs, fertilisation, zygote transport to the uterus, implantation in the uterus of the blastocyst and early embryonic development can be observed. The dose range is based on subacute toxicology data and normally 3 dose groups and 1 control group are used. This test can be carried out using the route of administration that is most relevant for the therapeutic application of the drug candidate. The tests are carried out in male as well as female animals and the species selected is usually the rat.

Embryo–fetal development toxicology

Embryo–fetal development toxicology tests are performed in two animal species, the rat and the rabbit. When it appears in a dose range-finding study that the rabbit does not tolerate well the drug candidate or the formulation, then the mouse is selected as a second animal species. In this test, dosing covers the period of organogenesis in the pregnant animal. Organogenesis is the phase of embryo–fetal development that is most sensitive for teratogens and is the interval between gastrulation and closure of the hard palate. This period corresponds with the days of gestation 6–17 for the rat, 6–19 for the rabbit and 6–15 for the mouse. The most sensitive period for humans is between the 2nd and the 8th week of gestation although hard palate closure is then still not complete. Normally, 3 dose groups and 1 control group are used and the route of administration is the one that is most relevant for the therapeutic application of the drug candidate. When a clear dose–effect relationship for birth abnormalities is established for the candidate drug in the two animal species tested, a specific warning for women of child-bearing age has to be mentioned in the label. Even if no indications of any embryo–fetal toxicity are found in these studies still precautionary measures should be taken when women of child-bearing age are admitted for participation in clinical trials in drug development. Only when sufficient clinical evidence becomes available later in development and post-marketing, can a drug be considered as safe for human embryo–fetal development.

Pre- and post-natal development toxicology

The full data set on fertility and embryo–fetal development is normally available before the end of the clinical phase of early drug development. As soon as these data are available, the planning can start for the conduct of a pre- and post-natal development study. This study can be initiated in late early development if nonclinical and clinical data at hand are promising for transfer to late development. A pre- and post-natal development toxicology study covers the complete period of organogenisis of the conceptus as well as the phases just before and after birth until weaning. The pups are allowed to be born and nursed by the maternal animals until the end of the lactation period and are observed for any signs of disturbance of normal development caused by the drug candidate when administered to the maternal animals. The dose range is based on the results from the fertility and embryo–fetal toxicology studies. Normally, 3 dose groups and 1 control group are used and the route of exposure is the one that is most relevant for the intended therapeutic application of the drug candidate.

Immunotoxicology

Any effects of the drug candidate on the normal functioning of the immune system such as suppression, enhancement, antigenicity (anti-drug response) and allergic reactions are addressed in immunotoxicology studies. Standard subacute toxicology studies can already provide quite a lot of information on the potential immunotoxicity of the drug molecule. Examples are changes in white blood cell populations (e.g. increase in eosinophils, decrease in leucocytes), changes in serum biochemistry parameters (e.g. globulin levels, albumin/globulin ratios) or changes in lymphoid tissues (e.g. thymus, spleen, lymph nodes, Peyer's patches in the small intestine, bone marrow). To specifically address certain effects on the immune system a proper immunotoxicology test has to be performed. The design of such tests is very flexible and is most of the time tailored towards the type of immune effects that need to be investigated. The pharmacological properties of the drug candidate (e.g. immunosuppressant, anti-inflammatory), the intended patient population, the known effects of the drug class on the immune system and the distribution of the drug and its metabolites in lymphoid tissues are all criteria that have to be taken into account. Other immunotoxicology assays that can be performed are the natural killer activity assay, the host resistance assay and assays assessing macrophage/neutrophil function. When effects on the functioning of the immune system are identified specific immunotoxicology parameters/assays are added to the longer-term repeated-dose animal studies.

Neurotoxicology

Repeated-dose toxicology studies already contain a well-developed observational battery for neurotoxicological effects such as home cage observations (e.g. posture, abnormal movements, convulsions), sensory observations (e.g. touch response, startle response, pain response, air righting reflex), handling observations (e.g. reactivity, salivation, piloerection, muscle tone), open field observations (e.g. mobility, rearing, gait abnormalities, bizarre behaviour) and neuromuscular observations (e.g. limb grip strength, limb foot splay, rotarod performance). In the event that one or more of such effects are observed in a single-dose safety pharmacology test (e.g. modified Irwin test) or repeated-dose toxicology tests (e.g. 3-month study) and that they are clearly dose related, further investigations are needed to better understand the underlying mechanism of action.

Mechanistic toxicology

In the event of any adverse effects that have been noted in nonclinical and clinical studies during early development and that constitute a cause of concern for the safety of the drug candidate, a mechanistic toxicology or pharmacokinetic study can be initiated. These studies are designed on an *ad hoc* basis and are conducted to better understand the underlying cause or mechanism of action of the toxicity observed and in how far that mechanism is also operative in man. An example of such an adverse effect is the sudden death of a dog during the course of a repeated dose gavage study. The cause of death was inflammatory lesions in the heart that were produced by the repeated passage of the gavage tube through the esophagus exerting pressure on the heart tip. In principle, any adverse health effect that is observed in the clinic and was not predicted by nonclinical testing needs to be addressed in the laboratory using new exploratory experimental models, if needed.

5.3.3   Clinical development

Early clinical drug development is focused on exploring and learning how the drug candidate behaves in humans (healthy volunteers and patients), and on demonstrating that it has some potential as a therapeutic agent in the target patient population.

In the traditional chronological approach, as adopted in this book, early clinical drug development is subdivided into:

–   Phase 1: first studies in humans with the objective to get a preliminary idea of the safety and tolerability of the drug candidate, its pharmacokinetics and, if possible, its pharmacodynamics. Phase 1 is sometimes further partitioned in phase 1a (single dose studies, including the First-in-Human or First-in-Man study) and phase 1b (repeated dose) studies. Most of these small-scale studies are conducted in healthy male volunteers in specialised phase 1 centres. In some exceptional cases the drug candidate is immediately administered to patients without a preliminary safety screen in healthy volunteers (e.g. for cytostatic anti-cancer drugs).

–   Phase 2a: early small-scale clinical studies in patients with the objective to get an idea of the preliminary efficacy and safety of the candidate drug in patients, to define the target population and to explore an appropriate dose range. This phase also includes the so-called Proof-of-Concept (PoC) study[1], verifying in patients with the disease of interest whether

---

[1] The term Proof-of-Concept is mostly used in relation to patients, either as PoC study (to prove that the candidate drug really works in the targeted population), as PoC strategy (the strategy used to prove it), or as the positive outcome of the approach (the first confident proof of its efficacy in patients) and therefore sometimes also called Proof-of-Confidence.

the drug candidate is active on the intended pathophysiological mechanism and shows early evidence of therapeutic potential on relevant surrogate or clinical endpoints.

5.3.3.1 Phase 1 studies

Phase 1 studies are generally the first clinical studies in humans. They are typically designed to obtain a preliminary idea of the safety and tolerability of the drug candidate in humans, its human pharmacokinetic profile, and as much as possible, to get early evidence of its pharmacodynamic activity in humans. By definition, these studies confer no therapeutic benefit to the study participants.

A phase 1 development programme generally foresees several small studies of short duration (1 day to 2 weeks), mostly in healthy volunteers rather than in patients, either after single (phase 1a) or repeated administration (phase 1b) of the drug candidate. The very first administration of the drug candidate is generally studied in the 'First-in-Human' (FIH) clinical trial (typically a phase 1a or single ascending dose study).

Not all phase 1 studies are carried out in the early stage of clinical drug development. They can be performed later, even in the late stage of clinical development, when they are designed, for example, to study drug-drug interactions, the bioavailability or bioequivalence of different pharmaceutical formulations, genetic polymorphisms, and pharmacokinetics of the drug in development in patients with impaired organ function (kidney or liver failure) or to explore potential differences among gender and age groups.

Phase 1 studies are usually conducted in specialised phase 1 centres by highly experienced investigators and staff.

General aspects

Participants

Phase 1 study participants are generally healthy volunteers. They are 'healthy' in the sense that they are overall in good health and disease free, even if some physiological variables deviate from the normal values within certain limits. In addition, they should not use chronic medication or other treatments that are critical for the study. They are 'volunteers', as much as any participant in any clinical study, because they are legally competent to freely give their informed consent to participate in the trial, and thus perfectly understand the objective, the risks and the requirements of the study.

Most phase 1 study participants are young healthy males. Young individuals tend to show less intersubject variability, take less concomitant treatments, and can better withstand the potential adverse effects of the tested drug candidates. As age may alter the function of some key organs involved in pharmacokinetics, e.g. kidney and liver, older subjects are typically included up to the age of 55 years. Women of child-bearing potential are generally excluded from these trials because of the risk that they could become pregnant during the study and that the experimental drug could harm their unborn child. To be able to include women in clinical trials sufficient securing information from reproductive toxicity testing in animals has to be available. As this is usually not the case in early clinical development, women can generally participate only if they are surgically sterilised or in a post-menopausal state. As regulatory agencies have encouraged the inclusion of women earlier on in the clinical development of new drugs, obviously because in later patient studies women will be exposed to the candidate drug, there is a trend of more participation of women in phase 1 studies, most often women who have no child-bearing potential.

For different reasons phase 1 studies can also be performed in specific groups of healthy volunteers, such as elderly subjects (as they may be more representative of the targeted patient population, and their aged liver and kidney functions may result in pharmacokinetic differences with young volunteers), ethnic groups with defined genotypes for metabolising enzymes (e.g. to study the difference in pharmacokinetics of the candidate drug between Caucasians and Asians, which may have consequences for the chosen dose range and/or dosing regimen to avoid potential side effects).

Some classes of drug candidates are only studied in patients because their intrinsic characteristics, typically toxicological concerns, preclude giving them to healthy volunteers. This is, for instance, the case with cytotoxic anti-cancer drugs that are only administered to patients with an advanced stage of cancer, either any type of cancer (so-called 'all-comers') or a specific type of cancer (e.g. breast or colon cancer), and who are resistant to the best-of-care treatment of their disease. Drugs with high immunogenic potential and drugs that target anti-coagulation factors are also usually studied in specific patient populations. Other examples are hypoglycaemic agents (in patients with type 2 diabetes) and bronchodilators (in asthma patients). In some cases, anti-viral drug candidates may also be directly administered to patients.

Phase 1 studies do not confer any therapeutic benefit to the participants, as they are not designed to explore the efficacy of the drug candidate. Participation in these trials is essentially motivated by fostering the idea that new innovative drugs might bring better care to future patients, and is thus greatly inspired by altruism. In this context it is generally accepted that participants in studies without therapeutic benefit are paid for their participation as compensation for the extra burden, time and inconvenience. This amount should remain reasonable in order not to be perceived as an incentive to participate and should be approved by the IEC/IRB. Regulations and customs on this principle may vary from country to country and it may be more easily accepted for healthy volunteers than for patients.

Setting
Phase 1 studies are generally carried out in specialised phase 1 centres. The investigators, normally clinical pharmacologists and their staff are all well trained and highly experienced in this type of studies. Phase 1 centres are mostly part of or situated in the campus of a hospital or clinic, in order to

benefit from the specialist medical environment and in particular to be close to an emergency or intensive care unit, if needed. The centres can either be a Clinical Pharmacology Unit (CPU) of a (university) hospital, or be run by a Contract Research Organisation (CRO) as a service provider to pharmaceutical companies, or be entirely owned by one pharmaceutical company for the exclusive testing of its own drug candidates (although this is less common today, as regulators have concerns about the independence of trial staff and participants in such centres).

Phase 1 study participants are very closely monitored, especially for safety. Therefore, these centres need to have the appropriate infrastructure, personnel and equipment (e.g. hospital beds with up-to-date (tele-)monitoring systems and research physicians and research nurses well trained in GCP and early clinical development). In addition, they need to have access to proper biological sampling and storage facilities as well as hospital pharmacy support for the management of the administered test substances, and some centres are also certified to work with radiolabelled drug candidates or have advanced laboratory facilities to enable pharmacodynamic assessments of ever-increasing complexity. Phase 1 units are also equipped with 'hotel' or 'home' facilities such as bedrooms, a cafeteria and relaxing rooms. This is required for studies in which participants have to stay for longer periods (days to weeks) of continuous safety follow-up.

Recruitment

Recruitment of healthy volunteers can be done in different ways. Phase 1 centres can contact subjects directly, either by using their proper database (although repeated participation in trials is usually limited by excluding participants to other clinical trials within the previous 3 months), or via call centres. Otherwise, they use advertisements that are posted in various places in the hospital or university buildings or announcements on websites, via social or classic media (magazines, papers). A lot of healthy volunteers are still recruited by word of mouth. Whatever the procedure and the material used, it needs to be approved by the IEC/IRB before the start of the study.

Before any study participant can undergo any procedure to check eligibility criteria to participate in a trial, they must first give and sign their informed consent (Section 3.5).

Once informed consent is obtained, potential study participants are screened for eligibility criteria to enter the trial. In the case of healthy volunteers, the objective is to ensure that they are 'healthy'. Although not all subclinical disease manifestations are (or can be) tested for, this is usually done during a screening or selection visit to the centre and typically includes:

– a full physical examination;
– recording of the medical history (if needed, with confirmation from the treating physician);

- clinical measurements such as height and weight (+ derived BMI), and vital signs (blood pressure, heart rate, respiration rate and temperature);
- a 12-lead ECG;
- blood sampling for testing routine haematology and biochemical variables, as well as serology for hepatitis and HIV (as they represent a safety hazard to study operators associated with the drawing and handling of blood samples of seropositive individuals); and
- urine sampling for standard urine analysis and screening for drugs of abuse;
- in addition, study-specific screening may be needed such as genotyping for metabolic studies or a pregnancy test whenever women can participate.

Before deciding to include the subject in the study, all the gathered information is reviewed against the inclusion and exclusion criteria as described in the study protocol. The most common exclusion criteria in phase 1 trials with healthy volunteers are:

- Age outside the range of 18–55 years.
- Clinically significant abnormalities in the screening tests mentioned above (minor deviations may sometimes be acceptable).
- History of clinically significant diseases with recurrence potential (such as malignancies).
- Risk of pregnancy in women.
- Known hypersensitivity or allergic reactions to drugs.
- Regular use of substantial quantities of alcohol, coffee/tea, grapefruit juice or tobacco (maxima as mentioned in the study protocol), as they may interact with the effects of the study drug.
- Blood donation in the previous 3 months, because blood sampling for pharmacokinetics and routine safety can require between 250 and 500 mL of blood during a phase 1 study.
- Participation in another clinical trial within the previous 3 months, because of the risk of interference with the new study. In addition, healthy volunteers should not participate too frequently in too many phase 1 trials (recommended maximum of 2–3 per year), in order not to expose them to excessive risks, and to prevent them from becoming 'professional' trial volunteers.

Finally, if the subject has given his/her informed consent and meets all inclusion and exclusion criteria, (s)he is ready to be included in the study.

Conduct
During the whole course of a phase 1 trial the participants are closely and intensively monitored, especially for signs and symptoms related to

drug tolerability (mild to moderate unwanted effects, transient or easily manageable) and toxicity (more serious side effects requiring adequate intervention and follow-up).

This includes effects on vital signs and ECG, adverse events and abnormalities in blood and urine analysis. Special attention should be paid to clinical signs or symptoms and biochemical variables that were pre-identified by the nonclinical safety team as items for particular follow-up during early clinical studies.

All along the conduct of phase 1 trials, the results are continuously monitored and step-wise reviewed in close collaboration between the principal investigator and the sponsor staff according to pre-agreed procedures. Also the clinical development team remains in permanent close contact with the chemical-pharmaceutical and the nonclinical development teams.

If needed, external advice is requested (either from the study's Data Safety Monitoring Board or external experts) and serious safety issues should be communicated as required by regulatory guidance and regulations, i.e. to other investigators, Ethics Committees and Regulatory Agencies involved in studies with the same drug. In fact, all safety findings are eventually communicated to these stakeholders via the final study report (and are later included in the revised Investigator's Brochure), but previously unknown serious adverse drug reactions are to be reported using specific expedited procedures.

Phase 1a studies (single-dose trials)
In phase 1a studies, single doses of the candidate drug are given to small cohorts of trial participants that are then followed over time to study its effects. The first full study of the drug candidate in humans, First-in-Human (FIH) or First-in-Man (FIM) study, is usually a Single Ascending Dose (SAD) study in healthy volunteers, whereby the first cohort receives the starting dose that has been determined to be safe based on the prior animal toxicology and pharmacokinetics studies, and each next cohort receives a higher dose than the previous one.

Other phase 1a studies just compare the effects of a single dose in one cohort of subjects (e.g. a mass-balance and metabolism study with a radioactive drug in 4 subjects), or in the same cohort under different circumstances (e.g. in the fed and the fasted state), or in several cohorts with different formulations (e.g. an intravenous versus oral bioavailability study in a crossover design).

First-in-Human (FIH) study
The first administration of the candidate drug to humans is an important milestone in the life cycle of the drug and needs careful preparation to limit the safety risks.

The primary objective is to study the pharmacokinetic profile, the safety and the tolerability of different doses of the drug after single administration.

An additional objective is the study of its pharmacodynamic activity as much as possible.

All the prerequisites prior to its start are described in Section 4.4.6.1 and are supposed to be met. Also, a structured risk analysis has been done and a strategy developed to manage these risks (Section 5.2.3.2). Here, we will focus on some important aspects of the design and conduct of the study [15, 18].

Investigator site   FIH studies should preferably be performed at a single investigator site. According to the GCP guideline, 'The sponsor is responsible for selecting the investigator(s)/institution(s)'. In the case of a FIH study, this comes down to the choice of one excellent phase 1 centre with experience in FIH studies.

Because of the flexible nature of the study protocol, procedures should be in place to allow regular review of safety and pharmacokinetics data by the principal investigator and the clinical team of the sponsor to take informed decisions on dose escalation, adverse drug reactions and stopping of the trial.

Some FIH studies may have to be performed in more than one centre, usually two or three. This is often the case for oncolytic drugs that are tested for the first time in cancer patients. Good communication between the different centres and the sponsor is then an even bigger challenge.

Study population   The choice of the study population (human volunteers or patients) should be fully justified in the study protocol taking into account the following factors:

- risks inherent to the type of drug, it is important that such risks, and their uncertainty are quantified and justified;
- molecular target;
- immediate and potential long-term toxicity;
- lack of a relevant animal model of the targeted disease;
- relative presence of the target in healthy subjects or in patients (e.g. cancer patients);
- possible higher variability in patients;
- ability of (healthy) volunteers to tolerate any potential side effects;
- potential differences in pharmacogenomics between the targeted patient group and healthy subjects;
- patients' ability to benefit from other products or interventions.

To be able to clearly assess the effects of the new candidate drug in humans, it is recommended not to allow any other medication to be taken by the study participants except in certain circumstances. Combination with other drugs may increase the variability of the study results such as plasma kinetics due to possible drug–drug interactions and may constitute an impediment to data interpretation.

Study design options The FIH study is usually a Single Ascending Dose (SAD) study, whereby a first cohort of participants receives the first dose and each next cohort receives a higher dose than the previous one until the Maximum Tolerated Dose (MTD) has been reached. The MTD in clinical trials is the highest single dose without significant safety or tolerability issues.

There are no regulatory recommendations about sample size and the use of placebo, but usually each cohort contains 8 to 12 subjects, with 6 to 9 of them receiving the active drug and 2 to 3 receiving the placebo in a randomised order and blinded to the investigator and the site and sponsor staff. The total number of participants may vary between 24 and 48 participants depending on the number of cohorts being tested and whether the doses are escalated between or within cohorts. The use of a placebo is important to be able to distinguish study-related effects (can be picked up in the placebo group) from potential drug-related effects (are only present or are more frequent or severe after drug administration).

Many different study designs are used. The most commonly used is a parallel group design, whereby each cohort is assigned one dose and the doses are escalated between each new cohort (Figure 5.6).

Alternatively, in a sequential cohort design, doses are escalated within a cohort and each participant receives 2 or 3 ascending doses of the drug or

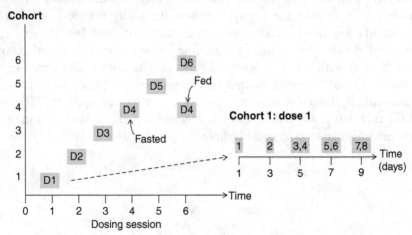

- Each cohort has, e.g., 8 participants receiving at random either the same dose of active drug (6) or placebo (2)
- In cohort 1, participants 1, 2, 3/4, 5/6, 7/8 receive the same first dose at, e.g., 48 h interval in order to allow proper safety evaluation after each (couple of) single administration(s)
- In the next cohorts, dose escalation from D1 to D6 progresses only when the response to the previous dose is considered safe
- Cohort 4 is tested twice with the same dose, once in the fasted and once in the fed state

Figure 5.6 Parallel group design for a SAD study.

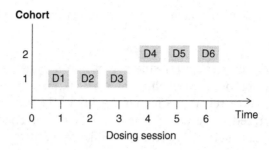

Figure 5.7   Sequential cohort design for a SAD study.

placebo at successive visits. The first cohort receives the lowest dose and the next cohort(s) the higher ones (Figure 5.7).

In this design, a wider dose range can be covered with fewer participants. This comes at the expense of a longer study duration to avoid the risk of carry-over effects especially for drugs with a long elimination half-life and a greater risk of subject dropouts. This can partially be prevented with an inter-locking cohort design, whereby the first cohort receives the lowest dose in period 1 and the second cohort the next dose in period 2. Then, the first cohort receives the next dose in period 3 and the second cohort the next one in period 4, etc. (Figure 5.8). This design increases the washout period within a cohort between doses whereby the risk of carry-over effects is reduced.

More and more flexible or adaptive study designs are used. Flexible designs in general use the results generated in the study to modify the study design *ad hoc*. In adaptive designs the rules for design modifications based on in-study evolving data are pre-specified in the study protocol, so that no amendments are needed. The type of adjustments can be, for example, changes of doses and timing of sampling or assessments, use of flexible cohort sizes and addition of optional cohorts. The nature and range of the adjustments must be pre-specified in the protocol, thus avoiding protocol amendments that need regulatory and ethics committee approval. Together with the fact that fewer data are needed to move to the next step in the dose escalation, this can lead to considerable time saving for the study.

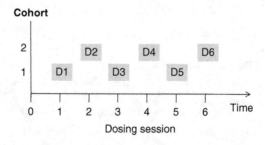

Figure 5.8   Interlocking cohort design for a SAD study.

Drug administration In FIH studies, the route of administration of the candidate drug should be identical to the one used in the nonclinical studies. In the
case of an intravenous administration, the authorities prefer the use of a slow
rate infusion instead of a slow bolus injection. This allows more careful monitoring of adverse reactions and – if necessary – a timely discontinuation of
the infusion to mitigate an adverse outcome. The estimation of a safe first dose
is of paramount importance and has been described earlier (Section 5.2.4).
Some precautions apply to dose administrations within a cohort receiving the
same single dose. For drugs with a higher risk for adverse effects such as a
steep dose–response curve for toxicity or acting on receptors of the immune
system, the first administration of each (new) dose level should be to one single subject of the intended cohort and sufficient time should be allowed to
observe and interpret any adverse events. The next subjects within the cohort
will only receive the same single dose respecting the same interval between
subjects (usually 24–48 h) when no adverse effects have been observed in
the first subject. This staggered dosing approach, has been introduced in the
European guidelines after the TeGenero incident where a cytokine storm was
triggered in subjects that were all treated at the same time with a CD-28 super
agonist monoclonal anti-body. For low risk drugs, the dosing interval can be
shorter (e.g. every 10–15 min).

Other precautions apply to dose administrations between cohorts receiving
higher doses. Progression to the next higher dose level should not take
place before the subjects who received the previous dose have all been
treated and their results reviewed according to pre-specified criteria including
comparison with the results of previous cohorts (e.g. safety, pharmacokinetics
or pharmacodynamics) and all nonclinical data. Observations that were
not anticipated may force the investigator to revise the dose escalation
scheme.

Dose escalation should proceed with caution and be based on nonclinical
data such as the pharmacokinetic profile, the slope of the dose–response curve
of toxicity and satisfactory safety data obtained at the previous dose level.

Typical dose escalation schemes are (starting with dose x):

–   Geometric progression ($x, 2x, 4x, 8x, 16x, 32x$), especially suitable for a
    drug with low toxicity in nonclinical studies.
–   Fibonacci series ($x, 2x, 3x, 5x, 8x, 13x, 21x$), more conservative and more
    appropriate for a drug with a smaller safety margin in animals (also
    widely used for cytotoxic agents).
–   Mixed progression ($x, 3x, 9x, 18x, 36x, 48x, 60x$), initially more aggressive
    with subsequently smaller increments around the expected therapeutic
    range.

The study protocol should clearly define processes and responsibilities for
making decisions about dosing in subjects, dose escalation and stopping a

cohort or the trial. To be sufficiently alert, an adequate communication system should be put in place between the centre and the sponsor staff.

Safety and tolerability As one of the primary objectives of a FIH study is to assess the initial safety and tolerability of the candidate drug in humans, all participants should be closely monitored throughout the study for any clinical signs or abnormal laboratory findings that may be related or not to the administration of the drug (Adverse Events, AE). Special attention is paid to any untoward clinical signs and laboratory findings that were identified in nonclinical safety testing and considered as potentially relevant to man.

In this context, the safety of a drug refers to the absence of damage or harm resulting from adverse events, while tolerability represents the degree to which these events can be tolerated by the participant.

All adverse events must be recorded by the site staff in the Case Record File (CRF) of each participant. The CRF was formerly a paper document but has today evolved into a web-based electronic format, stored in the clinical trial database and assessed for causality (in relation to the study drug) by a medically qualified person. If the association of an event and experimental treatment is labelled 'possible', 'probable' or 'certain', then the AE is considered to be an Adverse Drug Reaction (ADR).

Some AEs or ADRs are classified as serious (SAE or SADR), i.e. if the event/reaction results in death, is life-threatening, requires (prolongation of) hospitalisation, results in persistent or significant disability/incapacity, is a congenital anomaly/birth defect, or is medically important (e.g. epileptic fit or asthma attack not necessitating hospitalisation). These SAEs and SADRs, especially when they are 'unexpected' (i.e. not mentioned in the IB), require expedited reporting to Regulatory Agencies, Ethics Committees and investigators involved in the ongoing clinical development programme, within 7 days of death and the onset of a life-threatening condition or within 15 days in all other situations. Again, clear procedures for communication should be described in the study protocol to meet these criteria and deadlines.

In general, cardiovascular function is also closely monitored (blood pressure, heart rate, 12-lead ECG) and specific monitoring of other functions may also be indicated for specific safety reasons due to observations in pre-clinical studies.

Once the investigator considers that during the ascending course of the study the Maximum Tolerated Dose is reached, the trial is stopped.

When all the clinical and laboratory study data have been monitored, medically reviewed, and statistically analysed, the safety and tolerability profile after single administration of the candidate drug can be summarised according to the nature of the adverse events, their seriousness, severity, duration and outcome. In particular, the causal relationship between the adverse events and the administration of the drug candidate merit special attention.

According to the safety and pharmacokinetic results obtained in the FIH study, a safe dose range after single administration can be defined that should guide, together with the data from repeated-dose nonclinical toxicology and pharmacokinetics, the selection of the doses to be used in the phase 1b repeated-dose study.

Pharmacokinetics (PK) All FIH studies explore the pharmacokinetic profile of the candidate drug after single administration to humans. Therefore, blood samples are drawn from each participant before dosing and at specified intervals post-dose to measure the plasma concentration of the parent drug and its metabolites. A typical sampling schedule after oral administration of a single dose is: pre-dose, at 10, 20, 30, 45, 60, 90 min post-dose, and at 2, 3, 4, 6, 8, 12, 24, 36, 48 and 72 h post-dose. This schedule may have to be adapted according to the pharmacokinetic profile of the drug candidate identified in nonclinical experimental models (e.g. very long elimination half-life, entero-hepatic circulation or release kinetics from intramuscular or subcutaneous injection sites).

Urine is also collected during specified time periods to get a preliminary idea of the excretion of the parent drug and its metabolites by the kidneys. Faeces are collected to measure the fraction of unabsorbed parent drug and to determine drug metabolites that have been metabolised by the liver and subsequently excreted in the bile. To allow the reliable determination of parent drug and a selected set of metabolites in body fluids and excreta bioanalytical methods have to be developed and validated for each of the biological media used for analysis. From the plasma concentrations determined at each of the blood sampling points a plasma concentration (of parent and metabolites) versus time curve can be constructed allowing the derivation of a number of standard pharmacokinetic parameters such as C_{max}, t_{max}, AUC (0–24 h, 0–t, 0–∞), $t_{1/2}$, V_d, Cl_{tot}.

The plasma concentration versus time curves are established based on the plasma concentrations from each of the individual participants and on the mean concentrations of all participants. The pharmacokinetic analysis of the plasma concentrations versus time curve allows the estimation of the rate of absorption, the maximum plasma concentration reached, the rate of elimination, the number of pharmacokinetic compartments (e.g. a central compartment for blood and a peripheral compartment for certain tissues with drug retention), the area under the curve (AUC) and the relationship between the dose and the AUC to determine the linearity (proportionality) of the pharmacokinetics of the drug after single dosing. Nonlinear pharmacokinetics can be attributed to the saturation of metabolising enzyme systems or transporter systems involved in the absorption, distribution and excretion of drugs.

The analysis of the individual data provides an insight into the interindividual differences between subjects receiving the same dose.

For orally administered drugs, the presence of food in the gastrointestinal tract at the time of dosing can have an influence on the rate and extent of absorption. Therefore, this potential effect may already be tested in the FIH study. Near the end of the dose escalation, a safe single dose is given to another cohort, once in the fasted state (after an overnight fast) and once in the fed state (after a standard breakfast), with a sufficient washout period in between the two administrations. Comparison of the rate of absorption, peak plasma concentration (C_{max}) and the AUC provides an idea of the effect of food on the absorption of the drug and whether the drug should be given during or in between meals.

The pharmacokinetic results obtained from a single-dose administration study help to decide which doses can be explored in more specific pharmacokinetic studies in the phase 1a programme, and which dose regimen (e.g. once daily or twice daily administration, before or during meals) can be tested in the phase 1b repeated-dose study.

Pharmacodynamics (PD)   Although FIH studies do not confer any potential therapeutic benefit to the participants, they will also try to explore as much as possible whether single administrations of the candidate drug can demonstrate any pharmacological activity in humans in relation to the mechanism of action of the drug.

This is only possible in a number of instances, for example:

–   when the drug has an effect on a clinical sign, such as heart rate (e.g. reduction by beta blockers or sinus node inhibitors);
–   when the drug has an effect on a biomarker that is easily measurable in blood, plasma/serum or urine (or alternatively in cerebro-spinal fluid, a tissue/tumour biopsy or other biological matrix/specimen) or that can be visualised by imaging techniques.

Another option is to induce an effect with a challenge (agent) test, and investigate whether the induced effect can be suppressed or not by drug treatment. Well-known examples are the use of cold air (as the challenge) or methacholine (as the pharmacological challenge agent) to assess airway responsiveness.

When the new drug candidate is supposed to act by a new mechanism of action, the first demonstration of some pharmacologic activity in humans is called the Proof-of-Mechanism (PoM) or the Proof-of-Principle (PoP). Relevant pharmacodynamic biomarkers at this stage could be drug target oriented (receptor occupancy, ligand binding, enzyme inhibition) or be related to the mechanism of action of the drug (downstream signalling functioning).

When PK as well as PD data are available from the FIH study, preliminary PK-PD evaluations are possible. They explore the relationship between dose and pharmacologic effects (early dose-response curve) and between plasma concentrations and pharmacologic activity (early concentration-response data).

The results from PD and PK-PD data from FIH studies can be of great help in the selection of doses to explore in the next phases of early clinical drug development such as the repeated-dose studies in healthy volunteers (phase 1b) and the first drug administration in targeted patient populations (phase 2a studies).

Conclusion Once the FIH study is completed and all the results have been analysed and interpreted, the development team meets to discuss the next steps in early development. Either the development programme can be continued as planned, be revised or stopped because of safety or pharma-cokinetic issues. Without objection, other and more specific single-dose and repeated-dose studies can be started.

The Investigator's Brochure (IB) of the drug candidate is then updated as soon as possible and within one year after the end of the trial, a synopsis of the results is sent to the Authorities and the Ethics Committee, and the clinical study report is finalised.

Other phase 1a studies

Beside the classic FIH clinical trial, many other types of single-dose studies can be performed in the clinic. They are not necessarily all to be carried out in this phase of drug development but in all phases where they are necessary to help in deciding to go forward. This type of phase 1a studies are very flexible and are designed to address specific data requirements such as the:

- establishment of a mass balance with unlabelled (cold) or ^{14}C-labelled drug that provides an idea about the excretion of parent drug and metabolites (combined or separate) in urine and faeces;
- elucidation of the metabolic pathways with cold or ^{14}C-labelled drug by the isolation and determination of the metabolites in plasma, urine and faeces;
- investigation of the bioequivalence/relative bioavailability (by compari-son of the AUC) between new and previously developed drug formula-tions;
- investigation of food intake on newly developed drug formulations;
- investigation of drug-drug interactions;
- investigation of the influence of certain genotypes on the metabolism and the kinetics of the drug in the case of genetic polymorphisms of some metabolising enzymes or some transporter peptides (e.g. rate of metabolism in Asian versus Caucasian populations);
- investigation of certain disease states (e.g. impaired liver or kidney func-tion) on the pharmacokinetics of the drug;

– investigation of specific mechanisms of toxic or pharmacologic action using advanced biomarkers or noninvasive imaging techniques in translational medicine.

While it is customary to refer to these other trials as phase 1 trials, it is not very helpful and may lead to confusion. ICH terminology labels them rather as Human Pharmacology studies.

Phase 1b studies (repeated-dose trials)

After successful completion of the Single Ascending Dose (SAD) study, the planning can be initiated of repeated-dose studies in the clinic with trial participants who are usually healthy volunteers. Typically, a Multiple Ascending Dose (MAD) study is designed to study the drug's safety, tolerability, PK and PD profile after repeated administration at different dose levels. Other more specific repeated-dose trials (e.g. drug-drug interaction studies, cardiac safety studies, imaging studies) can also be conducted in healthy volunteers during this early clinical development phase. Although these studies can be defined as phase 1b studies, they can be performed at any stage of drug development. At the end of phase 1, sufficient information should be available to decide whether the drug candidate can be administered to patients, and if so, in which dose range what dosing frequency and for how long.

Multiple Ascending Dose (MAD) study

The objective of a MAD study is to explore the safety, tolerability, pharmacokinetics and pharmacodynamics of the candidate drug after the repeated administration of increasing doses in humans.

Study participants and setting   This study is mostly conducted in similar conditions as the FIH SAD trial, i.e. in healthy volunteers and in an experienced phase 1 centre, although patients can be considered for some drug classes (e.g. anti-viral drugs, oncology drugs) and more than one centre could be involved.

Study design   The classic design is in parallel groups of 8–12 subjects (6–9 on active drug, 2–3 on placebo) with each group receiving a fixed daily dose (or other dosing interval) that is repeated for several successive days (or other periods). The first cohort receives the lowest dose and the subsequent cohorts receive each of them escalating doses (Figure 5.9).

Different subject cohorts can receive different dose levels in the same dosing regimen, but different dosing regimens can also be compared, either at the same dose level or at different dose levels, which can lead to fairly complex study designs.

Here too, adaptive designs become more popular, where the study design is accommodated to the results obtained previously in the same study according

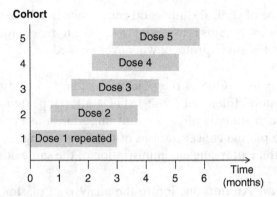

Cohort

5   Dose 5

4   Dose 4

3   Dose 3

2   Dose 2

1   Dose 1 repeated

   0   1   2   3   4   5   6   Time (months)

- Each cohort has, e.g., 12 participants, receiving at random either the same dose of active drug (9) or placebo (3), repeated at the same interval (e.g. daily in this example)
- Each next cohort at a higher dose is only started after proper safety evaluation of the repeated dosing in the previous cohort for a sufficiently long period (e.g. 20 days in this example of daily dosing for 3 months)

Figure 5.9 Parallel group design for a MAD study.

to procedures that are predefined in the study protocol (e.g. addition of optional cohorts, change of the number of subjects within the next cohort, change of the number of subjects on active drug versus placebo in a cohort, change of the dose regimen).

Drug administration The dose levels and the dosing regimens (i.e. the frequency and total duration of the repeated administrations) to be explored in the MAD study will be determined by the results of the SAD study as well as the safety and pharmacokinetic data from the nonclinical repeated-dose toxicology studies.

The frequency of administration can be once daily, several times per day, weekly, etc., while the treatment duration can vary from several days up to months. Both are dependent on the time needed to reach the 'steady-state' plasma concentration (time point from where the drug input rate equals the drug elimination rate) and the expected drug concentrations needed to exert a therapeutic effect. The pharmacokinetic behaviour of drugs at repeated dosing following different dosing regimens can be predicted using pharmacokinetic modelling based on single-dose pharmacokinetic data. Some precautions should be taken into consideration in dose escalation depending on the risk level of the drug under study. Within the first cohort, initial safety results from the first subject after a few repeated administrations (adapted to the estimated risk) should be available before administering the drug to the next subjects. Similarly, sufficient safety data should be available from the previous dose level before moving to the next dose level. Some overlap in time between the dose levels is commonly accepted especially for longer treatment durations and when no safety issues have been identified before (Figure 5.9). This overlap can also be modified in an adaptive design.

Also in this type of clinical study good communication between the investigator and the sponsor teams is essential to be able to react promptly to safety issues and adapt the study protocol whenever needed.

Safety and tolerability   One of the objectives of an MAD study is to determine the Maximum Tolerated Dose (MTD) after repeated dosing. Safety assessment in such study is of paramount importance as systemic exposure and steady-state plasma concentrations of the drug are higher after repeated administration than after single administration of the same dose.

Pharmacokinetics   An introduction to the analysis of plasma concentration versus time curves is given in Section 4.3.1.2. If the drug candidate shows no evidence of dose- or time-dependent nonlinear kinetics, i.e. when key pharmacokinetic variables do not change with dose or time, then the plasma concentration time curve is fairly straightforward (Figure 4.6).

When the drug is not completely eliminated within 24 h after the first dose, the second dose plasma concentration versus time curve of the second administration at 24 h after the first dose, is superimposed on the residual plasma levels of the first administration. The gradual building up of the plasma concentrations during successive doses continues until the steady-state plasma concentration is reached (C_{ss}). At steady state, the rate of absorption of the drug is then in equilibrium with the rate of elimination. The pharmacokinetic parameters which are derived from repeated dose plasma concentration versus time curves are the C_{max} (maximum plasma concentration in one dosing interval), C_{min} (minimum plasma concentration in one dosing interval), C_{av} (average plasma concentration of one dosing interval), the degree of fluctuation within a dosing interval ($(C_{max} - C_{min})/C_{av}$) and the AUC of a dosing interval at steady state (Figure 4.7).

The time needed to reach the steady-state plasma concentration is an important PK parameter for a drug as it conditions the speed of onset of action of a drug. If the drug has a linear kinetic profile, this steady state is usually attained after about 5 times the plasma elimination half-life of the drug. If it takes too long to reach the targeted plasma concentration range and this is incompatible with the therapeutic need, then a dual dosing regimen may have to be considered giving first a higher loading dose followed by a lower maintenance dose.

Another important characteristic of the PK profile of the drug and its metabolite(s) is its interindividual variability when administering the same dose/dose regimen. If this is high, it could be a serious drawback for the drug candidate to determine its most effective dose later in patients.

Repeated-dose pharmacokinetics will also reveal whether the PK parameters of the drug and/or its metabolite(s) change after repeated dosing in comparison with single dosing. It may well be that metabolising enzymes get gradually saturated as the plasma concentrations of the drug increase with each administration with a shift towards a nonlinear pharmacokinetic behaviour. On the other hand, the drug may induce its own metabolism with a gradual decrease in plasma concentrations that could lead to subtherapeutic levels and thus lower efficacy. This type of change in kinetic behaviour as a result of repeated dosing can be predicted on the basis of nonclinical pharmacokinetic studies.

Comparing the observed data with the data predicted by pharmacokinetic modelling based on single-dose kinetics will provide evidence of dose- or time-dependent kinetics of the drug or its metabolite(s). These findings are used to further refine the pharmacokinetic models to the kinetic behaviour of the drug.

Pharmacodynamics   If one or more validated biomarkers are available, their measurement during MAD studies can be very informative to get a first idea of the dose-response curve of the candidate drug after repeated dosing.

When these data can be linked to systemic exposure data in a plasma concentration-response curve (PK-PD analysis), they can be of great value to support the decision on the dose range and dosing regimen to be explored in phase 2a studies in patients.

Conclusion   The finalisation of the MAD study is a second important step in the early clinical development of the drug in healthy volunteers. All the safety, PK and PD data generated are then reviewed and this information together with the results of previous clinical and nonclinical studies are used to decide whether the database provides sufficient confidence to move to the next step, which is the exploration of the safety and efficacy of the candidate drug in patients.

Other phase 1b studies

Pharmacokinetics   Specific PK studies can be performed after repeated dosing if the study objective cannot be included in the MAD study. This is the case for studies with drugs with an extremely long elimination half-life or nonlinear PK, metabolism and drug-drug interaction studies. Quite a few phase 1a studies labelled as 'other' have also a phase 1b version. In contrast, the effect of age and gender can be included in the MAD study.

Pharmacodynamics   Early PD explorations in the MAD study can be supplemented with specific PD or PK-PD studies, for instance with more advanced imaging techniques such as PET or PET-CT and with a smaller window of safe and well-tolerated dose levels, to get a better idea of the interaction of the candidate drug with its target in humans. This type of study is commonly known as a Proof-of-Mechanism (PoM) or Proof-of-Principle (PoP) study after repeated dosing.

Also, more sophisticated PK-PD studies may be programmed using more advanced data-driven modelling techniques such as physiologically-based pharmacokinetic modelling (PBPK).

Cardiac safety Prolongation of the QT interval on the surface electrocardiogram (ECG) is a common side effect of many drugs that can induce potentially fatal ventricular arrhythmia or 'Torsade(s) de Pointes'.

The 2004 ICH E14 guideline [35] deals with the evaluation of the QTc (QT interval corrected for heart rate) prolongation liability of a drug during its clinical development, and focuses on the need to conduct a 'thorough QT study' (also known as a TQT study) conducted in healthy volunteers. This can only be performed when the repeated-dose pharmacokinetics and the therapeutic dose range of the drug are known, i.e. at the end of phase 2 studies in patients (see Section 6.2.3.3 for a more detailed description of the TQT study). For a number of years, there has been a tendency to try to evaluate the QTc liability of new drugs much earlier on in clinical development, and more particularly during the MAD study. This possibility was recently nicely reviewed by Shah and Morganroth [36].

If robust intensive ECG monitoring is included in the MAD study at 10–12 time points post-dose, together with the PK sampling and with an additional positive control cohort treated with moxifloxacin, a drug known to increase QTc intervals, the information gathered in this modified MAD study comes close to the information collected from a TQT study.

The MAD study offers the advantage of studying several high doses up to the MTD, whereas the TQT study only investigates cardiac effects at one therapeutic and one supratherapeutic dose of the drug of interest. This approach also permits making crucial go/no-go decisions earlier in the drug development.

Integrated phase 1 studies
The recent pressure to increase the efficiency of early clinical drug development has seen the rise of the combination of the single- and the repeated-dose escalation studies in one single trial in a seamless or interwoven design. The performance of such an integrated SAD-MAD FIH study significantly reduces the timeline to the go/no-go decision at the end of the phase 1 clinical testing programme. If this combined study also includes adaptive design features, the FIH study may become relatively complex needing extra vigilance in its execution.

An example of the design of such a combined phase 1 study is given in Figure 5.10.

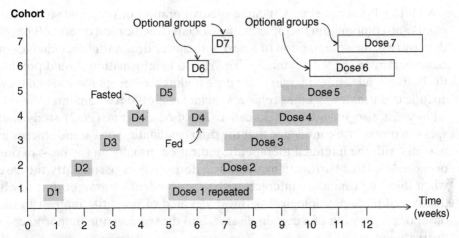

Figure 5.10   Design of an integrated phase 1 study.

- Cohort 1 starts with the SAD part
- Cohorts 6 and 7 are planned optional in the case the Maximum Tolerated Dose (MTD) after single administration is not reached before
- After cohort 4 has finished the fasted SAD part, all data are thoroughly reviewed for safety issues before the start of the MAD part in cohort 1
- This is an example of a combined interwoven SAD/MAD study in the same group of cohorts, where each cohort participates as well in the SAD as in the MAD part. If for safety reasons this is not feasible, this same design can also be performed with 2 different groups of cohorts, but needing twice as many study participants.

Go/no-go decision to start studies in patients

At the end of phase 1 of the clinical drug development programme that is essentially performed in healthy volunteers, all the results of single-dose trials (the FIH or SAD study and some specific studies), together with the results of the repeated dose trials (the MAD study and any specific studies), are formally reviewed and discussed with external experts.

In parallel, the essential design features of the first trial to be performed in patients, the so-called phase 2a or Proof-of-Concept study, are proposed (e.g. patient population, dose range, dosing regimen and treatment duration, evaluation criteria).

With this information, management will take the decision to study the drug candidate in phase 2a clinical trials.

5.3.3.2   Phase 2a studies

In the classic approach of clinical drug development, phase 2a studies are generally First-in-Patient studies. These are conducted in rather small groups of selected patients with the targeted disease of interest. Their objective is therapeutic exploratory and can be summarised as follows:

- explore in patients preliminary evidence of efficacy and safety;
- define the target population; and
- learn more about an effective and safe dose range and dosing regimen.

Additional objectives may include the exploration of potential study end-points and combination therapies with associated medication or other types of therapy (e.g. the combination of a new anti-cancer drug with other chemo- or radiotherapy in cancer treatment). The resulting information should provide the basis for subsequent larger-scale dose finding studies (phase 2b) and therapeutic confirmatory studies (phase 3) in late clinical development.

Phase 2a also includes the so-called Proof-of-Concept (PoC) study that seeks to prove with confidence that the drug candidate shows some efficacy in patients with the intended therapeutic indication, usually on the basis of one or more validated surrogate evaluation criteria. This is particularly the case when the drug candidate interacts with a newly identified target or a newly discovered pathophysiological pathway deemed of potential interest in the onset or progression of a certain disease, and thus of potential importance in its treatment.

Participants

Phase 2a study participants are patients with the targeted disease. Per study, their number can vary between several tens to several hundreds, according to the type of the disease and the level of confidence in the evaluation criteria. Each study recruits a fairly homogeneous study population with strict inclusion and exclusion criteria to allow the drug candidate to demonstrate its pharmacological activity in optimal conditions. Either all types of patients with a certain condition are included, or a subset with, for example, only severe patients or patients who test positive to a biomarker predictive of a better response. Typically for anti-cancer drugs, the activity of a drug candidate is tested in patients suffering from different types of cancers in separate studies.

Setting and conduct

In contrast to phase 1 studies that are usually performed in specialised phase 1 centres, phase 2a trials in carefully selected patients are usually performed in a hospital setting by clinical investigators (in general, medical specialists in the disease of interest) who are well experienced in (early) clinical drug development.

In this case it is common practice to also involve the patient's general practitioner (GP) in the trial who can help the investigator with referral of potentially suitable patients, document his full medical history, see to it that no forbidden medication is used during the trial, and follow-up events of interest that occur in-between visits to the study centre. In any case, the GP is always informed by the investigator when one of his patients is included in a clinical trial with an experimental treatment.

Just as in phase 1 trials with healthy volunteers, initial phase 2 trials in patients need careful follow-up by the investigator and clinical development teams with a tight collaboration between both of them.

Research tools

Phase 2a studies are of paramount importance in the decision-making process at the end of early drug development. Without having the possibility to evaluate the effect of the drug candidate on hard clinical endpoints, the clinical investigators as well as the clinical development team have to rely on the availability of validated research tools and surrogate evaluation criteria to help them make decisions about the therapeutic potential of the candidate drug.

In this context, some of the tools discussed in Chapter 4 are very useful in early drug development in patients. Biomarkers allow the identification of specific patient populations or can be used as prognostic factors for disease progression. Some can also serve as predictive factors for drug activity and are thus to be considered as a substitute or surrogate for clinical endpoints.

Imaging techniques such as computer tomography (CT), positron emission tomography (PET) or magnetic resonance imaging (MRI) are often used as pharmacodynamic activity indicators in early clinical drug development.

PK and PK-PD analyses are instrumental in describing and understanding the relationship between drug exposure and drug effects. These tools help to select the dose range and dosing regimen(s) to be tested in patients from the results of earlier studies in healthy volunteers.

Study design

Phase 2a studies are usually randomised controlled trials (RCT) with parallel design including placebo and several dose or dose regimen arms of the candidate drug. Initial trials may lack an active control arm, while later trials may also include it to increase assay sensitivity.

The dose range is generally selected on the basis of the safety and pharmacokinetic data from the phase 1 studies. Doses can either be fixed or titrated during the course of the study. Dose titration can be forced up or down for an entire study group, or on an individual basis within a group according to pre-specified response criteria (adaptive trial design).

Other critical study design issues are the dose interval and dosing regimens to be tested, as well as the duration of the study periods at a given dose. Dose interval and dose regimens are selected on the basis of the pharmacokinetic characteristics of the drug candidate after single and repeated dosing in phase 1. For example, drug candidates with a very short half-life will have to be administered several times per day to maintain sufficiently high systemic concentrations to exert a pharmacological effect. The total duration of the study on the other hand is conditional on the repeated-dose toxicology data that are available by that time. At least 2-week or one-month toxicology studies in rat and dog have been finalised in the pre-clinical phase which allows the conduct of clinical studies of up to 2 weeks or one month. Depending on the duration of phase 1 also data of 3-month toxicology studies may be available before the design of a phase 2a study, which provides opportunities for a clinical trial of more than one month (but not exceeding 3 months). Critical in the design of a phase 2a study is the selection of the blood sampling times for pharmacokinetic analysis. These are based in the first place on the experience gathered during trials with healthy volunteers but should also provide sufficient room to capture possible changes of pharmacokinetic behaviour of the candidate drug due to the disease state of the patients. For example, patients suffering from chronic liver inflammation may show a decreased rate of liver metabolism and biliary excretion of the drug resulting in higher plasma concentrations with higher activity and/or toxicity as a consequence.

The choice of the right design of a dose-response study depends on a multitude of factors, including the type of disease (acute versus chronic, mild versus life threatening, risk to lose future treatment options, e.g. because of resistance, etc.), the type of the desired response (numerical like blood pressure decrease or categorical like cure or death), as well as the onset of the therapeutic response (rapid or late).

Evaluation criteria

As the primary aim of these studies is to explore therapeutic efficacy, a lot of effort goes into finding the best available way to do this at this early stage of drug development in patients. Again, this is highly dependent on the type of disease studied. In most cases hard clinical endpoints such as survival, myocardial infarction or bone fracture cannot be applied. At best, a surrogate or intermediate endpoint can be used (e.g. tumour regression, exercise tolerance, bone mineral density), and most of the time pharmacodynamic criteria are the only ones available (e.g. tumour marker, cardiac output, bone degradation marker). The robustness of the analysis of the dose–response curve depends heavily on the validity of the evaluation criteria used. Therefore, it is not uncommon that dose-response information from phase 2a trials solely based on pharmacodynamic data is not confirmed later when based on clinical observations.

Safety evaluation is also very important especially when it concerns the First-in-Patient study with a somewhat longer duration and the maximum tolerated dose in patients has still to be established. In some instances, an MTD can best be established in patients (and may be higher than in healthy volunteers), as the risks are balanced by benefits in patients.

This is also the time to evaluate whether the pharmacokinetic profile of the new drug candidate is different between patients and healthy volunteers, and whether the dose range derived from studies with healthy volunteers doesn't have to be adapted to avoid toxicity or lack of a therapeutic effect. The availability of pharmacokinetic data also allows study of PK-PD relationships, such as the plasma concentration-response curve.

Proof-of-Concept (PoC) approaches

A Proof-of-Concept or PoC study is a phase 2a trial that generates sufficient evidence of a positive benefit/risk ratio for a new drug in patients with the targeted indication. It is performed to prove that the interaction of a drug candidate with the supposedly important pathophysiological pathway (the concept) is indeed effective and safe in patients. The term Proof-of-Concept is also used as the strategic approach or as the outcome of the approach.

The strategy for PoC testing is quite different whether the drug candidate is intended to become a 'First-in-Class' or a 'Best-in-Class' drug, or whether a new indication has to be investigated for an established drug. A First-in-Class drug is a full innovator, with a new mode of action without any proof of its therapeutic effect in patients. A Best-in-Class drug is a 2nd or later follower in an existing class with proven therapeutic benefit.

For a First-in-Class drug candidate the preferred PoC approach is to try to know as quickly as possible whether it has any beneficial effects at all in man, without knowing whether the best drug candidate, the best formulation, the best route of administration or the best potential target population are selected for these initial studies.

In contrast, for a Best-in-Class candidate, the PoC strategy focuses on the removal of the weaknesses of the earlier molecules of this drug class. Possible improvements can be a better safety profile, a higher bioavailability, easier to formulate or a change in pharmacokinetic profile allowing a better dosing regimen. As the intention is to find the best possible candidate, this development can be rather time and resource consuming with a lot of iterations between the clinical, nonclinical and chemical/pharmaceutical development. In this case, the phase 2a PoC study may also have to include the innovator (i.e. the First-in-Class molecule) as a comparator, i.e. when published data on the innovator are not available. This may be an issue if the innovator drug is not marketed yet or otherwise readily available.

When the drug already has a marketing authorisation for one or more indications and it is the intention to add yet another one, the PoC approach will probably be easier to manage as a lot of dose-response information is already available from the development(s) for earlier indication(s).

In conclusion, phase 2a studies including the PoC study are considered as the cornerstone and the final step of early drug development and merit special attention. Sometimes, initial studies may miss the dose range of interest (e.g. all tested doses show equally low or maximum activity) and further studies have to be initiated to demonstrate a clear dose-response relationship. Because it is common practice to try to demonstrate a relevant therapeutic effect in phase 2a clinical studies, doses are sometimes pushed to the limits so that in later confirmatory trials (or even when the drug is already on the market) it is shown that lower doses have a better benefit/risk ratio. Typical examples are the use of diuretics in hypertension (some doses have come down 5- to 10-fold) and the low dose of aspirin used in the secondary prevention of coronary artery disease (it took years to get the dose right). In general, extra time spent on the careful exploration of the dose-response curve will reduce the time spent on subsequent confirmatory studies.

5.3.4   Integration and decision making

The results of all the studies performed by chemical/pharmaceutical, nonclinical and clinical development during early development from the pre-clinical phase up to and including the Proof-of-Concept constitutes the knowledge base on the drug candidate necessary to make a decision to proceed to late development. A careful evaluation of all data is required before such a decision is taken as the resources needed for the next step of development up to marketing authorisation will increase exponentially.

The compilation, evaluation and integration of all available data is first done by each development stream separately and discussed at the level of the project team with representatives of other corporate disciplines such as drug safety, regulatory affairs, marketing and finance. If needed, scientific or strategic advice is obtained from external consultants (e.g. individual experts, an advisory board, regulatory agencies). At the same time, a detailed late development plan is made with a proposal for a budget to cover the resource and financial needs of the late development phase. Finally, the strengths and weaknesses of the project are weighted against the opportunities and threats in the market (SWOT analysis) and summarised in a go/no-go recommendation to management who takes the final decision. The most important basis for this decision is the outcome of the phase 2a clinical study that clearly should demonstrate the efficacy of the drug candidate in patients at systemic exposure levels that don't produce any adverse effects in the clinic after repeated dosing. In the meantime, data have already been produced by chemical/pharmaceutical development on the feasibility of the upscaling of manufacturing and the availability of promising pharmaceutical formulations to be tested at larger scale in late development. Nonclinical data on longer-term toxicology (e.g. up to 3 months), male and female fertility effects and embryo-fetal development effects are also available for review and can contribute to the confidence management should have in deciding to continue the development of the drug.

If the project teams and management feel comfortable about proceeding to the next step in development, this is considered as the 'Proof-of-Confidence' that the data generated are sufficiently solid and promising to bring the candidate drug ultimately to the market. As from this moment on the drug candidate will then be referred to as the 'drug in development'.

If the decision is taken to stop the project at this early stage (e.g. because of embryo-fetal toxicity, lack of therapeutic response, lack of a suitable drug formulation), this should not necessarily be considered as a failure. Indeed, it has been shown that the most successful innovative drug companies stop unsuccessful drug development projects earlier than others, thus saving money for their more successful projects [37]. According to the problems encountered, either initial research hypotheses can be dropped or revised and new ideas can be generated to come up with a solution and save the project.

References

[1] Amidon GL, Lennernas H, Shah VP *et al.* (1995) A theoretical basis for a biopharmaceutic drug classification: The correlation of in vitro drug product dissolution and in vivo bioavailability. *Pharmaceutical Research* **12**, 413–420.

[2] Rowe RC, Sheskey PJ, Quin ME (eds). (2009) *Handbook of Pharmaceutical Excipients*, 6th edn. Pharmaceutical Press and the American Pharmacists Association, RPS Publishing, UK, USA.

[3] ICH Guideline Q6A: Test procedures and acceptance criteria for new drug substances and new drug products: Chemical substances, October 1999.

[4] OECD Guidelines for the testing of chemicals, Section 4: Health effects, OECD, Paris.

[5] ICH safety guidelines http://www.ich.org/products/guidelines/safety/article/safety-guidelines.html.

[6] OECD SERIES ON PRINCIPLES OF GOOD LABORATORY PRACTICE AND COMPLIANCE MONITORING (1998), Number 1, OECD Principles on Good Laboratory Practice (as revised in 1997), ENV/MC/CHEM(98)17, OECD, Paris.

[7] ICH guideline M3(R2): Guidance on non-clinical safety studies for the conduct of human clinical trials and marketing authorisation for pharmaceuticals, 15 July 2008.

[8] EMA CHMP. Position paper on non-clinical safety studies to support clinical trials with a single microdose. EMEA CHMP/SWP/2599/02/Rev 1.

[9] US FDA-CDER Guidance for Industry. Exploratory IND studies, 2006.

[10] Federal Agency for Medicines and Health Products, Belgium (FAMHP), Guidance to the conduct of exploratory (phase 0) trials in Belgium, version 2, January 2012.

[11] Garner R and Lappin G. (2006) The phase 0 microdosing concept. *British Journal of Clinical Pharmacology* **61**(4), 367–370.

[12] Vogel JS. (2005) Accelerator mass spectrometry for quantitative in vivo tracing. *BioTechniques* **38**, S25–S29.

[13] Dollery CD and Bankowski Z. (1983) Safety requirements for the first use of new drugs and diagnostic agents in man. Council for international organizations of medical sciences (CIOMS), Geneva.

[14] Suntharalingam G, Perry MR, Ward S *et al.* (2006) Cytokine storm in a phase 1 trial of the anti-CD28 monoclonal antibody TGN1412. *The New England Journal of Medicine* **355** (10), 1018–1028.

[15] EMA/CHMP Guideline on strategies to identify and mitigate risks for first-in-human clinical trials with investigational medicinal products, July 2007.

[16] Kenter MJH, Cohen AF. (2006) Establishing risk of human experimentation with drugs: lessons from TGN1412. *The Lancet* **368**, 1387–1391.

[17] FDA Guidance. Estimating the maximum safe starting dose in initial clinical trials for therapeutics in adult healthy volunteers, July 2005.

[18] ABPI. (2011) First in human studies: Points to consider in study placement, design and conduct. The Association of the British Pharmaceutical Industry (ABPI), London (www.abpi.org.uk).

[19] ABPI. (2012) Guidelines for phase 1 clinical trials. The Association of the British Pharmaceutical Industry (ABPI), London (www.abpi.org.uk).

[20] EPA Guidance: (1992) A Cross-species scaling factor for carcinogen risk Assessment based on equivalence of mg/kg $^{0.75}$/Day. *Federal Register* **57**, 24152–24173.

[21] Lowe MC, Davis RD. (1998) The Current Toxicology Protocol of the National Cancer Institute, in K Hellman and SK Carter (eds.), *Fundamentals of Cancer Chemotherapy*, pp. 228–235, McGraw Hill, New York.

[22] Reagan-Shaw S, Nihal M, Ahmad N. (2007) Dose translation from animal to human studies revisited. *The FASEB Journal* **22**, 659–661.

[23] ICH Guideline Q11: Development and manufacture of drug substances (Chemical entities and biotechnological/biological entities), May 2012.

[24] ICH Guideline Q1A(R2): Stability testing of new drug substances and products, 6 February 2003.

[25] ICH Guideline Q1B: *Stability testing*: Photostability testing of new drug substances and products, November 1996.

[26] ICH Guideline Q8(R2), Pharmaceutical development, August 2009.

[27] Dobo KL, Greene N, Cyr MO *et al.* (2006) The application of structure-based assessment to support the safety and chemistry diligence to manage genotoxic impurities in active pharmaceutical ingredients during drug development. *Regulatory Toxicology and Pharmacology* **44**, 282–293.

[28] Kenyon MO, Cheung JR, Dobo KL *et al.* (2007) An evaluation of the sensitivity of the Ames assay to discern low-level mutagenic impurities. *Regulatory Toxicology and Pharmacology* **48**, 75–86.

[29] Munro IC, Kennepohl E, Kroes R. (1999) A procedure for the safety evaluation of flavouring substances. *Food and Chemical Toxicology* **37**, 207–232.

[30] Kroes R, Kozianowsky G. (2002) Threshold of toxicological concern (TTC) in food safety assessment. *Toxicology Letters* **127**, 43–46.

[31] Kroes R, Renwick AG, Cheeseman M *et al.* (2004) Structure-based threshold of toxicological concern (TTC): guidance for application to substances present at low levels in the diet. *Food and Chemical Toxicology* **42**, 65–83.

[32] EMA Guidance on the limits of genotoxic impurities. CPMP/SWP/5199/02, London, 28 June 2006.

[33] US DHHS-FDA-CDER Guidance for Industry: Genotoxic and carcinogenic Impurities in Drug Substances and Products, Recommended Approaches, December 2008.

[34] Mueller L, Mauthe RJ, Riley CM *et al.* (2006) A rationale for determining, testing, and controlling specific impurities in pharmaceuticals that possess potential for genotoxicity. *Regulatory Toxicology and Pharmacology* **44**, 198–211.

[35] ICH Guideline E14: The clinical evaluation of QT/QTc interval prolongation and proarrhythmic potential of non-antiarrhythmic drugs, May 2005.

[36] Shah RR, Morganroth J. (2012) Early investigation of QTc liability: the role of Multiple Ascending Dose (MAD) study. *Drug Safety* **35**(9), 695–709.

[37] Frantz S. (2006) Study reveals secrets to faster drug development. *Nature Reviews Drug Discovery* **5**, 883.

6

The Late Development of a New Drug

6.1 Introduction

When early drug development has shown with a sufficient level of confidence that the drug candidate has the potential to become an efficacious and safe drug that can be manufactured with a high level of quality, the late development phase is initiated. Late drug development is essentially confirmatory in nature and is divided into 2 parts: pre-approval and a post-approval development. This corresponds to the terminology used by the US FDA, whereas in the EU they are described as the 'pre-marketing authorisation' and 'post-marketing authorisation' development periods. Both these terminologies refer to the fact that the two phases of late drug development are centred around a focal point in time, i.e. the time of approval (for sale) or marketing authorisation of a new drug.

As from the start of late development, the active pharmaceutical ingredient is referred to as 'drug in development' instead of 'drug candidate', which is assigned to drugs that are still in early development. Once the drug candidate in early development has reached the stage of drug in development, it means that there is growing confidence about the potential benefit of the drug. During the pre-authorisation or pre-approval part of late development, the objective is to prove by means of clinical studies in larger groups of patients that the drug is indeed efficacious and safe, and that the health benefits outweigh the known risks. In parallel, nonclinical studies are performed to deliver in due time the prerequisites for the initiation of clinical trials of longer duration and to further support the marketing authorisation claims.

Global New Drug Development: An Introduction, First Edition.
Jan A. Rosier, Mark A. Martens and Josse R. Thomas.
© 2014 John Wiley & Sons, Ltd. Published 2014 by John Wiley & Sons, Ltd.

In the meantime, the development of a high-quality chemical and pharmaceutical production process is fine tuned for approval.

When the clinical studies show that the drug is efficacious and safe, and that it can be produced with sufficient quality, a marketing authorisation (MA) application is submitted to the regulatory authorities worldwide. After careful evaluation of the benefit/risk ratio, the drug is eventually granted a MA in its first indication(s) and becomes available on the market.

However, once the new drug has obtained access to the pharmaceutical market, the development of the new drug does not stop. In the post-marketing authorisation or post-approval phase of late drug development the objective is to refine the use of the new medicine in its approved indication(s) in day-to-day clinical practice, to study its safety profile under real-life conditions (known as 'post-marketing pharmacovigilance'), and to invest in new innovative developments (e.g. new indications, new formulations, associations with other drugs).

Pre-approval and post-approval late drug development takes many years and requires, as much as the early phase, intensive collaboration and interaction between the 3 development streams.

6.2   Pre-approval development

6.2.1   Chemical and pharmaceutical development

The major objective of chemical and pharmaceutical development during late development is to consolidate all the knowledge collected during the previous phases. This means that the technical know-how generated during early development reaches a level that is sufficient to 'freeze' the knowledge such that the manufacturing process, quality specifications and methods can be used to manufacture active ingredient and drug product for use in confirmatory clinical trials. This is important because the drug product used in these trials should be identical to the drug product that will be introduced in the market. If the drug product developed for the market is different from the drug product used in confirmatory clinical trials, a bio-equivalence study has to be conducted comparing the phase 2b/3 formulation and the market formulation.

While early development is about change, control of change and intense development, late development is about trying to keep changes to an absolute minimum. Frequent manufacturing campaigns are set up during clinical phases 2b and 3 to respond to the demand of the large amounts of active ingredient and drug product that are needed for these clinical trials. These frequent campaigns of increasing output generate a large number of batches of both active ingredient and drug product. In order to maintain control over these changes, the upscaling of manufacturing will only be allowed when other changes are kept to a minimum. The newly produced batches are submitted to formal long-term stability studies to allow the accurate prediction of shelf life. In addition, a considerable amount of analytical data from quality testing becomes available whereby active ingredient or drug product quality specifications can be fixed, tightened, relaxed or removed. In other words, late pre-approval development can only be effective if the preliminary data obtained during early development can be used as a sound basis for the further accumulation and experience in manufacturing and quality testing of active ingredient and drug product.

6.2.1.1   Development of the active ingredient

When sufficient experience is gained with the chemical synthesis process and it is shown to consistently yield active ingredient with high quality and purity, the decision can be taken to manufacture what are called 'registration batches' that will be 'put on stability' [1–4]. Registration batches are crucial in the chemical development project because they represent the batches that are manufactured using the final manufacturing process and from which the final stability characteristics will be derived. Because a minimum of 1 year stability data is required to obtain regulatory approval, registration batches need to be manufactured well in advance of the submission date of the registration dossier (NDA or MAA). It is therefore impossible to have full-scale production batches put on stability for 12 months because these are only manufactured near the end of the late pre-approval development process, prior to the launch of the new product. The regulatory authorities (e.g. FDA, EMA) accept stability data of 3 batches (the 'registration batches') if they are manufactured at a minimum of 10% of the full-scale batches when using the same manufacturing process. During the many years that the chemical development process takes, different batches of an active ingredient are manufactured (with increasing batch size) and most of them are put on stability to collect as much information as possible about the stability characteristics of the active ingredient.

The final phase of a chemical development project consists of an intensive collaboration with full-scale manufacturing units and involves process validation that proves that the manufacturing process is doing what it is purported to do, i.e. manufacturing an active ingredient with a consistent yield, quality and purity. This is achieved by the manufacturing of three consecutive batches of active ingredient according to a detailed 'validation protocol' that includes process descriptions, in-process controls with limits/ranges and the expected yield in terms of quality, purity and amount of material produced. Rework and reprocess procedures are also included in the validation process. Reprocess procedures consist of the re-introduction of an intermediate or the active ingredient into the process from which it first emerged while rework procedures consist of chemically treating the intermediate or active ingredient with

the objective to obtain a product of better quality. Also, purification procedures have to be introduced to remove specific impurities, reduce the overall
impurity level or to remove solvents, reagents, catalysts etc. from intermediates or the active ingredient.

6.2.1.2   Development of the drug product

At the interface between early and late development and to allow phase 2a/b
clinical trials to be conducted, a formulation is developed that can be manufactured at a relatively large scale and that is stable enough for the duration
of the trial. In some (very rare) cases phase 2a formulations are identical to
phase 3 formulations [5]. In most instances, however, phase 2a formulations
still need to be optimised to improve, for example, organoleptic properties and
to assure manufacturability on a larger scale for phase 3 trials and the market.
Regulatory approval of a phase 2 drug product is based on the submission to
and review by the authorities of an IND (USA) or IMPD (EU).

A phase 3 formulation resembles the formulation to be marketed as closely
as possible. The organoleptic properties, the bioavailability of the active ingredient, the specifications and stability of a phase 3 formulation and the market
formulation should be very similar (and ideally identical). The quality requirements of phase 3 drug product are the same as those expected of the product
that will be available on the market. Before phase 3 clinical trials start, the
phase 3 formulation must be approved by the regulatory authorities using a
similar procedure as for a phase 1 or a phase 2 clinical trial. The quality and
performance (including bioavailability) of the formulation used for phase 3
clinical trials must be equivalent to the quality and performance of the market formulation to ensure the same therapeutic efficacy. An overview of the
characteristics of a phase 3 formulation is given in Table 6.1.

Because clinical trials in phases 2b and 3 are conducted according to an
appropriate clinical trial design such as placebo-controlled studies, placebo

Table 6.1 Phase 3 formulation characteristics.

	Objectives of formulation	Characteristics of formulation
Phase 3	Used for phase 3 trials to confirm a proposed dosage strength	– Quality specifications are final – Manufactured on pilot scale to full scale and assures consistency of output – Semi-final supply chain up and running in preparation of market supply – Analysed by means of validated analytical methods and similar to market methods – Stable for the duration of the phase 3 trial and similar to stability of market drug

formulations are used that have the same characteristics as the drug product with the exception that they do not contain the active ingredient. If clinical trials are conducted in a double blind design, placebo and active formulations are 'blinded'. This means that it is not possible to distinguish between the drug product containing the active ingredient and the placebo. In some clinical studies comparative medication is used, i.e. medication that is already on the market and is introduced into a clinical trial, for example, in an attempt to prove superiority or non-inferiority of the new drug.

6.2.1.3 Development of the final quality specifications

The approach taken in the development of the final specifications of the active ingredient and the drug product that will be submitted to the regulatory health authorities as part of the marketing authorisation application (MAA, NDA) is presented in the following sections [6, 7]. First, the development of quality specifications for the active ingredient will be discussed, followed by a discussion on the quality specification setting for the drug product.

The focus in late development is on the full validation of the analytical method [8]. Analytical validation is the scientific process that shows that the analytical method is doing what it purports to do. The validation characteristics that are required for an analytical method are shown in Table 6.2.

Each quality specification needs to be justified. Questions such as 'why are these specifications proposed?', 'why are these limits set and can they be tightened?' are raised in anticipation of questions posed by regulatory reviewers and to increase the quality of the active ingredient. It should be emphasised that the first specifications assigned to the active ingredient and later to the drug product at the start of development are preliminary in nature and change continuously during the course of development until they become final.

Quality specifications for the active ingredient

Impurity profiling and reporting Establishing an impurity specification for an active ingredient is one of the most important specification-setting activities in analytical development. During the clinical trial approval procedure of a new drug candidate or drug in development, experts from the regulatory authorities critically examine the proposed impurity specifications in the CMC/quality section of the IND/CTA or an NDA/MAA and assess whether the proposed limits are justified. They base their judgment on what is called an 'impurity profile overview'. An impurity profile overview is a tabular summary of all the impurities that are detected in the batches manufactured since the manufacturing campaign for the first nonclinical study. An example of an

Table 6.2 Analytical method validation parameters.

Parameter	Definition
Reproducibility	The precision that is attained when the analytical test is carried out between laboratories, e.g. in the context of collaborative studies.
Specificity	The degree to which an analytical method is capable of unambiguously determining the level or the presence of a compound in a mixture in the presence of other components such as impurities. If a method's specificity is high for a specific impurity, it means that the method is capable of identifying and measuring the given impurity in a mixture of the active ingredient and other impurities or degradants.
Detection limit	The smallest amount of an active (or inactive) ingredient that can be detected in a matrix, but is not quantifiable at that level. For example, impurities may be present at a very low level and can be "seen" on, e.g. a chromatogram, but they are beyond the quantification range of the analytical method. The detection limit contrasts with the quantification limit as the quantification limit is the validation characteristic of an analytical method that indicates what the smallest amount of a substance is that can be assayed with acceptable precision and accuracy. The quantification range is linked to the concept of linearity.
Linearity	The validation characteristic that indicates the extent to which the test results, within defined limits, are directly proportional to the concentration or amount in the sample of the substance that is to be determined.
Accuracy	The validation characteristic that indicates the degree to which the observed value approaches a reference value such as a proposed content of an active ingredient in a drug product
Precision	The degree to which the measured result, after repeated measurements with the same analytical method, are close to one another. Precision is expressed by means of the standard deviation. The precision of an analytical method has two dimensions: – Repeatability or intra-assay precision: the precision achieved under identical operational conditions during a short period. – Intermediate precision is the precision of an analytical method that indicates the variation of an analytical test result in the same analytical environment (i.e. the same laboratory) but conducted on different days, by different analysts, and with different equipment.
Range	The interval between the highest and the lowest concentration of an amount of a substance in a sample.

Table 6.2 (*Continued*)

Parameter	Definition
Robustness	The degree to which test results of an analytical procedure are unchanged by small but deliberately introduced changes to the parametric conditions of the method. It serves as an indicator for reliability with normal use. Robustness, as the term implies, means that if an analytical method is transferred from one laboratory to another, it is still capable of generating the same test result. This is important when technology is transferred between one manufacturing/QC site to another manufacturing/QC site. For example, when a product is developed at a European site but – for logistical reasons need to be transferred to another site in, e.g. China, it must be shown that the method is still capable to do what it purports to do. The validation of analytical procedures is described in ICH guidelines and describes the requirements that apply to the validation of analytical methods that are used for release and stability testing. It draws attention to four conventional analytical procedures: identification tests, qualitative determinations for the impurities assay, limit tests for the control of impurities, and qualitative methods for the assaying of APIs and products.

(Source: Adapted from ICH Guideline Q2(R1)[8]. Reproduced with permission of ICH.)

impurity profile overview is presented below for the imaginary batches A0101 to A1001 (Table 6.3):

- 10 batches of active ingredient have been manufactured. Batch A0101 is a development batch manufactured using synthesis method A shortly after the transfer from medicinal chemistry to chemical development. This batch was used in early toxicology studies, was put on stability but was not used in clinical studies. Batches A0201 to A0401 were manufactured by means of a new synthesis process (process B) and the output was increased from 5 kg to approximately 50 kg. Then, 2 batches (A0501 and A0601) were manufactured using synthesis process C at a production scale of approximately 100 kg, and finally, 4 batches (A0701 to A1001) were manufactured using the final manufacturing method D that is the commercial (COM) method of manufacture,
- 8 batches (A0201, A0301, A0401, A0501, A0601, A0801, A0901 and A1001) were used for clinical studies of which batches A0801, A0901 and A1001 were used in pivotal clinical trials in phase 3,
- The majority of batches were introduced in stability studies.

Table 6.3   Impurity profile of a fictive series of production batches of an active ingredient.

Batch number	Synthesis method	Type of batch	Tox	Clin	Stab	0.15	0.25	0.65	0.7	0.88	0.9	1.95
			Use of batch			Impurity profile (RRT)						
A0101	A (5 kg)	Devpt	√		√	0.066	-	0.143	-	-	-	0.044
A0201	B (52 kg)	Pilot	√	√		-	-	0.102	-	-	-	0.045
A0301	B (50 kg)	Pilot	√	√	√	-	-	0.100	-	-	-	0.25
A0401	B (51 kg)	Pilot		√	√	-	-	0.152	-	-	-	0.28
A0501	C (108 kg)	Pilot	√	√		-	0.15	-	0.08	0.12	0.075	-
A0601	C (112 kg)	Pilot		√	√	-	0.16	-	0.10	0.15	0.065	-
A0701	D (105 kg) COM	Scale-up	√			-	0.10	-	0.15	0.123	0.065	-
A0801	D (312 kg) COM	Scale-up		√	√	-	0.098	-	0.16	0.21	0.075	-
A0901	D (305 kg) COM	Scale-up		√	√	-	0.1	-	0.12	0.10	0.05	-
A1001	D (299 kg) COM	Scale-up		√	√	-	0.12	-	0.10	0.09	0.04	-

If a new impurity appears in batches intended to be used for pivotal clinical trials, it can be questioned whether the safety conclusions based on the toxicology studies using batches that did not contain these impurities are still relevant. Table 6.3 shows that when the synthesis method changes from method B to C, four new impurities appear at LC (Liquid Chromatography) relative retention times (RRT) 0.25, 0.7, 0.88 and 0.9. These impurities were not present in the previous batch (A0401) that was tested in a toxicology study and are therefore not covered by a nonclinical safety study. If these new impurities are present in concentrations equal to or greater than 0.15% w/w, they should be toxicologically qualified [9, 10]. Consequently, the batch containing these new impurities (A0501) should be tested in a new toxicology study and the toxicity profile (toxic effects, NOAEL, LOAEL) compared to that of former batches. In most cases 2- to 4-week toxicology studies are carried out in rats or dogs for the toxicological qualification of new impurities. When the new impurities can be isolated or newly synthesised, the batch preceding the new batch can be 'spiked' with higher concentrations of impurities (e.g. 5% w/w) to increase the confidence in the safety testing.

The process of generating safety data on a new impurity is called 'impurity qualification' and the safety/toxicology study is called a 'qualification study'. It means that all impurities observed during the manufacturing campaigns of the active ingredient are to be 'qualified' such that the batches that enter the next clinical development phase or the market only contain impurities and/or impurity profiles that have been assessed for their safety. The concentration at which an impurity appears in the active ingredient and at which it has been 'qualified' is called the 'qualified level' of the impurity. The concentration of an impurity in an active ingredient for which toxicological data have been generated can be considered as safe. The qualification of genotoxic impurities is addressed in the toxicology section of the clinical phase of early development (Section 5.3.2.2).

If, as a result of a change in the manufacturing process, the concentration of an existing impurity increases, as is the case for the impurity at RRT 0.88 (from batch A0701, 0.123% (w/w) to batch A0801, 0.21% (w/w)) it is no longer considered as 'qualified' and an investigation needs to be conducted as to whether this increase poses a safety risk. It is therefore crucial that the impurity profiles of all batches are 'tracked' and that all batches are re-analysed when new and improved analytical methods become available. Therefore, the impurity specification setting of the active ingredient proceeds by means of a continuous evaluation of batch impurity profiles. If the result of a qualification study shows that the new impurity and/or the increase of an existing impurity may result in a concern for human safety, these impurities have to be removed or an alternative synthesis method developed.

If an impurity present at the level of, e.g. 0.1% (w/w), in an active ingredient is safe, then the impurity specification limit can be set at that level. However if, after several manufacturing campaigns, it can be demonstrated that this impurity appears at levels far below 0.1% (w/w), then the specification limit can be lowered to the level that can be reached by the manufacturing process. A stable production process leads to impurity levels that are situated consistently within well-defined limits and it is inappropriate to 'relax' these limits.

Not only the actually observed impurities but also the 'potential impurities', which could appear in theory as a result of side reactions during synthesis, should be reported. Knowledge of the chemical synthesis process and stress stability studies allows the theoretical prediction of potential impurities. At the end of late pre-approval development, the impurity profile of the batches produced for the market is compared with the impurity profile of the batches that are used in nonclinical and clinical research. The impurity profiles should be similar from a quantitative and qualitative point of view.

Impurities are specified by their LC relative retention time (RRT) and they are therefore called 'specified impurities'. Specified impurities may be identified or remain unidentified. Unspecified impurities are impurities that are limited by a general acceptance criterion but are not individually listed in a quality specification of the active ingredient. The presence of unspecified impurities is limited by a criterion that limits the total content accounted for by these impurities. The importance of controlling impurities in the active ingredient during the development of a new drug cannot be overemphasised. To a considerable degree, the final success of both the nonclinical and clinical development depends on the control of impurities in the active ingredient.

The official approach that is used for establishing acceptance criteria for specified impurities that have been qualified at a given concentration is presented in Figure 6.1 and starts with an analysis of the impurity profile in 'relevant' batches, i.e. batches used during development, pilot phase and

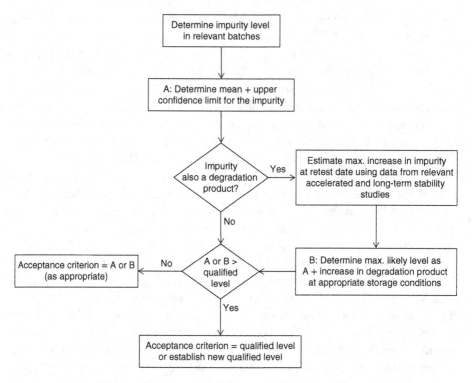

Figure 6.1 Impurity specification setting (Source: Adapted from ICH Guideline Q6A [6,7]. Reproduced with permission of ICH).

scale-up. For each impurity, a mean and upper confidence limit is determined. If the impurity is not a degradation product but appears as a result of a side reaction of chemical synthesis, the question should be raised whether this observed level is greater than the qualified level. If it is not, the acceptance criterion can be set at this level. If it is greater, then the acceptance criterion is either the qualified level or a new qualification study should be conducted. If the impurity in the active ingredient is a degradation product, then an estimate is made of the maximum increase in impurity level that will be observed at a re-test date of the active ingredient as determined from relevant accelerated and long-term stability studies. This results in the determination of a maximum likely level calculated as the sum of the mean level for that impurity and the increase found or expected during the accelerated and long-term stability studies. This level should then be compared with the qualified level of this impurity. If the level is identical to the qualified level, then this level can be set as the acceptance criterion. If it is not, a new qualified level needs to be considered and a qualification study initiated.

Reporting of impurities in the API Impurities in the active ingredient and in the drug product must be reported because they constitute an important parameter to determine the quality and the safety of an active ingredient. It is therefore crucial to address the principles that should be followed for the reporting of impurities. The reason for putting forward reporting principles is a very practical and straightforward one. When a sample of an active ingredient is analysed by means of, for example LC, the resulting chromatogram shows a series of peaks beside the main peak representing the active ingredient (Figure 4.5). The clearly visible peaks – ranging from minute 'blips' on the chromatogram to clearly visible and distinguishable small peaks – constitute the 'fingerprint' of the active ingredient. Some peaks are not identified, while others have been identified but appear at such a low level that their importance can be questioned in view of the dosage strength of the active ingredient. Therefore, the impurities are categorised according to threshold values that depend on the projected dose of the active ingredient. These threshold values are therefore called 'dose-adjusted threshold values'. This categorisation takes place in accordance with the level at which impurities should be reported, identified and qualified. In addition, although impurities present in the active ingredient also constitute synthesis impurities as degradation products, they are generally referred to as 'impurities'. On the other hand, the synthesis impurities in the active ingredient are normally not tested in the drug product as the focus is on the degradation of the active ingredient. In this section, the reporting principles for impurities in active ingredients is presented first followed by the reporting principles of degradants in the product.

An adjusted threshold value for the purpose of reporting impurities (the reporting threshold) is determined as a function of the maximum daily intake. For a maximum daily intake of 2 g per day (≤ 2 grams/day), the reporting threshold is 0.05% (w/w) and for a daily intake higher than 2 g per day (>2 grams/day), the reporting threshold is 0.03% (w/w). This means that each peak that occurs in a chromatographic analysis of an active ingredient and that is greater than 0.05% or 0.03% (w/w) of the main peak (the peak of the active ingredient) must be reported. However, not all peaks on a chromatogram that are reported need be identified. The threshold value for which the observed impurities must be identified (the identification threshold) is respectively 0.10% (w/w) or 1.0 mg of the daily intake (whichever value is lower) and 0.05% (w/w), respectively, for a daily intake ≤ 2 g/day or >2 g/day. The maximum daily intake also determines the value from which an impurity must be qualified (the qualification threshold). Qualification of an impurity is expected from 0.15% or a daily intake of 1.0 mg of the impurity (whichever value is lower) and 0.05% for respectively a daily intake ≤ 2 g/day or >2 g/day (Table 6.4). An example is given in Table 6.5 [9].

To report impurities in the quality specifications of an active ingredient, a distinction is made between identified impurities, the molecular structure of which has been elucidated, and non-identified impurities, the molecular

Table 6.4   Reporting of impurities.

Maximum daily dose	Reporting threshold (% w/w)	Identification threshold (% w/w)	Qualification threshold (% w/w)
< or equal to 2 g/day	0.05	0.10 or 1.0 mg per day intake (whichever is lower)	0.15 or 1.0 mg per day intake (whichever is lower)
>2 g/day	0.03	0.05	0.05

(Source: ICH Q3A(R2).)

Table 6.5   Example of reporting of impurities.

0.5 g maximum daily intake-reporting threshold 0.05% (w/w) – identification threshold 0.10% (w/w) – qualification threshold 0.15% (w/w)

"Raw" result (% w/w)	Result Reporting (% w/w)	Calculated total daily intake of the impurity (mg)	Action	
			Identification (threshold value of 0.1% (w/w) exceeded?)	Qualification (threshold value of 0.1% (w/w) exceeded?)
0.044	No Reporting	0.2	None	None
0.0963	0.10	0.5	None	None
0.12	0.12	0.6	Yes	None
0.1649	0.16	0.8	Yes	Yes

(Source: ICH Guideline Q3A(R2) [9]. Reproduced with permission of ICH.)

structure of which is not known, or for which the attempts to establish the molecular structure have been unsuccessful. These impurities are identified solely, for example, by means of their relative retention time, during a chromatographic separation. In summary, the quality specifications of a starting material contain a list of organic impurities as follows:

– each specified – and identified-impurity with a limit value in % (w/w);
– non-specified impurities with an acceptance criterion of not more than the identification threshold value in % (w/w);
– total content of all impurities and a limit value in % (w/w).

It goes without saying that the analytical methods that are used for the detection and quantification of impurities must be validated at least at a level that is appropriate for the phase of development.

Pharmaceutical evaluation   It is the responsibility of chemical development to look for ways to remove impurities. This can be done either by introducing additional purification steps or by considering alternative steps in chemical synthesis. If the impurity arises as part of a pharmaceutical manufacturing process, a similar approach has to be followed. The approach whereby techniques or processes are developed to minimise the level of the impurity to levels as low as practicably possible is known as the 'ALARP' approach, 'As Low As Reasonably Practicable' [11]. This approach must show, for example, that sufficient efforts have been made to reduce the content of genotoxic impurities and that there is no alternative to the production of the active ingredient or the drug product without a genotoxic substance. When it is practically impossible to completely remove genotoxic impurities from the active ingredient, a risk assessment is conducted following the principle of the threshold of toxicological concern (TTC). The application of this principle is explained in Section 5.3.2.2. Since this approach requires the monitoring of impurities down to the parts per million (ppm) level, very sensitive and specific analytical methods have to be applied to detect and quantify these impurities or to evaluate their transformation during storage. The ALARP efforts must be described in detail (e.g. use of other starting materials, other reaction conditions, other excipients or treatment conditions, purification techniques) and submitted to the authorities for assessment.

Residual solvent determination The problem of the residual solvent in the active ingredient and in the drug product is a problem of impurities but is dealt with separately because of the importance of solvent residues in the active ingredient and in the drug product. The analytical methods used to quantify residual solvent levels in the active ingredient and/or the drug product are based on gas chromatography techniques. The use of solvents used during the pharmaceutical production processes (for example, the use of methylene chloride to dissolve poorly soluble active ingredient for further processing), is a matter of concern for analytical scientists and toxicologists. In many cases, it is a challenge to choose a suitable solvent during a pharmaceutical process; especially in the case of poorly soluble drugs. In ICH guideline Q3C(R3) "Impurities: Guideline for Residual Solvents", solvents are classified into three classes [12].

Class 1 solvents should not be used in drug manufacturing because of their unacceptable toxicity or their deleterious impact on the environment. In exceptional cases, for example, for the production of a drug with a significant therapeutic value, the use of these solvents is permitted provided that their levels in the drug product are restricted to a maximum level. Examples are 2 ppm for benzene as a carcinogen, 4 ppm for carbon tetrachloride as a human and environmental toxicant and 1500 ppm for 1,1,1-trichloroethane as an environmental toxicant.

Class 2 solvents should only be used to a limited extent because of their toxicity. These solvents have a permitted daily exposure (PDE) ranging from 0.5 mg/day (methylbutyl ketone) to 38.8 mg/day (cyclohexane) that corresponds with a limit concentration in the drug product of respectively 50 ppm and 3880 ppm. Some well-known solvents that belong to this class are acetonitrile, 1,2-dichlorethene, dichloromethane, ethylene glycol, methanol and toluene.

Class 3 solvents are less toxic in acute and short-term studies and are negative in genotoxicity studies. It needs to be mentioned, however, that there are solvents in this class for which there are no long-term toxicity and carcinogenicity data available. It is considered that a daily exposure of 50 mg per day or less would be acceptable without justification. Some well-known solvents in this class are acetic acid, isobutyl acetate, propyl acetate, ethanol, ethyl acetate, formic acid and 1- and 2-butanol. For some solvents there is not sufficient toxicology information available for the calculation of the permitted daily exposure (PDE). These solvents include petroleum ether, isooctane, isopropyl ether, trifluoroacetic acid and trichloroacetic acid.

Other impurities   Heavy metals or other metallic impurities, inorganic salts, activated carbon, etc. may appear in the active ingredient. These inorganic impurities are determined and their presence in an active ingredient are limited by means of a pharmacopoeial monograph. Whether these impurities are included in the final quality specification of a starting material or active ingredient depends on the levels at which they are observed during development and production. If it can be shown that certain metallic impurities, such as lead, appear below a pharmacopoeial limit in batches of active ingredient obtained after consecutive manufacturing campaigns, a removal of this test in a set of specifications can be justified. The starting material(s), the intermediates during the synthesis, the reagents, ligands and catalysts may also appear as impurities in the active ingredient.

Particle size   It has been shown that the particle size of an active ingredient is a potential driver of bioavailability. Therefore, the setting of a specification for particle size (distribution) is not only important from a quality point of view but even more so from a performance point of view. If the drug product is a solid dosage form, a suspension or a formulation that contains an undissolved active ingredient, the particle size of the active ingredient may be critical for dissolution, solubility or bioavailability, product processability, drug product stability, drug product content uniformity and/or product appearance. If particle size has been shown to potentially impact these parameters then it is necessary to put forward a particle-size specification. This should be done preferably by means of a particle-size distribution and appropriate analytical methods. A schematic overview and a decision tree [6] that presents the development of particle-size specification is presented in Figure 6.2.

Polymorphic modifications   If an active ingredient exhibits polymorphism and analytical technology is available to allow the determination of the

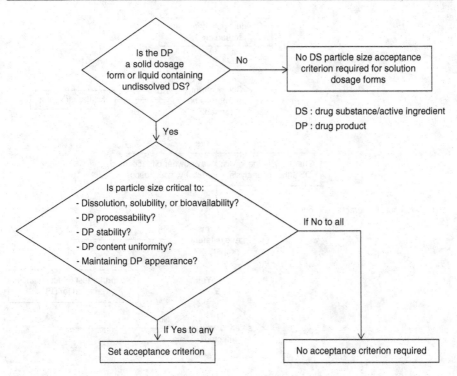

Figure 6.2 Particle-size specification setting (Source: Adapted from ICH Guideline Q6A [6,7]. Reproduced with permission from ICH).

polymorphic forms of the active ingredient in a drug product, a number of approaches can be followed [10]. It depends on the availability of an appropriate analytical technology whether it is capable of 'tracing' the polymorphic character of the active ingredient and whether the polymorphic character of the active ingredient has an impact on the performance of the drug product. If this is the case, appropriate acceptance criteria have to be established. If polymorphic modifications are observed, these should be formally characterised by means of e.g. X-ray powder diffraction, differential scanning calorimetry (DSC), thermo-analysis, microscopy etc. In addition, it should be explored whether these polymorphs impact the safety and/or efficacy of the drug in development and if so, whether their presence and content should be specified as part of acceptance criteria (Figure 6.3).

Microbial purity specifications Whether or not it is required to assign a microbial quality attribute to an active ingredient depends on the capability of the active ingredient to support microbial growth [6, 7]. If it cannot support microbial growth, then there may be no need to assign an acceptance criterion. However, if microbial growth can be supported by the active ingredient,

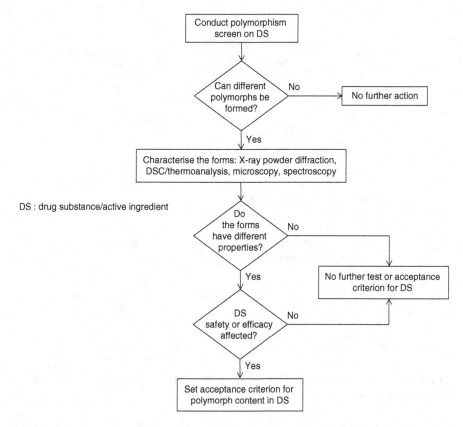

Figure 6.3   Polymorphism specification setting (Source: Adapted from ICH Guideline Q6A [6,7]. Reproduced with permission from ICH).

the question needs to be asked whether it is sterile before introduction into a finished dosage form. If so, no further microbial testing is required. However, for active ingredients that are not sterile, microbial organisms may or may not be removed by means of the synthesis procedures used during the manufacturing process. In this case, appropriate pharmacopoeial monographs may be used to establish microbial acceptance criteria. The ICH guideline [7] offers two approaches in the quality specification setting for the active ingredient.

Either the synthetic procedure leads to microbial levels below the acceptance criterion limit (including the absence of compendia indicator organisms) and data of the microbial/indicator levels show that these are consistently below the acceptance criteria limits, microbial limits acceptance criteria and testing may not be necessary. If reduction of microbial limits by means of synthesis procedures consistently results in data below the microbial limit, then these data should be included in the registration dossier as justification for not conducting continuous and repetitive batch microbial testing.

However, if investigative data show that the synthesis procedures do not result in an active ingredient that is falling within the microbial acceptance criteria limits, each batch has to be tested separately (for microbial limits and freedom from compendial indicator organisms). If data show that batches consistently show microbial levels below the acceptance criteria level, test lots on a skip-lot basis can be conducted for microbial limits and freedom from compendia indicator organisms. The above processes can be used as well for active ingredients (DS) as for excipients (Exp) (Figure 6.4).

Enantiomeric purity In the section on the development of chiral drugs, it is mentioned that optical purity is a requirement for a number of drugs as the other enantiomer may exhibit unfavourable or even adverse effects. It is therefore necessary to develop specifications for the identity, assay and optical purity of chiral drugs. If the active ingredient is chiral and is an enantiomer [6], the specifications should include a chiral identity test and assay and an enantiomeric impurity determination (for the drug product a chiral assay and enantiomeric impurity test should be introduced in the specifications). A schematic overview is presented in Figure 6.5.

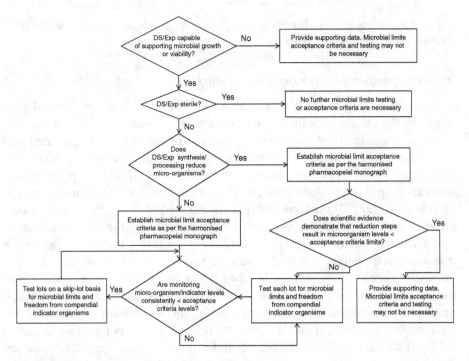

Figure 6.4 Microbial purity specification setting (Source: Adapted from ICH Guideline Q6A [6,7]. Reproduced with permission from ICH).

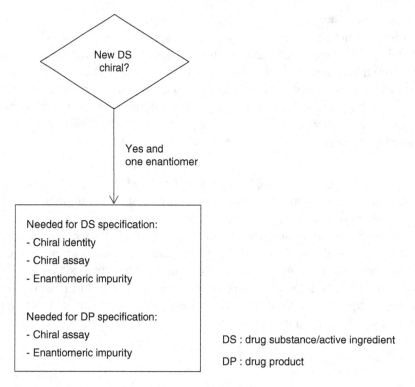

Figure 6.5 Enantiomer specification setting (Source: Adapted from ICH Guideline Q6A [6,7]. Reproduced with permission from ICH).

Quality specifications for the drug product

Degradation Degradation products in the drug product are formed as a result of the influence of light, temperature, pH or water or due to a reaction of the active ingredient with an excipient and/or with the packaging material [10]. The same principles are applied as those that were used when the impurities in the active ingredient were discussed. Organic impurities may appear during the production of an active ingredient but they can also appear during its storage. The impurities that appear during storage are more appropriately called 'degradants' because they result from degradation processes of the active ingredient. It may be possible that the active ingredient present in the drug product degrades during storage and it is therefore important to put forward limits to the potential level of degradation. The degradation of the active ingredient may start at the moment the active ingredient is introduced into the manufacturing process, resulting in an amount of degradation product at the moment of the final QC release. If this is the case, the level of degradation should be measured and reported in the regulatory dossier. If this is not the case, the stability studies will need to address degradation by means of appropriate stability indicating analytical methods and determine the maximum level of degradation that occurs up to the shelf life of the drug product by means of accelerated and long-term stability studies. These maximum degradation levels in the product (either through manufacturing or through stability studies) should be combined with the maximum degradation levels observed in the active ingredient. If the total degradation level (of the active ingredient and of the active ingredient in the product) is above the qualified level of that degradation product, then a qualification study should be conducted, or the acceptance criterion can be set at the qualified level. Alternatively, the shelf life may be shortened or the storage conditions modified. The process for the specification setting of degradants in drug products is given in Figure 6.6.

Reporting of degradants in the drug product Both specified and non-specified degradation products and specified identified and specified non-identified degradation products are reported. In analogy with the reporting principles for impurities in the active ingredient, an identified degradation product is a degradation product whose molecular structure is known. A non-identified degradation product is a degradation product whose structure is not known

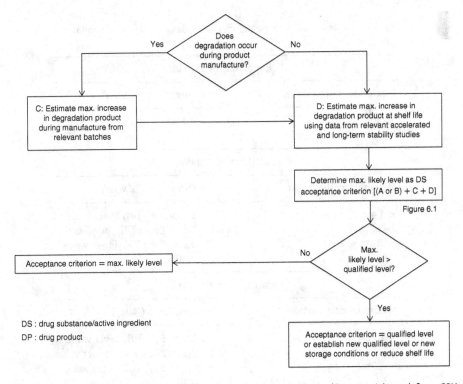

Figure 6.6 Specification setting of degradants in drug products (Source: Adapted from ICH Guideline Q6A [6,7]. Reproduced with permission from ICH).

but that can be specified by the retention time in a chromatographic analysis. The qualification of a degradation product should be carried out as a function of the daily intake of the medicine. When, for example, the daily intake is lower than 10 mg, the threshold value is 1.0% or 5 µg of the total daily intake, depending on which value is lower (Table 6.6). An example of the reporting of degradation profiles of a drug with a maximum daily intake of 50 mg daily and 1.9 g is presented in Table 6.7 [10].

Polymorphism   If an active ingredient is found to exhibit polymorphism and if the analytical technology allows measurement of the polymorphic content in a drug product a number of approaches can be followed [6]. It depends on the availability of an appropriate analytical technology whether the 'tracing' of the polymorphic character of the active ingredient in the drug product is possible and whether the polymorphic character of the active ingredient impacts the performance of the drug product. If this is the case, appropriate acceptance criteria have to be established. If it is not possible to provide proof of adequate control of drug product performance as a result of polymorphic changes, there is a need to monitor the polymorphic form during the

Table 6.6   Threshold values and maximum daily intake for degradation products.

Reporting threshold	
Maximum daily intake	**Threshold (% w/w)**
≤1 g	0.1
>1 g	0.05

Identification threshold	
Maximum daily intake	**Threshold (% w/w)**
< 1 mg	1.0 or 5 µg TDI, lower value
1–10 mg	0.5 or 20 µg TDI, lower value
>10 mg – 2 g	0.2 or 2 mg TDI, lower value
>2 g	0.10

Qualification threshold	
Maximum daily intake	**Threshold (% w/w)**
< 10 mg	1.0 or 5 µg TDI, lower value
10–100 mg	0.5 or 200 µg TDI, lower value
>100 mg – 2 g	0.2 or 3 mg TDI, lower value
>2 g	0.10

(Source: ICH Guideline Q3B (R2) [10]. Reproduced with permission of ICH.)

Table 6.7 Examples of maximum daily intakes of degradation product.

Example 1: 50 mg Maximum Daily Intake – Reporting Threshold 0.1% (w/w) – Identification Threshold 0.2% (w/w) – Qualification Threshold 200 μg

"Rough" result (% w/w)	Result reporting (% w/w)	Calculated total daily intake of degradation product (μg)	Identification (threshold value of 0.2% (w/w) exceeded?)	Qualification (threshold value of 200μg TDI exceeded?)
0.04	No Reporting	20	None	None
0.2143	0.2	100	None	None
0.349	0.3	150	Yes	None
0.550	0.6	300	Yes	Yes

Example 2: 1.9 g Maximum Daily Intake – Reporting Threshold 0.05% (w/w) – Identification Threshold 2 mg – Qualification Threshold 3 mg

"Rough" result (% w/w)	Result reporting (% w/w)	Calculated total daily intake of degradation product (mg)	Identification (threshold value of 2 mg TDI exceeded?)	Qualification (threshold value of 3 mg TDI exceeded?)
0.049	No Reporting	1	None	None
0.079	0.08	2	None	None
0.183	0.18	3	Yes	None
0.192	0.19	4	Yes	Yes

(Source: ICH Guideline Q3B (R2) [10]. Reproduced with permission of ICH.)

stability studies. If these stability studies indicate that that these polymorphic changes may influence the safety or efficacy of the drug, then criteria should be established that clearly link polymorphic levels with safety and/or efficacy characteristics. If this is not the case, no polymorphic acceptance criteria should be set for the drug. The specification setting process for polymorphism is given in Figure 6.7 [6, 7].

In vitro dissolution *In vitro* dissolution tests are applicable to solid oral dosage forms such as coated and uncoated tablets, hard capsules and also soft capsules and granules. These tests allow the measurement of the release of the active ingredient from the drug product. The *in vitro* dissolution of a drug product can be considered as being predictive of the *in vivo* performance, i.e. bioavailability, of a drug product, although clear *in vivo–in vitro* correlations are rare.

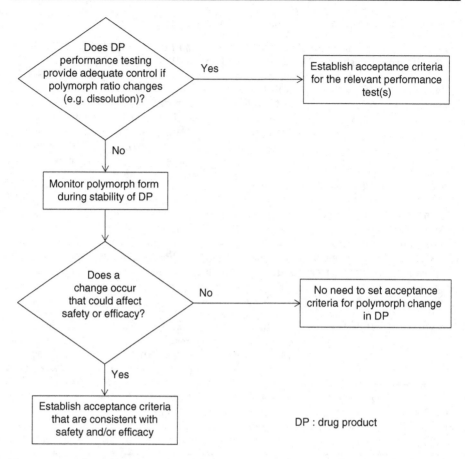

Figure 6.7 Polymorphism specification setting in drug product (Source: adapted from ICH Guideline Q6A [6,7]. Reproduced with permission of ICH).

There are 3 aspects that require attention from an analytical method development point of view:

−   the type of drug release acceptance criteria;
−   the specific test conditions; and
−   the appropriate acceptance criteria.

An important point in addressing the acceptance criteria for *in vitro* dissolution is whether the dosage form is intended to generate a modified release behaviour such as extended release or delayed release. Multiple time-point measurements are appropriate for extended release dosage forms and two-stage testing for delayed release dosage forms. In two-stage *in vitro* dissolution testing, two different media (e.g. artificial gastric fluid and artificial intestinal fluid) are used in sequence or in parallel.

For immediate release forms, the dissolution of the active ingredient determines whether a single-point dissolution acceptance criterion is acceptable or not. The dissolution rate of immediate release dosage forms has been demonstrated to affect bioavailability to a great extent and the test conditions should be such that a distinction can be made between batches of different bioavailability. If the solubility of the active ingredient at 37°C is high throughout the physiological pH range of pH 1.2 to 6.8, i.e. the dissolution is greater than 80% in 15 min at pH 1.2, 4.0 and 6.8, and there is a relationship between disintegration and dissolution, then a disintegration acceptance criterion with an upper limit is an acceptable approach. If these criteria are not met, the drug product should be tested using a single-point dissolution criterion (Figure 6.8). It is not an easy task to develop *in vitro* test conditions and acceptance criteria allowing the identification of batches of a drug product with an unacceptable performance. Nevertheless, regulatory authorities have requested – as part of

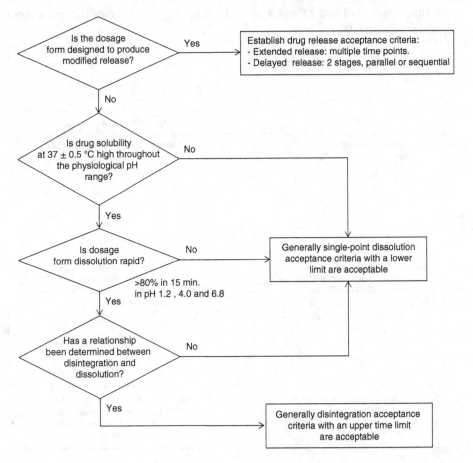

Figure 6.8 *In vitro* dissolution specification setting in drug product (Source: Adapted from ICH Guideline Q6A [6,7]. Reproduced with permission from ICH).

an approval procedure – to develop and manufacture development batches with a low performance to assess the predictive and discriminative power of an *in vitro* dissolution test.

If there is no (apparent) effect of *in vitro* dissolution on bioavailability, the possible impact of changes of the formulation or manufacturing process on the *in vitro* dissolution of the active ingredient in the physiological pH range needs to be investigated. If no effect is found then appropriate test conditions and acceptance criteria can be proposed without concern for their discriminating power, i.e. whether or not the method is capable of making a distinction between 'good' (bioavailable) and 'bad' (less bioavailable) batches. On the other hand, if changes in the manufacturing process do have an impact on *in vitro* dissolution, the question should be asked whether these changes can be controlled by other procedures or acceptance criteria. If this is the case, then appropriate test conditions/criteria can be proposed. If not, then test conditions and acceptance criteria should be developed that can distinguish between these changes, generally as single-point acceptance criteria (Figure 6.9).

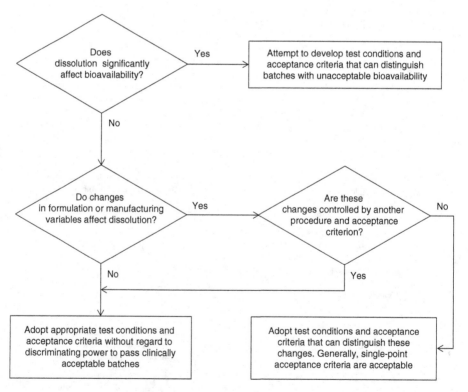

Figure 6.9   *In vitro* dissolution specification setting in drug product (Source: Adapted from ICH Guideline Q6A [6,7]. Reproduced with permission from ICH).

One of the most difficult issues to be resolved in analytical development is the definition of appropriate acceptance ranges for *in vitro* dissolution testing of drug products with extended release profiles. For these drug products, acceptance ranges can be established if human bioavailability data are available for dosage forms with different release rates and data are available that show *in vitro–in vivo* correlations. If not, acceptance ranges can be established using all available stability, clinical and bioavailability data. If the total variability acceptance ranges are greater than 20% of labelled content, appropriate human bioavailability data can be used to validate the acceptance ranges. If not, other ranges need to be put forward [6] (Figure 6.10).

Chiral active ingredients If the drug product contains a chiral active ingredient, stereoisomeric specific testing may not be required if racemisation has been shown not to occur during drug product manufacture and during storage of the drug product [6].

Microbial purity The microbiological attributes of a drug product should be investigated and specifications put forward. For liquid formulations such as solutions and suspension, the effectiveness of preservative systems need to be investigated and for those formulations that are intrinsically anti-microbial

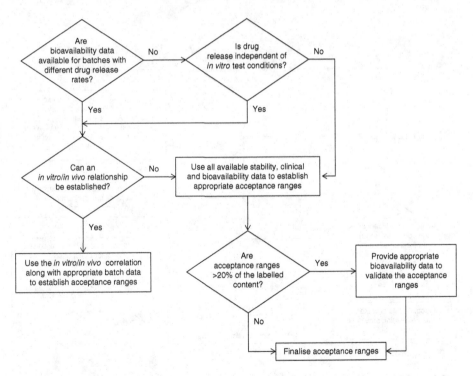

Figure 6.10 *In vitro* dissolution specification setting in drug product (Source: Adapted from ICH Guideline Q6A [6,7]. Reproduced with permission from ICH).

it should be assessed whether these are sufficiently protective to prevent microbial growth. The level of anti-microbial preservative should be sufficient to prevent microbial contamination and validated by means of a preservative efficacy test (PET). It should function in real-life conditions (e.g. after having opened the container several times in conditions that simulate conditions under which patients are likely to use the dosage form). The concentration of the preservative should also protect the formulation with respect to microbial purity as the patient with respect to the safety of the ingested dose of the preservative agent. When a container is used that is to be sterile, its integrity with respect to preventing microbial contamination needs to be shown. The question is whether the drug product requires either no microbial limit acceptance criterion and – hence – no testing, a lot-by-lot microbial testing of the acceptance criteria or a skip-lot testing approach. There is no need for the development of acceptance criteria and lot testing for microbial purity, if the drug product is a dry dosage form (solid oral or dry powder) and if there is sufficient scientific evidence that the drug product by itself inhibits microbial growth [6]. The specification setting process for microbial purity is given in Figure 6.11.

However, if the drug product is not a dry solid dosage form or it is a dry dosage form that by itself does not inhibit growth, microbial limit acceptance

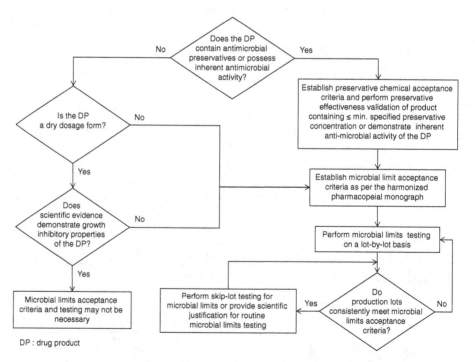

Figure 6.11 Microbial purity specification setting in drug product (Source: Adapted from ICH Guideline Q6A [6,7]. Reproduced with permission from ICH).

criteria will have to be established in line with pharmacopoeial monographs. If the drug product contains anti-microbial preservatives or possesses inherent anti-microbial activity then preservative chemical acceptance criteria will need to be established together with the conduct of PET validation at or below the level of the minimum specified preservative concentration or, alternatively, the anti-microbial activity of the product will need to be established. To these products, a microbial limit acceptance criterion will need to be assigned and a lot-by-lot testing of each batch will need to be conducted. If the batches of manufactured drug product consistently meets these requirements skip-lot testing may be considered if sufficient data are available to justify such a decision.

6.2.1.4 Final stability testing: registration batches

When a registration dossier is submitted with a view to commercialisation, the authorities, as a minimum, expect stability data collected over a period ranging from 6 to 12 months depending on the storage conditions. For materials that have to be stored in the refrigerator or that have to be frozen, specific storage conditions apply. Analysis of stability data is conducted in line with ICH guidelines. A number of requirements will need to be fulfilled with respect to the nature of the stability studies, these are as follows:

– the quality specifications of the stability batches should be identical to the quality specifications of the market batches and the quality specifications that are potentially subject to change will need to be introduced into the stability protocol as stability test parameters;
– the three batches have been produced at pilot scale as a minimum and reflect the full-scale manufacturing process of the market batches;
– the manufacturing process that was used for the manufacture of the stability batches should be identical to the manufacturing process used for the manufacture of the market batches;
– the three batches have been produced – preferably – with three different batches of active ingredient;
– each dosage strength (e.g. 1, 10, 20 mg) and container (e.g. 100, 200 mL bottle) should be tested in the stability study.

The stability conditions are identical to these used during early development, i.e. they are those of the ICH stability guidelines [13–17].

6.2.1.5 Changes during development

It goes without saying that – by definition – changes occur frequently during the process of drug development and especially in chemical and pharmaceutical development. While clinical development consists of conducting clinical trials that take place in line with an approved protocol and where the objective is not to change the protocol but to execute it with little or no modification, the essential characteristic of chemical and pharmaceutical development is that of continuous change and modification of processes, methods, parameters, specifications, etc. in order to obtain the best high-quality product. This means that in line with the obligation to inform and communicate these changes to the authorities (Chapter 3), procedures need to be followed to comply with these requirements. As argued above, these changes are more frequent in early development than in late development.

A clinical trial is supplied with drug product that is manufactured according to a process, tested according to specifications and methods and with stability data that are available at the time of the start of phase 2b or 3 clinical trials. Chemical and pharmaceutical development takes place in the background and all changes that are found to improve the quality of the drug product are communicated to the authorities at pivotal time points during development such as the start of a phase 3 clinical trial. At that time, the new processes, specifications, methods, etc., are communicated through a regulatory process of IND modification (in the US) or a modification of the original IMPD (EU). Some of these changes are critical and their implementation cannot be delayed until the start of a phase 3 clinical trial or marketing authorisation when they have been developed in a previous stage in development. Changes such as the removal of a synthesis step that may impair the safety of manufacturing workers or the removal of a new impurity in the active ingredient are/should be implemented immediately.

In accordance with Good Manufacturing Practice (GMP), for each investigational medicinal product there should be a product specification file on site where the clinical trial is being conducted. This file should be kept updated as new information on the product becomes available as presented in the EMA guideline on 'The requirements to the chemical and quality documentation concerning investigational medicinal products in clinical trials' [18]. The guideline provides a non-limitative overview of changes of chemical and pharmaceutical data originally supplied in the IMPD as part of a clinical trial application:

- importation of the medicinal product;
- change of name or code of IMPs;
- immediate packaging material;
- manufacturer(s) of drug substance;
- manufacturing process of the drug substance;
- specifications of active substance;
- manufacture of the medicinal product;
- specification (release or shelf life) of the medicinal product;
- specification of excipients where these may affect product performance;
- shelf life including after first opening and reconstitution;

- major change to the formulation;
- storage conditions;
- test procedures of active substance;
- test procedures of the medicinal product;
- test procedures of non-pharmacopoeial excipients.

These changes are considered to be 'substantial' when they are likely to have a significant impact on:

- the safety or physical or mental integrity of the patients;
- the scientific values of the trial;
- the conduct or management of the trial; and /or
- the quality or safety of the investigational medicinal product used in the trial.

In general, any amendment or change in the chemical and pharmaceutical data that have a potential effect on safety are to be considered a substantial amendment to the originally submitted regulatory dossier. Changes other than the ones presented above may also have a substantial impact on the safety of the patients enrolled in the clinical trial. Other examples of changes that are considered substantial are, for example, stability issues whereby a new degradation product is formed, microbial contamination and new impurity profiles. If the change in the chemical and pharmaceutical data is implemented at the time of a new phase of clinical trial such as the start of a phase 2 or 3 trial, then the notification of a substantial amendment becomes part of the clinical trial application and its IMPD. Notifications of substantial amendments are only necessary for changes in ongoing clinical trials.

According to FDA, changes to the chemical and pharmaceutical development data are to be divided into two main regulatory pathways: information amendments that include safety information linked to the CMC section and corroborating information that can be submitted through an annual report. While an annual report to the IND needs to be submitted at the anniversary date of the original IND and contains new – modified – development data that were implemented during the previous year and did not cause any concern for the safety of the patient, an 'information amendment' contains prior-approval CMC data. The annual report to the IND (Chapter 1) includes:

- a summary of CMC safety information submitted as part of the 'information amendments' during the past year and, when applicable, corroborating information;
- updates of corroborating information; or
- corrections to information that was provided to the IND but cannot be considered significant enough to warrant an information amendment.

6.2.2 Nonclinical development

During early development all nonclinical data were generated to allow the conduct of clinical trials in healthy volunteers and patients [19]. Before transfer to late development, sufficient nonclinical data must be available to be able to start therapeutic confirmatory trials (phase 2b and 3). It concerns data from 90-day toxicology studies in the rat and the dog or in any other appropriate animal species, fertility studies in male and female rats and embryo–fetal development toxicology studies in the rat and the rabbit or the mouse. By the end of early drug development longer-term toxicology studies are also started such as the 6-month study in the rat and the 9-month study in the dog in the event that the drug is projected to be used for long periods of time. At the same time the pre- and post-natal development toxicology study in the rat can be initiated or continued in late development. The pre-approval phase of late development is the last phase of drug development before market authorisation. By the end of this phase definitive evidence needs to be presented regarding the safety, efficacy and quality of the drug. To support the clinical trials (phases 2b and 3) and depending on the projected therapeutic use of the drug nonclinical development has to focus on long-term toxicokinetics, drug–drug interactions, long-term toxicity, carcinogenicity, mechanistic toxicology and extended reproductive and development toxicology studies in the event of possible paediatric development.

6.2.2.1 Pharmacokinetics

Toxicokinetics
The main focus of pharmacokinetics in this phase of development is on the refinement of the understanding of the pharmacokinetic behaviour of the drug in different treatment regimes and longer treatment times and during the critical phases of the reproductive cycle. Pharmacokinetics also play an important role in the elucidation of the mode of toxic action of the drug in experimental animals and in man. This is done by the inclusion of toxicokinetic satellite groups in toxicology studies with a very careful design of blood sampling. In such way data are produced that help in understanding, for example, the transfer of the drug and its metabolites to the developing fetus, the metabolic handling of the drug by the fetus in the pre-natal and post-natal phases of development and the transfer of the drug and its metabolites to the pups through lactation. Toxicokinetic data from long-term toxicology studies and clinical pharmacokinetic data are essential in the selection of a dose range for carcinogenicity studies with a sufficiently high margin of safety. During late development there is also a continuous interaction between nonclinical and clinical pharmacokinetics to help in further refining treatment regimes and drug-delivery systems and to better understand adverse

effects observed in the clinic (e.g. jaundice in the case of interaction with hepatic transporter peptides).

Drug–drug interactions

In early development, the metabolic pathways of the drug were identified in several animal species and in man as well as the effects of the drug on the metabolising enzyme systems involved in its own metabolism but also of that of other drugs. This provides the knowledge to investigate interactions with drugs that might be taken in combination with the drug under development. In drug–drug interaction studies the effect (e.g. inhibition or induction of metabolism, inhibition/occupation of transporter peptides) of the other drugs on the pharmacokinetic behaviour of the drug under study as well as the effect of the drug on the kinetics of the other drugs are investigated. If one or more of the enzymes or transporter peptides involved in drug metabolism, distribution and excretion is genetically polymorphic, specific attention is paid to those patient populations that exhibit different pharmacokinetic profiles due to a deficient enzyme or transporter activity. In such cases there is a lot of interaction between nonclinical and clinical pharmacokinetics for the conduct of studies to identify the vulnerable patient populations and adapt the treatment regimes to their pharmacokinetic profile.

6.2.2.2 Toxicology

Repeated-dose toxicology

Late development is the phase where longer-term (chronic) toxicology studies are either started or continued when they were started already in early development. It concerns a 6-month toxicology study in the rat and a 9-month toxicology study in the dog. These studies are required when the drug is intended for use for long periods of time (more than 6 months) up to lifetime. The design of the test protocols is based on the findings of the 3-month toxicology studies where the incidence and severity of the adverse effects at the higher-dose levels play a role in the selection of the high-dose level. This dose should exert overt toxicity but not severe enough to impact survival. The lowest dose should stay free of any adverse effect findings. The mid-dose level is situated in between and normally differs with a factor of 2 to 5 with the high and the low dose. The toxicological parameters are similar to those of the 3-month toxicology studies with the exception that ophthalmology and neurobehavioural testing are no longer included. Instead, more endpoints can be added based on the findings in the clinic, 3-month toxicology studies or as a result of more specific nonclinical investigations in early development (e.g. immunotoxicity, neurotoxicity, endocrine effects). Chronic toxicology studies contain a satellite group for toxicokinetic analysis to establish the AUC at the end of treatment that is an important parameter

Table 6.8   Repeated-dose toxicology studies required to support marketing.

Duration of indicated treatment	Rodent	Non-rodent
Up to 2 weeks	1 month	1 month
>2 weeks to 1 month	3 months	3 months
>1 month to 3 months	6 months	6 months
>3 months	6 months	9 months

(Source: ICH Guideline M3(R2) [19]. Reproduced with permission of ICH.)

for the design of carcinogenicity studies. The minimum duration of nonclinical studies required to support marketing of the drug in all regions of the world are shown in Table 6.8 [19].

The dose range finding study and the subacute toxicology study in the mouse performed in early development serve as a basis for the design of the 3-month toxicology study in the mouse that is normally carried out at the beginning of late development. The outcome of this study is important for the design of the carcinogenicity study in the mouse.

Genotoxicology

The genotoxicology database of the drug is complete at this stage of development but further genotoxicology testing may be required to address possible genotoxic impurities in the event of a change of the drug manufacturing process [11]. During the upscaling of the manufacturing process that is needed to provide sufficient drug compound for the larger clinical trials, it may occur that different starting materials or different reactants and intermediates are used to accommodate the larger scale of production. Such a change in the synthesis process gives rise to different impurity profiles that require the re-definition of the drug specifications. The molecular structure of impurities that are present in concentrations of equal to or greater than 0.1% (w/w) have to be identified. If it appears that these structures contain molecular moeities that are recognised as 'mutagenic alerts', then action is required. Either manufacturing tries to eliminate the impurity or a bacterial mutagenicity test (Ames test) is carried out. If this test is negative then there is no problem, if positive, manufacturing has to try to reduce the impurity below an acceptable level that is called the threshold of toxicological concern (TTC). The TTC is addressed in Section 5.3.2.2.

Carcinogenicity

Since it is impossible to assess any carcinogenic effect in the clinic, nonclinical studies in rodents are the only way to address this type of effect [20–22]. However, it should be emphasised that rodent carcinogenicity studies with treatment times of up to 24 months are not always a good predictor of human carcinogenicity. There are many possible mechanisms of carcinogenicity and they can be roughly subdivided into two main mechanistic groups: genotoxic and non-genotoxic. The genotoxicological database of the drug obtained so far should be sufficiently robust to exclude the first category of mechanisms of carcinogencity. The second category concerns mechanisms based, for example, on cell damage, nuclear receptor activation, mitogenesis and inhibition of programmed cell death (apoptosis). The initial steps of these mechanisms (e.g. cell death, cell proliferation, enzyme induction) can already be revealed in shorter-term toxicology studies.

Carcinogenicity tests are required when the drug is intended to be used either for continuous treatment for at least 6 months or for intermittent treatment of chronic or recurrent diseases (e.g. allergic rhinitis, depression). Carcinogenicity studies may also be recommended for drugs for which there is a cause of concern because of:

- previous demonstration of carcinogenicity of drugs belonging to the same pharmacological class;
- structure-activity relationships suggest an increased risk of cancer;
- evidence of preneoplastic lesions in subchronic and chronic toxicology studies; and
- long-term tissue retention of the drug and/or its metabolites producing pathological responses.

The conduct of carcinogenicity tests of drugs for the treatment of very serious chronic diseases and for which there is an urgent unmet need (e.g. HIV) may be postponed until after marketing authorisation. In certain cases, and in consultation with the regulatory authorities, the use of alternative carcinogenicity models such as 6-month studies with transgenic rodents may be considered (e.g. p53+/− deficient model, Tg.AC model, TgHras2 model).

A critical aspect of the design of carcinogenicity studies is the dose selection. The most critical studies that help in the dose selection of carcinogenicity studies in rodents are the 6-month chronic toxicology study in the rat and the 3-month toxicology study in the mouse. The data that play an important role in dose selection are toxicity endpoints, pharmacodynamic endpoints, plasma kinetics, saturation of absorption and the maximum feasible dose. Any specific target organ toxicity such as chronic inflammation, hypertrophy and hyperplasia should be a point attention in the design of a cancer study. The ratio between the AUC of the highest dose level at the end of a rodent chronic toxicology study and the AUC of the projected therapeutic dose at the end of the longest clinical trial is an important criterion to understand the margin of safety in terms of carcinogenicity (if the concerned tumours are relevant to man). This margin of safety should, preferably, be at least 25-fold. Saturation of absorption is an important factor. It does not make sense to continue exposing experimental animals to still higher dose levels if their drug blood levels are no longer increasing. The dose at which saturation of absorption is reached after repeated dosing should be taken as the high-dose level even in the event of low toxicity. The maximum feasible dose is largely influenced by the physicochemical characteristics of the active ingredient, the formulation and the mode of administration. As gavage is the most applied mode of administration in oral carcinogenicity studies in pharmaceutical development, the viscosity of the drug formulation is a critical factor. It doesn't make a lot of sense to further increase the dose when the drug formulation becomes too viscous to be injected by gavage or solidifies in the stomach of the animals. In the case of dietary studies, the maximum feasible incorporation in the diet is 5% (w/w) to avoid nutritional imbalances in the animals. An appropriate limit dose is 1500 mg/kg body weight/day where rodent systemic exposure (as AUC) is at least 10-fold greater than human systemic exposure at the intended therapeutic dose.

The high dose of a carcinogenicity study should not be greater than the maximum tolerated dose (MTD). The MTD should not cause a reduction of body weight gain of more than 10% and not produce histopathological changes of a severity that would interfere with the interpretation of the study. The estimation of the best possible high-dose level of a carcinogenicity study based on the data from a chronic toxicology study (e.g. 6 or 12 months) is quite straightforward and might in many cases be the same. It is much more difficult to estimate a high-dose level when only data are available from a subchronic toxicology study where the extrapolation from 3 to 24 months is difficult and may entail the risk of missing the right dose range. Sometimes, 4 dose levels may be selected to avoid this problem. If it appears that the dose range selected is not optimal, too many animals may die before the end of the study or the MTD may be largely exceeded. In the first case, the number of animals at the end of the study is not enough for statistical analysis and in the second case the tumour incidence may shoot up because of a severe disturbance of homeostasis due to too much toxicity.

In the interpretation of carcinogenicity data only those tumours can be taken into consideration that:

– show a clear dose–effect relationship;
– are statistically significantly different from control;
– are present at dose levels not higher than the MTD; and
– have an incidence that is beyond the historical control range of the test laboratory for the same species and strain within the same timeframe.

The interpretation of cancer studies in rodents is difficult since many tumour types are either based on a mechanism of action that is of no relevance to man or are spontaneous in nature and typical for the species and strain of experimental animals under investigation. In order to be able to dismiss certain tumour types in the analysis of carcinogenesis study results, the carcinogenic mode of action of the drug or one of its metabolites in the rodent (rat, mouse) should be understood and its non-relevance to man should be proven. If there is insufficient evidence to prove that the tumours found in the rat or the mouse are of no relevance to man they cannot be dismissed in human cancer risk assessment.

A typical example of a tumour in the rat that is not relevant to man is thyroid follicular adenoma. When the drug induces the conjugation of the thyroid hormones thyroxine (T4) and triiodothyronine (T3) with glucuronic acid it enhances the excretion of these hormones into the bile. Since the elimination half-life of T4 and T3 is very short in the rat their concentration in the blood drops very quickly as a result. Through a feedback mechanism, the pituitary is then stimulated to produce more thyroid-stimulating hormone (TSH) which in turn stimulates the thyroid follicular cells to produce more thyroid hormone to restore blood levels. Chronic stimulation of the thyroid by TSH produces hyperplasia of the follicular cells that ultimately results in tumour formation [23]. This mechanism is well known in the rat and generally recognised to be of limited relevance in man. To be able to dismiss this tumour the presence of this mechanism of action has to be proven in the rat. This can be done by the conduct of a subacute or subchronic toxicology study with emphasis on the histopathology of the thyroid, induction of glucuronyl transferase, determination of TSH, T3 and T4 in serum and excretion of T3 and T4 glucuronides in the bile. Another example of a tumour that is not relevant to man is the tubular carcinoma of the kidney in the rat based on a mechanism of binding with α2 μ-globulin. This protein is very species specific and is produced in the liver of the male rat and excreted in the urine (pheromone function) and has a high affinity for lipophilic substances such as d-limonene and hydrocarbons. Normally, this protein is degraded in lysosomes of the proximal tubular cells of the kidney after reabsorption but this process is slowed down by binding to lipophilic substances. The consequence of this interaction is that the ligand–protein complex accumulates in the tubular epithelium causing nephropathy, cell death and regenerative cell proliferation ultimately leading to the production of kidney tumours [24]. Recently, a lot of progress has been made in the understanding of the mechanism of action of the formation of hepatocellular tumours in the mouse and the rat and their limited relevance to man [25]. Such liver tumours are often found in rodents and are reported as such in the label of the drug.

Apart from the incidence of tumour production at the end of the study the latency of tumour formation is also taken into account. The latency is the time it takes for the tumour to become detectable. Since no interim groups are included in carcinogenicity studies conducted in pharmaceutical development only an idea of latency can be obtained through the detection of tumours in animals that died before termination of the study. In the interpretation of carcinogenicity studies special attention should be paid to tumours with a short latency time or that have a very low spontaneous tumour rate in the species under investigation.

Reproductive toxicology

All data in relation to fertility and embryo–fetal development are available at the start of late development and the results obtained form the basis for the dose setting of the pre- and post-natal development toxicology study. When a pre- and post-natal toxicology study has already been started in early development it continues its course in late development. The results from this study can already be used for the design of a paediatric development programme. If more data are required on the development of specific target organ systems as a function of well-defined treatment periods during the development of a child, juvenile toxicology studies are designed to meet that purpose before starting a paediatric development programme in the clinic.

Juvenile toxicology

Structural and functional characteristics of many organ systems differ significantly between children and adults because of growth and development during post-natal maturation [26–28]. Examples of such organs/systems are the brain, the kidneys, the lungs, the immune system, the reproductive system, the skeleton, the gastrointestinal system and organs/systems involved in the absorption and metabolism of drugs. Post-natal growth and development can affect drug disposition and action. Examples include changes in metabolism (maturation rate of Phase I and Phase II metabolising enzymes), body composition (water versus lipid content), maturation of receptor expression and function, growth rate and organ functional capacity.

Juvenile toxicology studies are often initiated to support paediatric development and focus on aspects of growth and development from weaning to sexual maturity that have not been addressed in previous reproductive toxicology studies. Since young animals have in general developing characteristics similar to paediatric patients, they are considered as adequate models for assessing drug effects in this population. The conduct of a juvenile toxicology study should be considered on a case-by-case basis and only initiated to address specific questions on growth and development that have not been resolved yet by previous nonclinical and clinical studies.

Juvenile toxicology studies may be useful for the assessment of:

– age-specific differences in sensitivity to toxicity between adult and immature animals;
– the sensitivity of organs/tissues to drug toxicity that undergo significant post-natal development and which have been identified as target organs/tissues in toxicology studies with adult animals;

– developmental effects that cannot be assessed in an adequate, safe and ethical manner in paediatric patients.

Important aspects that have to be taken into consideration for the design of juvenile toxicology studies are:

– intended use of the drug in paediatric populations;
– timing of the dosing in relation to the phases of growth and development;
– potential differences in pharmacological, toxicological and metabolic profiles between mature and immature organ systems and tissues;
– established temporal development differences between animal species and paediatric populations;
– findings from previous toxicology studies in adult animals;
– findings from clinical studies with adult patients;
– findings from pre- and post-natal development studies including the extent of pup exposure in relation to the expected therapeutic exposure;
– juvenile animal data from drugs having similar molecular structures or belonging to the same pharmacological class;
– similarity of development processes in target organ systems in experimental animals and the intended paediatric population.

Rats and dogs are the species of the first choice and the use of both sexes of one species is normally sufficient. The route of administration should be the same as that of the intended paediatric population. In most studies 3 dose groups and 1 control group are used in combination with a toxicokinetic satellite group. Pharmacokinetic data in juvenile animals are very useful for the interpretation of the toxicology data and for the understanding of differences in sensitivity to toxicity between juvenile and adult animals.

The toxicological endpoints of a juvenile toxicology study are in general:

– overall growth (e.g. body weight, growth rate, tibial length);
– clinical observations;
– hematology and serum biochemistry (limited because of limited blood volume);
– organ weights (absolute and relative to body weight);
– gross pathology;
– microscopic pathology of target organs;
– sexual maturation landmarks (age of balano-preputial separation, vaginal opening);
– reproductive performance (mating, fertility);
– developmental neurotoxicity, similar to the battery used in pre- and post-natal development studies (reflex ontogeny, sensorimotor function, locomotor activity, reactivity, social behaviour, learning and memory).

The study results of a juvenile toxicology study should be available before the initiation of clinical studies with paediatric patients. The knowledge gathered in relation to the sensitivity of certain organ systems and tissues to toxicity in different stages of development and the corresponding systemic concentrations of the drug and its metabolites is of great help in the design of clinical paediatric studies. If it appears from juvenile toxicology studies that the drug severely interferes with the normal development of the organism at systemic drug concentrations of therapeutic importance, a decision may be taken not to embark on paediatric development.

6.2.2.3   Environmental risk assessment (ERA)

Active ingredients of pharmaceuticals are widely established as ubiquitous contaminants in the environment. They have been detected in various compartments of the environment such as sewage, surface waters, ground water, marine water, drinking water, sediment, sewage sludge, aquatic organisms, crops and vegetation. The most important routes by which drugs are introduced into the environment are the excretion of unabsorbed and unmetabolised drugs, release from the skin of topically applied drugs and the improper disposal of drugs in waste and sewage systems. Some metabolites of drugs that are excreted in urine such as glucuronic acid conjugates can release the active drug through microbial metabolic activity in waste water treatment sludge (e.g. ethinylestradiol glucuronate).

Drug products also contain excipients that may be present in even larger amounts than the active ingredient. Most excipients belong to the regulatory domains of chemicals, food constituents or food additives and the assessment of their impact on the environment is covered by specific regulations. Many of the excipients used in pharmaceutical formulation are natural products or have the regulatory status of GRAS (Generally Recognised As Safe) compounds. If this is not the case and the release into the environment is significant, a separate environmental risk assessment may have to be considered.

Since most drugs are designed to be resistant to mammalian metabolism in order to achieve high systemic exposure, they are in most instances also more resistant to biodegradation in the environment and show a tendency to accumulate. It is therefore important that before a drug is placed onto the market drug development organisations are well aware of the consequences of the accumulation of the drug in the environment. The European Medicines Agency (EMA) issued a guideline in 2006 [29] to help drug development organisations to perform an environmental risk assessment. An environmental risk assessment (ERA) is required for all marketing authorisation applications in Europe. If an increase of environmental exposure is expected, for example, in the case of the introduction of a new indication (type II variation) of a marketed drug then a new environmental impact assessment should be made. Medicinal products such as vitamins, electrolytes, amino acids, proteins, carbohydrates, lipids, vaccines and herbal preparations are exempt from environmental risk assessment.

In the United States, an environmental assessment (EA) is required for those drug applications that don't qualify for categorical exclusion or that are suspected to have a significant effect on the environment [30]. Categorical exclusions are, for example, applications that don't increase the use of the active ingredient and as a consequence the release into the environment and when the estimated concentration of the active ingredient at the point of entry into the aquatic environment remains below 1 µg/L.

Environmental risk assessment of drugs in Europe

The environmental risk assessment of drugs in Europe is a step-wise process that consists of two phases. The first phase is a first estimate of the exposure of the environment to the drug. The second phase is started when exposure is above a pre-set threshold concentration in surface water. The second phase is divided into two parts, tier A and tier B.

ERA Phase I   This phase is a pre-screening phase where all existing data are used for a first estimation of environmental exposure to the drug. This rough estimation is only based on the active ingredient irrespective of its route of exposure, pharmaceutical formulation, metabolism and excretion.

When the predicted environmental concentration (PEC) is calculated the following assumptions are made:

–   the fraction of the overall market penetration is within the range of the existing medicinal products;
–   the predicted amount of drug used per year is evenly distributed over the year and throughout the geographic area of use;
–   the sewage system is the main route of entry of the active ingredient into the surface water;
–   there is no biodegradation or retention of the active ingredient in the sewage treatment plant;
–   there is no metabolism of the drug in the patient.

When the drug development organisation has data that can be used to refine the PEC they can be used. An example is a more accurate estimate of the market penetration of the drug based on epidemiological data.

When the PEC of surface water is less than 0.01 µg/L and there are no other environmental concerns (e.g. no risk for persistence or bioaccumulation) the medicinal product is unlikely to be a risk for the environment when it is used as intended. An overview of the ERA phase I process is given in Figure 6.12.

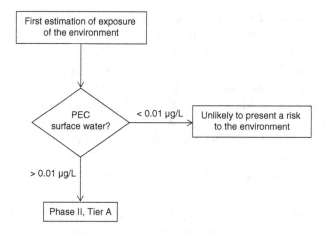

Figure 6.12   ERA phase I (Source: adapted from EMA/CHMP, 2006 Guideline [29]).

ERA Phase II   When the PEC value for surface water is equal to or greater than 0.01 μg/L, phase II assessment is initiated that is based on the evaluation of the ratio of the predicted-environmental-concentration (PEC) over the predicted-no-effect-concentration (PNEC). A more extensive environmental testing programme is then started to further refine the PEC and to produce data on the effects of the active ingredient on environmental organisms. In this phase all relevant data should be taken into account for the environmental risk assessment such as physicochemical properties, primary and secondary pharmacology, toxicology, pharmacokinetics, biodegradation and persistence. The ecotoxicology and environmental fate studies should preferably follow the guidelines issued by the EU Commission [31] the Organisation for Economic Co-operation and Development (OECD) [32] or the International Organisation for Standardisation (ISO) [33]. All studies conducted should be in compliance with the OECD guidelines on GLP [34].

ERA Phase II, Tier A   To refine the PEC data it is necessary to gain more insight into the environmental fate of the active ingredient in sewage treatment plants. The first test that can be performed is the ready biodegradation test to have an idea on how quickly the active ingredient can be degraded to CO_2 by the microbial flora of sewage sludge. If the drug is not ready biodegradable then it should be investigated in a water sediment study. The tendency of the active ingredient to adsorb to sewage sludge particles is described by the adsorption coefficient (K_{oc}) and is defined as the ratio between the concentration of the drug adsorbed onto the sludge and the concentration in the aqueous phase at equilibrium (measured as organic carbon). When the K_{oc} is high (e.g. 15 000 L/kg) then this is an indication that the active ingredient is retained by sewage sludge. As this sludge is often used as a fertiliser on agricultural land it is then necessary to test the active ingredient for its possible toxicity to terrestrial organisms in tier B.

For the determination of the $PNEC_{water}$ of the active ingredient standard long-term toxicity tests are performed on fish, daphnia and algae. Preference is given to long-term tests since in the case of human medicines a continuous exposure of environmental organisms to the active ingredient is assumed.

The PNEC is derived from the no-observed-effect concentrations (NOEC) obtained from each of the aquatic organisms tested. The NOEC from the most sensitive and relevant species is selected and divided by an assessment factor (AF). In most instances, an AF of 10 is used and covers interspecies variability, intraspecies variability and laboratory to field extrapolation. Next to the $PNEC_{water}$ the $PNEC_{microorganism}$ and the $PNEC_{groundwater}$ are also calculated. The $PNEC_{microorganism}$ is based on an anti-microbial effect study and the $PNEC_{groundwater}$ is estimated to be 0.25 times the $PNEC_{water}$. The latter is considered for active ingredients that have a low affinity for adsorption onto soil particles and that are not ready biodegradable. An overview of the phase II tier A process for surface water is given in Figure 6.13.

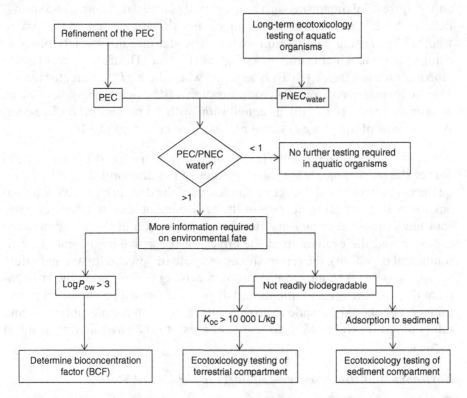

Figure 6.13 ERA phase II, tier A for surface water (Source: adapted from EMA/CHMP, 2006 Guideline [29]).

When the ratio PEC/PNEC for the active ingredient is less than 1 no further testing of the aquatic environment is required and the drug is considered unlikely to present a risk to the environment. When the ratio is equal to or greater than 1 then further testing is required in tier B. This is also the case when the log of the partition coefficient octanol/water ($logP_{ow}$) is greater than 3, and/or the K_{oc} is greater than 10 000 L/kg and/or the active ingredient is not ready biodegradable. The additional testing that is required to address this outcome is performed in tier B.

ERA phase II, Tier B In this part of the environmental risk assessment the PEC is further refined using the environmental fate data that have been produced during tier A (e.g. adsorption to sewage sludge, ready biodegradability). These data together with more refined information on demographics, production of waste water per inhabitant and the capacity of waste water treatment plants of the relevant geographic area are introduced into sewage treatment plant (STP) models such as the SimpleTreat model of the EU.

Depending on the data obtained in tier A, ecotoxicology testing can be performed on sediment dwelling organisms (if there is partitioning to sediment), specific micro-organisms (if a risk for micro-organisms is identified) and on terrestrial organisms such as terrestrial plants, earthworms and springtails (if there is adsorption onto sludge). For the assessment of the risk to wildlife the existing database on mammalian pharmacology, safety pharmacology, pharmacokinetics and toxicology can be used. The measurement of the bioconcentration factor (BCF) is required when the $logP_{ow}$ is greater than 3. The BCF is derived from the concentration of the active ingredient in an aquatic organism (e.g. fish) in equilibrium with its concentration in water. An overview of the phase II tier B process is given in Figure 6.14.

Environmental risk reporting The environmental risk report is an integral part of the marketing authorisation dossier of the drug and should be based on the characteristics of the active ingredient of the drug product, its potential environmental exposure, its fate in the environment and its effects on relevant environmental organisms. Beside the estimation of the environmental exposure and the evaluation of the effects of the active ingredient on environmental organisms, the report should propose the precautionary and safety measures to be taken into consideration regarding the release in the environment through the use by patients and disposal of unused products. Proposals for labelling should be made to provide information on the precautionary and safety measures to be taken to reduce the risk to the environment as much as possible.

Environmental risk assessment of drugs in the United States

Tiered approach to fate and effects testing For drug applications that don't qualify for categorical exclusions a tiered process that is based on the same

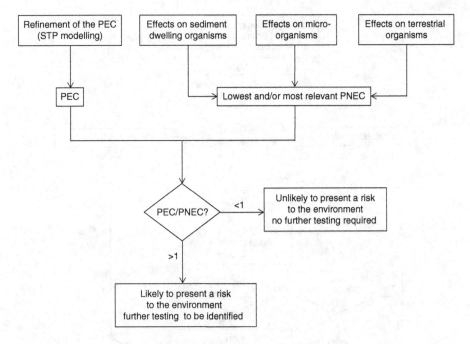

Figure 6.14   ERA phase II, tier B (Source: adapted from EMA/CHMP, 2006 Guideline [29]).

principles as the European process has to be followed in the United States. First, the environmental compartments of potential concern are identified (atmospheric, aquatic, terrestrial), then the depletion of the active ingredient in the environment is investigated. Depletion or dissipation mechanisms in the environment can be chemical such as hydrolysis and photolysis or biological such as microbial biodegradation. When the dissipation of the drug in the environment is slow and/or incomplete, a tiered system for effects assessment is initiated. The first step is the microbial inhibition test. This step is performed independent of the rate of dissipation of the drug in the environment and provides an indication whether the drug is capable of interfering with the normal functioning of the sludge in waste water treatment plants. If the compound has the tendency to accumulate in the environment based on the $\log P_{ow}$ or $\log K_{ow}$, immediately, chronic toxicity tests are carried out on aquatic and terrestrial organisms (Tier 3). When the compound shows less tendency to accumulate in the environment, Tier 1 acute toxicity testing is initiated. Depending on the ratio of the effect concentration (EC_{50}) or the lethal concentration (LC_{50}) over the maximum expected environmental concentration (MEEC), the evaluation process is either stopped or continued with Tier 2 or Tier 3 testing [30]. An overview of this evaluation process is given in Figure 6.15.

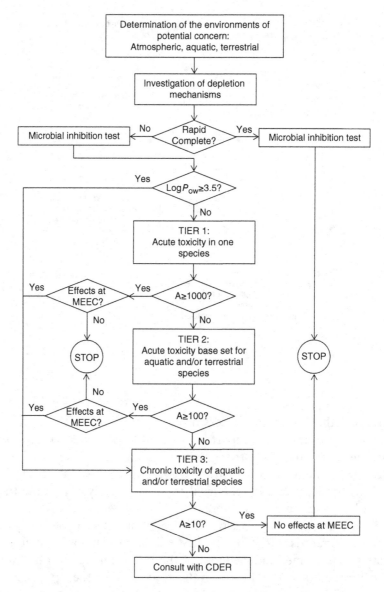

Figure 6.15   Tiered approach to fate and effects testing. A: EC_{50} or LC_{50} /MEEC; MEEC: maximum expected environmental concentration (Source: adapted from DHHS-FDA-CDER-CBER, 1998 Guidance [30]).

Environmental assessment reporting In general, the EA should include the intended use and the location of use and the disposal sites of the drug, the characterisation of the active ingredient, a short description of the environmental issues and the mitigation measures. If potential environmental effects have been identified for the proposed application, alternatives should be proposed to reduce the risk for the environment. For environmental issues that are not specifically addressed in the guidance, the applicants are encouraged to enter into dialogue with the experts of CDER before preparing the EA.

6.2.3 Clinical development

According to the traditional chronological approach, the pre-approval part of late clinical drug development is subdivided in:

- phase 2b: medium-sized, well-designed clinical trials in patients with the targeted indication, with the objective to find the optimal dose to use in the next phase on a larger scale;
- phase 3: large-scale studies in patients to provide an adequate basis for assessing the drug's benefit/risk ratio to support marketing authorisation.

These studies are considered 'pivotal' for marketing authorisation and should be prepared and conducted with the greatest methodological and organisational care. Because of their considerable strategic importance, both these phases are generally separated by a stage gate meeting, also known as the end-of-phase 2 meeting, where again all the available data are analysed and discussed (often also with regulators) in order to check whether the late development programme of the new drug is still on the right track or needs adjustment.

According to the ICH E8 guideline [35], most of the studies performed in the pre-authorisation phase are known as 'therapeutic confirmatory', with several objectives such as to establish the dose–response relationship, to demonstrate/confirm the drug's efficacy, and to establish its safety profile. Additionally, a number of 'human pharmacology' trials are conducted during this phase (e.g. drug–drug interaction studies, specific safety studies, drug metabolite studies), as well as the first 'therapeutic use' trials (including outcome variables such as Quality of Life and cost effectiveness), in order to get a better idea about the optimal use of the drug in future clinical practice.

6.2.3.1 Phase 2b trials

The primary objective of phase 2b trials is to study the dose–response curve of the drug in development in more detail, allowing selection, with confidence, of the optimal dose for introduction in the large-scale phase 3 trial(s).

In order to permit firm statistical and clinical conclusions to be drawn, a typical phase 2b study that is pivotal for dose finding should respect a number of sound methodological principles, such as:

- The usual design is a randomised placebo-controlled parallel group trial, whenever possible also including an active comparator. The placebo group permits to determine the drug's absolute efficacy and safety at different doses, whereas the active comparator drug arm provides information on relative efficacy and safety and increases the assay sensitivity of the trial. An example is shown in Figure 6.16 (period P2).

–   The target population to be included (with still fairly strict inclusion and exclusion criteria), the number of doses and the selected doses to be tested, the frequency of drug administration, the duration of the trial, as well as the study endpoints to be evaluated, are all carefully selected in agreement with the results of earlier phase 1 and 2a trials, using as much as possible quantitative (pharmacometric) methods to substantiate the decisions.

–   The study should include a sufficient number of patients (generally several hundreds), properly calculated by a statistician based on the variability of the primary endpoint and the treatment effect size considered clinically meaningful. However, the number of patients in the placebo arm should be kept to a minimum (with uneven randomisation), especially when an active comparator can be used.

The parallel group period can be preceded by a placebo run-in period, with the objective to eliminate non-stable patients or placebo responders, thus increasing the trial's ability to demonstrate the true drug effects. For example, in a trial where maximum exercise capacity is chosen as primary endpoint (1° EP), an exercise tolerance test (ETT) can be repeated twice during the placebo run-in period, so that patients showing a too big change in the 1° EP between the 2 readings (pre-defined in the protocol) can be excluded from randomisation in the parallel group part of the study (Figure 6.16, P1.).

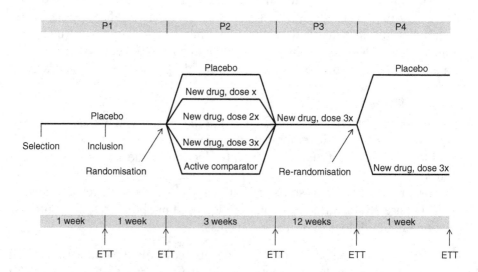

Figure 6.16   Example of a phase 2b study design, P: period; ETT: exercise tolerance test.

A classical phase 2b trial as described before is often extended to include additional objectives. For example, all patients can be switched to the highest tolerated dose of the drug in development and followed-up for longer-term safety assessment (Figure 6.16, P3), or they can be re-randomised in 2 groups (placebo and one selected dose) to study potential drug withdrawal symptoms (Figure 6.16, P4). In certain therapeutic areas, such as the development of anti-cancer and anti-HIV drugs, the use of a seamless phase 2b/3 adaptive design is popular, allowing all patients who finish the phase 2b part to move smoothly into the phase 3 part, thus gaining considerable development time and efficiency.

Dose-finding phase 2b trials need to be well prepared in advance and can be discussed with regulatory agencies in an end-of-phase 2a meeting. Currently, quantitative drug development or pharmacometric methods (e.g. PK–PD modelling, quantification of disease variability, clinical trial modelling) are used to improve dose selection and trial design in order to increase the likelihood of a successful study.

Although several hundred patients need to be included in these trials, because of the many methodological constraints, they are mostly performed in a restricted number of countries (e.g. 5 to 7, sometimes limited by the number of languages in which a validated evaluation scale is available) with a minimal number of centres (e.g. recruiting at least 20 patients).

In addition to finding the optimal dose of the drug in development for most patients, other objectives of phase 2b trials include:

- the definition of the target patient population with the best chance of success for a positive response, e.g. with mild, moderate or severe disease, or biomarker-positive versus biomarker-negative patients;
- the determination of the drug's optimal therapeutic regimen for further study, e.g. as a single treatment option or rather combined with other treatment modalities such as other medication, radiotherapy or surgery;
- the exploration of different study endpoints in order to select the ones with the best potential to discriminate the drug's effects from placebo or active comparator in later large-scale phase 3 studies.

Also at this stage, the decision can be taken to switch to an improved formulation for use in phase 3 and for the market. Therefore, one or more bio-equivalence studies may also be part of the phase 2b trial programme.

6.2.3.2 End-of-phase 2 meeting

The end of phase 2 is another important milestone. Once again, all available results from the different development stream studies are put together and carefully analysed within the drug development organisation. If considered sufficiently convincing to proceed further, the phase 3 trials are planned as well as all additional studies needed to support the marketing authorisation application.

If appropriate, scientific advice can be sought with regulatory agencies during a formal meeting (the so-called end-of-phase 2 meeting) where the following items may be discussed:

–   a summary of all the data currently available supporting the decision to proceed to phase 3;
–   the phase 3 development plan, the pivotal study protocols, and planned primary endpoints;
–   plans for additional nonclinical, pharmacokinetic and paediatric studies (or waivers or deferrals);
–   the proposed 'to be marketed' formulation.

At the end of the process, all data, plans and advice are summarised by the project team with arguments for and against further development. The final decision is taken by the corporate top management of the drug development organisation via the usual procedure that has been described before (Chapter 3). This stage gate decision opens or closes the door to the final step of drug development before application for marketing authorisation.

6.2.3.3   Phase 3 trials

In phase 3, the final phase of clinical drug development before marketing authorisation, every activity is focused on gathering clinical data to support the marketing authorisation application and to successfully launch the medicine in the pharmaceutical market. According to their objective, phase 3 trials can be subdivided as follows:

–   large-scale therapeutic benefit studies, seeking to confirm efficacy and safety of the drug in development in larger, simpler and longer trials than before;
–   clinical safety studies, either to study a specific potential safety issue (e.g. QT prolongation), or to assess the overall clinical safety of the new drug (e.g. by meta-analysis of all the available data);
–   other studies, such as drug–drug interaction studies, trials in special patient populations (elderly, children, ethnic groups, patients with renal or hepatic failure), bridging studies, and seamless phase 2/3 trials.

Some of these studies or data are labelled as 'pivotal' when they have been prepared and conducted to demonstrate the efficacy and safety of the drug (and hence its benefit-risk balance) in the intended indication, or otherwise known as 'supportive' when they add (long-term) information to the clinical safety database or support additional marketing claims mentioned in the Summary of Product Characteristics (SmPC) or the Prescribing Information (PI).

Large-scale therapeutic benefit studies

The primary aim of these studies is to confirm the efficacy and the safety of the drug in development in large patient groups with the targeted indication. According to ICH guideline E8 terminology they are labelled 'therapeutic confirmatory' trials and they provide pivotal evidence for marketing authorisation.

As evidence for approval, it is sufficient to demonstrate a positive benefit/risk ratio for the drug (the beneficial effects outweigh the harmful effects) with data from at least one pivotal trial versus placebo, thus demonstrating absolute efficacy and safety. However, in order for the new drug to be successful on the market, it should be better than existing therapy in the intended indication. To prove such a claim, the new drug will also have to be compared to an active comparator, thus demonstrating comparative efficacy and safety.

A three-arm trial including the new drug, placebo and an active comparator is considered the gold standard of phase 3 trials to demonstrate therapeutic benefit of the newcomer, but is not always needed nor feasible for various reasons, so that some strategic choices have to be made before starting these expensive studies.

Strategic choices   Regulatory agencies provide methodological as well as therapeutic area- or indication-specific guidance, and offer product-specific scientific advice (end-of-phase 2 meeting), but it is up to the drug development organisation to decide how they want to position the new drug in the market, taking into account a number of considerations such as:

–   the intended indication: acute or long-term treatment, prevention of future exacerbations or relapse;
–   the targeted patient population: all patients with the disease or a subset;
–   the potential competitive advantage(s): if superiority to existing therapy can be demonstrated, this is certainly the best starting position, but often drug development organisations have to be satisfied with demonstrating non-inferior or equivalent efficacy and advantages related to safety, acceptability or cost-effectiveness;
–   the therapeutic strategy: as monotherapy or combined with existing therapy (as' add-on' or 'on top of'), as first-, second- or third-line therapy.

All these elements, determine the type and the number of therapeutic confirmatory studies in phase 3. Some of these considerations will be discussed further.

Absolute efficacy and safety   Absolute (or true) efficacy and safety of the new drug are demonstrated in a randomised parallel group design trial versus placebo. This is only possible in therapeutic areas where the use of placebo is deemed ethical and feasible. For example, in patients with an episode of depression, placebo should be used with caution, because of the risk of suicidal ideation or suicide. During a short period (e.g. 4–8 weeks) this can be justified when accompanying measures are foreseen such as regular contact with the patients and the possibility to use rescue or escape medication in the case of treatment failure (the use of rescue medication can even be an outcome variable). On the other hand, in post-menopausal women with osteoporosis who have to be treated for several years in phase 3 trials, sufficient well-established therapies are available so that the use of placebo becomes problematic even on top of associated treatments like calcium and vitamin D. In patients with coronary heart disease, new drugs can only demonstrate long-term efficacy and safety versus placebo on top of the current best medical care, which is already a combination of several active drugs.

Previous results will justify whether just one arm with one fixed dose of the test drug is sufficient, or whether 2 fixed dose groups need to be compared to placebo, or whether the dose is best up- and downtitrated to an optimal response.

The (double-blind) randomised treatment period is often preceded by a (single-blind) placebo run-in period to be able to eliminate instable patients and placebo responders prior to randomisation, based on criteria for disease stability and placebo response that are pre-defined in the study protocol. Patients who (after informed consent) have to be screened or selected, but can finally not be included in the trial and randomised, are called screen or selection failures. In some therapeutic areas the screen failure rate can be quite high, so that (a lot) more patients need to be screened or selected in order to include and randomise the amount proposed by the statistician.

During the randomised period, there might first be an evaluation of the short-term efficacy and safety of the new drug, followed by a second evaluation point after longer-term treatment to demonstrate maintenance of efficacy and safety. Attention should be paid to the choice of study endpoints, with a preference in this phase of development for hard clinical endpoints (survival, bone fractures) over surrogate endpoints (biomarker, blood pressure reduction, bone mineral density). In most trials, evaluation is focused on identifying treatment responders, by looking at response rate, response duration, relapse rate, and predictors of response in the different treatment arms. Some trials may pay more attention to the development of resistance (with antibiotics or antivirals).

In large-scale and long-term trials, an independent data monitoring committee (DMC/DSMB) is responsible for intermediate statistical analyses, to be performed either when a certain number of patients have been included or when a certain number of primary events have occurred (in the case of an 'event-driven' trial). According to the results, the committee concludes whether the study should be continued as foreseen or amended or stopped prematurely.

After the randomisation period, the remaining patients are sometimes switched to the new drug and followed for one or several extra years, especially to get a better idea about the drug's long-term safety profile. In study patients where a clear beneficial response is maintained over time, the extension or follow-up period can be prolonged until the drug is available on the market so that they are not deprived of the benefits of a promising new drug.

Relative efficacy and safety The need for an active control in a placebo-controlled trial must be considered on a case-by-case basis. In therapeutic areas like depression, anxiety, cognitive decline, otitis media, where the demonstration of a new drug's efficacy versus placebo is not very consistent when the studies are repeated, the addition of an active comparator arm can be useful. If the comparator does not produce the expected effect (being significantly better than placebo), than the study becomes inconclusive because of lack of assay sensitivity instead of wrongly concluding that the new drug is better (false positive) or no better/worse (false negative) than placebo.

The gold standard of comparative trials is a design with three parallel groups, where the new drug, placebo and active control are directly compared within the same trial. In some therapeutic areas such as depression, where outcome measures are subjective (e.g. the Hamilton depression rating scale), it is not uncommon that comparative trials when repeated do not show consistent results. So even adding an active control arm to the study doesn't necessarily solve the problem. Analysis of a number of FDA or EMA public assessment reports (PARs) of anti-depressants [36] shows that when 5–7 placebo-controlled trials are presented in the marketing authorisation file (some with active control that can be different between trials), the majority demonstrate a therapeutic benefit for the new drug, but others are negative or inconclusive, making it difficult to reach a final conclusion.

In phase 3, direct 'head-to-head' comparison is also possible between the new drug and the active control, both designs allowing to study relative efficacy (and safety), also known as 'comparative efficacy research' (CER[1]) before marketing authorisation, which regulatory agencies increasingly appreciate [37, 38]. They are also favoured by many drug development organisations because they allow to show convincingly that the new drug is better than or

---

[1] Comparative Efficacy Research (CER) studies the relative efficacy of treatments in the context of clinical trials (including patients with strict inclusion and exclusion criteria), whereas Comparative Effectiveness Research (also abbreviated to CER and more used in the USA) studies the relative effectiveness of treatments in the context of usual clinical practice (including a much wider range of patients with all sorts of problems who were excluded from clinical trials). The effectiveness of a new drug in clinical practice is often lower than its efficacy demonstrated in clinical trials.

at least 'as good as' the comparator. This can be done by demonstrating that the new drug is either:

– superior to the existing one (in a superiority trial, or even in a non-inferiority trial wherein the new drug finally shows superiority);
– non-inferior (in a non-inferiority trial) or equivalent (in a bio- or therapeutic equivalence trial).

When superiority cannot be demonstrated, it is important that the new drug has some other advantage over existing drugs, such as a better safety profile, a better patient acceptability or compliance, or a potentially better cost-effectiveness ratio.

In this context, non-inferiority trials merit special attention. In a non-inferiority trial, the new drug can be somewhat less effective than the comparator, but only within a pre-defined (non-inferiority) margin that is considered as clinically irrelevant (between 5 and 20%, most commonly 10%).

However, if the new drugs turn out to be significantly superior or are really inferior to the comparator, then superiority or inferiority can also be concluded. (Figure 4.19). This type of clinical trial is prone to several methodological pitfalls, such as:

– The choice of the active control, as there might be a tendency not to select the best available therapy to compare with in order to increase the chance of the new drug to be non-inferior.
– The choice of the non-inferiority margin, i.e. the margin within which a lesser efficacy is considered not to be clinically relevant. If it is too wide, than one can erroneously conclude that the new drug is at least as good as the comparator, whereas in reality this may not be the case.
– When the active comparator does not show its expected effects, then any further comparison with the new drug becomes completely meaningless.
– Introduction of progressive bias, by misjudging a true inferior new drug as non-inferior and then accept it as active control in future non-inferiority trials. This phenomenon is known as biocreep and leads to a progressive decline in the quality of best care in the intended indication.

Because of these drawbacks, regulatory agencies have become more conservative and rigorous in evaluating evidence based on non-inferiority trials.

When direct comparison (in the same trial) between new drug and active control is not possible, indirect comparison may be considered. In this case, several similar clinical trials are compared in a network meta-analysis (Section 4.4.5.7). The evidence thus generated provides less confidence than the results obtained with direct comparisons.

Comparative therapeutic benefit studies are not only performed in phase 3 to support the marketing authorisation of the drug in development, but are also important to prepare the successful launch of the new drug on the market. In this context, these studies have additional objectives such as supporting:

- the future price setting, by a judicious choice of the comparator treatments being tested (being better than the standard treatment with a low price is a must, but being better than a more expensive treatment can be more interesting);
- the reimbursement of the drug, by gathering information about the patient's quality of life and health care costs, allowing pharmacoeconomists to calculate cost-effectiveness of the new drug compared to existing treatment;
- marketing claims, by demonstrating some competitive advantage or unique selling property (USP) of the new drug over current standard treatment. This can be anything from a broader indication, over a better response rate in a subset of patients, to the only drug showing a survival benefit.

In order to facilitate the generalisation of clinical trial data to routine clinical practice, some phase 3 trials are designed in a more pragmatic way, including large groups of less selected patients, with a simpler protocol, for longer treatment periods, and with the focus on practical morbi-/mortality outcomes useful in real life.

Because of their pivotal role in supporting not only marketing authorisation but also future marketing claims worldwide, all therapeutic benefit studies in phase 3 need to be well prepared by the clinical development team in agreement with corporate regulatory affairs and marketing teams, taking into account regional differences in regulatory and marketing strategies. Results obtained in one region of the world may be difficult to extrapolate to other regions, because of regional differences in 'intrinsic' factors (such as different genetic polymorphisms in cytochrome P450 drug metabolising enzymes), or 'extrinsic' factors (such as diet and clinical practice). For example, standard therapy can be different, so that several studies need to be conducted with different active comparators.

Clinical safety studies

Demonstration of safety of a new drug during its pre-marketing authorisation phase is considered to be more complex than demonstrating efficacy. The degree of uncertainty is higher as important side effects can be missed for various reasons, such as the relative small size of the clinical safety database (underestimating infrequent side effects) or the absence of long-term safety data. Regulatory agencies can accept a certain degree of residual uncertainty about the new drug's safety when granting marketing authorisation, provided that all reasonable efforts were made to study the drug's safety profile in sufficient detail, and that the applicant commits to continue to invest in safety studies in the post-approval phase of drug development.

As cardiovascular safety risks have become the most common cause of the withdrawal of newly introduced drugs on the market, we will focus on the clinical evaluation of:

- the potential for QT prolongation and hence fatal arrhythmia of non-anti-arrhythmic drugs, and the role of the thorough QT study; and
- the cardiovascular (CV) risks of anti-diabetic drugs, and the role of an integrated meta-analysis of all available data.

Pro-arrhythmic risk assessment of non-anti-arrhythmic drugs   Prolongation of the QT interval of the surface ECG is a currently used predictor of the pro-arrhythmic potential of a drug, especially for a potentially fatal ventricular tachyarrhythmia 'Torsade(s) de Pointes' (TdP). During recent decades, several interesting drugs have been withdrawn from the market because this liability was not recognised before granting marketing authorisation. Therefore, in 2005, regulatory agencies worldwide issued harmonised ICH guidelines for the nonclinical (S7B) [39] and clinical [40] evaluation of the QT prolongation liability of new drugs in development (especially non-anti-arrhythmic drugs). When nonclinical studies identified the potential for QT prolongation, the clinical evaluation of this drug safety aspect should be tackled as early as possible. Already during the multiple ascending dose study in phase 1b, a lot of useful information can be gathered (Section 5.3.3.1). A positive signal during this stage can trigger the need for intensive cardiac monitoring in all the later phases of the drug development, and in particular the conduct of a more rigorous 'thorough QT' (or TQT) study.

A TQT study is generally programmed before phase 3 in healthy volunteers. It tests both a therapeutic and a supratherapeutic dose of the new drug, versus placebo and a positive control (usually a single oral 400 mg dose of moxifloxacin) to establish assay sensitivity. The design can be in parallel groups (approximately 50–60 participants per arm or 200–240 in total) or more widely used in a crossover (only 50–60 subjects who receive all treatments consecutively). Without getting into too much detail the following information may help in interpreting the results of such a trial (Figure 6.17):

- the measured QT interval is corrected for changes in heart rate (QTc), as there is an inverse relationship between heart rate and QT;
- the primary endpoint is the maximum time-matched placebo-corrected change in QTc interval ($\Delta\Delta$QTc);

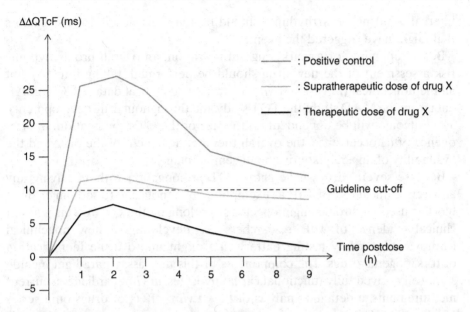

Figure 6.17 Example of a 'borderline' thorough QT study outcome. ΔΔQTcF: maximum time-matched placebo-corrected change in QT interval corrected according to Fridericia (Source: Adapted from Malhotra *et al.* 2007 [41], figure 3, p. 380. Reproduced with permission of Nature Publishing Group).

- a drug is deemed devoid of concern if the upper limits of the one-sided 95% confidence intervals around the mean ΔΔQTc are below 10 ms (milliseconds) at all the time points post-dose, whether therapeutic or supratherapeutic ('negative' TQT study).

If the TQT study demonstrates a significant prolongation of QT for the drug in development, the risk of a pro-torsadogenic potential in the clinic is real, but there are still different possibilities:

- if the results are clear-cut, this means the end of the development of the new drug;
- if the results are 'borderline' (between 5 and 15 ms of prolongation), it is recommended to study more closely the dose- and concentration-effect relationships using PK–PD modelling techniques.

In the latter case, it is of utmost importance to collect additional (ambulatory) ECG data and specific adverse event data from large patient groups in the phase 3 trial programme (and possibly also during the post-authorisation phase of drug development) to demonstrate that the risk, if real, is manageable with significant labelling restrictions once marketing authorisation is granted. Patients who develop marked QT/QTc prolongation (e.g. with QT interval >500 ms) or arrhythmia should be followed closely for risk factors that might have triggered the event.

Before applying for a marketing authorisation, an overall pro-arrhythmic risk assessment of the new drug should be performed, taking into account all the nonclinical (*in vitro* and *in vivo* tests) and clinical data (ECG and AE data from the MAD study, the TQT study and throughout drug development). The outcome will be dependent on the size of the QT prolongation, the frequency of its occurrence, the overall therapeutic benefit of the drug and the availability of an adequate risk management plan.

Because several drugs have shown QT prolongation without having any apparent clinical risk of TdP, as exemplified by ranolazine (a sodium channel blocker used in chronic angina pectoris) prolonging the QT by 8 ms without clinical evidence of TdP, researchers are developing a new nonclinical cardiovascular safety testing battery that might improve the identification of torsadogenic drugs. The components of this new assay paradigm include stem-cell derived fully functional cardiomyocytes, *in vitro* cardiac ion current measurements, a detailed analysis of the *in vitro* effect of drugs on a series of more than five functional ion channels including K, Na and Ca channels and computational models of cardiac cell electric activity. Once validated, it is hoped that costly TQT studies might become redundant and that the current overkill of promising drugs in development without causing fatal arrhythmia might be prevented. The FDA has shown interest in this approach and works closely with a consortium of interested parties to validate these new assays [42].

Cardiovascular risk assessment of anti-diabetic drugs The first oral anti-diabetic agents for the treatment of type 2 diabetes mellitus (sulfonylureas) have long been associated with increased cardiovascular (CV) risks. More recently, rosiglitazone has been linked to negative CV outcomes after the drug was already 10 years on the market [43]. Soon after that, the FDA (2008) and the EMA (2010) issued guidelines [44, 45] for the clinical evaluation of the CV risk of new anti-diabetic drugs. They stressed that the evaluation should be performed throughout the drug development programme and through an integrated meta-analysis. These new guidelines profoundly changed the way new anti-diabetic drugs should be developed. The key elements are as follows:

– diabetic patients with higher risk should be studied (with more advanced disease, elderly patients, and patients with renal impairment);
– a minimum of 2 years clinical CV safety data must be provided;
– relevant major adverse cardiovascular events (MACE), such as overall or cardiovascular mortality, non-fatal myocardial infarction, acute coronary syndromes, cardiac intervention (CABG or PCI), stroke or leg revascularisation, should be used as study endpoints;

  – all CV outcome events in phase 2 and 3 trials should be centrally
    reviewed by an independent adjudication committee of clinical experts,
    thus guaranteeing more confidence in the reality of the diagnosis;
  – and last but not least, the FDA guideline imposes statistical hurdles for
    marketing authorisation.

According to the results of a meta-analysis of all available phase 2 and 3
data, based on the pooled estimated risk ratio (RR) or hazard ratio (HR) and
the upper limit of the two-sided 95% confidence interval (CI) for the occurrence of relevant cardiovascular risk outcomes (stroke, myocardial infarction,
mortality, etc.) with the new drug versus control treatment (active or placebo),
there are several possible scenarios as shown in Figure 6.18:

  – when the upper limit of the 95% CI is below 1.0 (as in scenario A,
    indicating superiority of the new drug), or below 1.3 (as in B, indicating
    non-inferiority), then the new drug is approvable without the need for
    an additional post-marketing study;
  – when the upper limit of the 95% CI is between 1.3 and 1.8 (as in scenario
    C), then the drug is approvable if the overall benefit/risk ratio is positive,
    but an adequately powered post-marketing study should be performed
    in order to gather definite proof of an upper limit below 1.3;

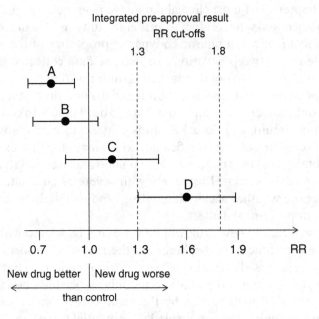

Figure 6.18 FDA hurdles concerning the cardiovascular risk assessment of new anti-diabetic
drugs. RR: Relative Risk or Risk Ratio for important CV events of the new drug versus control;
⊢●⊣: point estimate with lower limit (left) and upper limit (right) of the 95% confidence
interval.

–   when the upper limit of the 95% CI is over 1.8 (as in example D), additional studies are required before marketing authorisation can be granted.

It goes without saying that in order to respect this statistical guidance, many more outcome events need to be targeted than before, so that the number of (high-risk) patients with type 2 diabetes to be included in phase 2/3 trials is much larger than before. In addition, these studies also have to be longer (minimum 2 years), implicating that the costs of the clinical development of anti-diabetic drugs has risen considerably [46]. A first quantitative analysis of the long-term impact of these more stringent pre-approval requirements for new anti-diabetic therapies, focusing heavily on reducing their cardio-vascular risks, suggests that this policy change may not be as beneficial as expected [47].

Other phase 3 studies

In order to better characterise the optimal use of the new drug in clinical practice, many other studies have to be carried out before marketing authorisation application.

When the drug is approved it may be given to patient populations that have not been (extensively) studied up to this stage. Depending on the targeted indication, specific studies may have to be performed in children and elderly (Chapter 7). If most clinical data have been generated in Caucasians, it might be necessary to conduct a 'bridging study' in Asians, verifying that the pharmacokinetic and pharmacodynamic properties of the new drug are comparable in the two populations, so that the data collected in Caucasians can be used in Asians to obtain marketing authorisation.

According to the pharmacokinetic profile of the new drug, studies in patients with renal or hepatic insufficiency may have to be planned. In general, a single- (or sometimes multiple-) dose PK study is done in patients with different degrees of renal or hepatic insufficiency to evaluate to what extent the drug (and its metabolites) may be less well eliminated and accumulated, potentially giving rise to toxic effects. In patients with severe renal insufficiency, it can also be checked whether accumulated drug (and metabolites) can be cleared by haemo- or peritoneal dialysis.

Once approved, the new drug will be far more associated with other medications than in clinical trials. Therefore, the risk of drug–drug interactions will have to be assessed carefully. When there is a theoretical basis for such an interaction, e.g. the new drug and a commonly associated one in the targeted indication are both metabolised by the same cytochrome P450 isoenzyme, and nonclinical studies have confirmed the potential for interaction, a specific clinical drug–drug interaction study may be required to quantify the effect. In general, such trials are done in healthy volunteers ('human pharmacology studies' according to ICH guideline E8 [35] but also still called phase 1 studies), and either programmed in phase 2 (when the associated medication cannot be withheld from study patients) or in phase 3 in order to be able to restrict the labelling information when the interaction turns out to be clinically relevant.

As an alternative to planning specific studies in different subpopulations, population pharmacokinetics can be used. In a more pragmatic approach, higher-risk patients are not systematically excluded from the large-scale clinical trials. Few blood samples drawn from several patients at various time points, allowing linkage of pharmacokinetic data with clinical benefit data in subpopulations of interest, can be very helpful to demonstrate efficacy and safety in subpopulations such as elderly patients. The data thus generated can also be very useful in optimising the drug's prescribing information.

6.2.4 Integration and decision making

At a certain point in time during late development, the question arises whether sufficient data, information and knowledge has been gathered on the new drug allowing marketing authorisation (MA) to be applied for. This is again an important milestone in the life cycle of a new drug that merits careful reflection and preparation. The whole process is initiated and coordinated by the drug development project team and includes the following steps:

- gathering and evaluation of the available evidence;
- overall quality, safety and efficacy assessment;
- benefit-risk assessment;
- final decision making; and
- preparation of the marketing authorisation file(s).

6.2.4.1 Available evidence gathering and evaluation

When the results from the confirmatory clinical trials meet the objectives of the clinical development programme and all chemical/pharmaceutical and nonclinical data are considered sufficient for application for a marketing authorisation, the three development streams compile and summarise all available data. They check with representatives from the regulatory and marketing departments whether the data match all relevant regulatory requirements and are in conformity with the intended marketing strategy. Today, international requirements for drug marketing authorisations are quite harmonised, but regional differences in marketing strategy may need specific data to support specific marketing claims.

During these last phases of the drug development programme the chemical/pharmaceutical development teams will hold pivotal meetings during which the following questions are raised:

- Does the current manufacturing processes lead to an active ingredient and a drug product with high quality and within the specifications?

- Are the manufacturing processes reproducible, i.e. do they lead to a consistently high quality product output, are they valid(ated)?
- Are the analytical methods used to test the quality fully validated?
- Do all stability studies support the proposed shelf life and storage conditions?
- Are all impurities and/or ingredients qualified?

The answers should be satisfactorily to be able to confidently argue that all data support the claim of a high-quality, stable and safe drug. If affirmative, then the chemical and pharmaceutical development team gives the green light for data compilation and dossier preparation.

All nonclinical data on pharmacokinetics, safety pharmacology and toxicology generated during the course of development are critically evaluated and integrated and the results compared with the data from clinical development. The nonclinical safety studies for which there is no clinical investigation possible during drug development such as fertility, embryo–fetal development, pre- and post-natal development and juvenile development are carefully analysed for possible effects in humans. To that end use is made of data on comparative kinetics and metabolism and physiologically based pharmacokinetic modelling. In the event that certain risks cannot be ruled out certain groups in the human population should be excluded from the use of the drug such as women of child-bearing age if birth anomalies cannot be excluded. If the drug has to be used for long periods of time, carcinogenicity studies are carried out in rats and mice. The outcome of such studies is carefully analysed and the relevance to man evaluated. Beside the generation of safety data necessary for drug development, the nonclinical team also has the responsibility of the generation of data for the setting of occupational exposure limits (OELs) for the drug, relevant manufacturing intermediates and excipients. According to the structure of the drug development organisation, the nonclinical team either organises or liaises with environmental sciences to produce and report all the data that are essential for the environmental risk assessment of the active ingredient.

The clinical development team verifies that the available clinical evidence is sufficient to prove with confidence that the new drug is efficacious and safe for use in the intended therapeutic indication(s). Therefore, the pivotal clinical trials have to be positive, i.e. demonstrate superiority versus placebo and at least non-inferiority or better superiority versus comparative active treatment, while the supportive trials have to confirm the long-term safety and efficacy of the drug in a sufficiently large number of patients. The clinical database should demonstrate that the therapeutic benefits outweigh the potential harms, that the drug has some added value over existing treatment in the targeted indication(s), and that additional marketing claims can be substantiated by clinical evidence.

The available clinical evidence should also be sufficient to support essential elements of the Summary of Product Characteristics (SmPC) or Prescribing Information (PI), such as:

- the characteristics of the patient (sub-)population with the best guarantee of a positive clinical benefit-risk balance, allowing the careful description of the targeted therapeutic indication(s), the contra-indications, the special warnings and precautions for optimal use, as well as the special subsection for the paediatric population;
- whether the drug should best be used as monotherapy or in combination with life-style changes, dietary restrictions or other treatments, either as first-, second- or third-line treatment for the targeted disease;
- the standard optimal dose, dose regimen and duration of treatment, as well as dose (regimen) adjustments in special patient populations (e.g. elderly or patients with renal or hepatic function impairment) or in particular circumstances (e.g. risk of interaction with drink or food intake or concomitant treatments);
- advice on preventive measures to avoid potential side effects (e.g. co-administration of an anti-emetic in patients treated with anti-cancer drugs) or on monitoring the optimal use of the drug (e.g. by regular monitoring of the International Normalised Ratio or INR in blood of patients treated with classic anti-coagulants, in order to keep the INR within certain safe limits).

Once considered sufficient for MA application, all clinical evidence is summarised in specific reports that will become part of the submission file.

6.2.4.2   Overall quality, safety and efficacy assessment

As the marketing authorisation for a new drug is granted on the basis of 3 criteria, i.e. the quality, efficacy and safety of the product, it is also essential to analyse all the available data from this perspective.

The overall quality, safety and efficacy assessment of a new drug is not only a matter of gathering and summarising all the available evidence across the different development streams (e.g. for safety), but also to estimate the degree of uncertainty that goes with it. Product *quality* is essentially a matter of the chemical pharmaceutical stream. During the many years needed to develop a new drug sufficient evidence can be gathered to support this MA criterion with a high degree of confidence. Compiling evidence about drug *efficacy* is mainly the responsibility of the clinical team. At the time of MA application, it is accepted (also by regulatory agencies) that not everything is known yet about the drug's efficacy. For example, for an anti-hypertensive drug, MA can be acceptable on the basis of blood pressure lowering as a surrogate for cardio-vascular risk reduction (that can later be demonstrated in the post-MA phase of drug development with a morbi-/mortality trial). Finally, the knowledge about drug *safety* that has been gathered by the nonclinical and clinical development streams by the end of phase 3 has the highest degree of uncertainty of the three criteria for approval. But again, drug developers and regulatory authorities acknowledge that nonclinical safety studies and pre-authorisation clinical trials have only limited value to predict drug safety once the drug is on the market (in clinical trials, the inclusion criteria are too restrictive and too few patients are treated for insufficiently long periods). In order to compensate for this lack of knowledge without retaining an interesting drug from MA, regulatory agencies are somewhat more indulgent to grant MA in these circumstances provided that additional safety studies are performed once the drug is on the market, and that an adequate risk management plan (RMP) is available (Section 6.3.2) and regularly updated post-approval (Section 6.4.4).

6.2.4.3   Benefit-risk assessment

The ultimate criterion upon which to decide whether a new drug is ready for MA application (the development organisation's view) or is ready for MA granting (the regulator's view) is its benefit-risk balance.

Until recently, the way to assess the benefit/risk ratio of a drug was not well structured. The current model is still based on balancing the desired effects versus the adverse effects in a qualitative way, or at best with the help of a semi-quantitative method. The final assessment is done relatively 'intuitively' after discussion in a panel of experts (within the company or within the medicines agency) and ultimately decided by consensus or by voting if needed.

For a number of years, however, several individual initiatives were taken – either by regulatory agencies, academic experts or pharmaceutical company associations – to develop a more scientifically sound benefit-risk analysis methodology, also including more quantitative models. These methods take into account both the available evidence as well as the uncertainty surrounding it, and balance the conflicting beneficial effects versus the harmful ones by trying to weigh the different elements as is done in a multi(ple)-criteria decision analysis (MCDA), hopefully leading to more informed and ultimately better decisions.

Most of these initiatives are now coordinated under the Unified Methodologies for Benefit-Risk Assessment (UMBRA) Initiative by the Centre for Innovation in Regulatory Science (CIRS), allowing the accelerated development of a common framework and a common toolbox for a more structured, unified and internationally accepted benefit-risk assessment methodology for new drugs. This would not only be useful during the regulatory review of a MA application of a new drug, but equally during drug development from the early stages on till the post-approval late stage part of the drug life cycle. The interested reader is referred to the websites of CIRS [48], the EMA [49] and the FDA [50], where background information on structured benefit-risk assessment is available as well as other information on the current initiatives in this context.

6.2.4.4   Final decision making

Within the development project team, all three development streams present their conclusions and discuss them with other team members, mainly regulatory and marketing representatives. The team then evaluates the drug's benefit-risk balance and prepares the necessary summary documents to allow integrated decision making. An essential element of this process is the worldwide MA application strategy: in which country or region the first MA application will be submitted, which procedure will be followed, and when and in which order the other countries will follow.

At some stage during the process, the separate and/or overall conclusions are often discussed with individual external experts. Procedural and regulatory advice can also be sought from regulatory agencies during a pre-submission (EMA) or pre-NDA (FDA) meeting.

When in the end the project team is comfortable with the result of all previous discussions and consultations, it presents its proposal to apply for a MA to the top R&D and corporate management, who will take the final decision.

6.2.4.5   Preparing the MA application file(s)

Once it has been decided to apply for marketing authorisation, the final step is to prepare the MA application file or registration dossier, according to an internationally agreed reporting format (i.e. the ICH Common Technical Document or CTD as discussed in Chapter 3), allowing for worldwide submissions to regulatory agencies with minimal country- or region-specific adjustments.

The preparation of the MA application file is in fact an ongoing process initiated long before its final submission is foreseen. The individual study reports are prepared in real time after the end of each study, while the critical assessment reports integrating all results related to chemical/pharmaceutical development (Quality Overall Summary, QOS), nonclinical development (Nonclinical Overview, NCO), clinical development (Clinical Overview, CO) and overall safety assessment (OSA) are usually written before the start of the overall quality, safety, efficacy and benefit-risk assessment. All these documents are typically drafted and finalised in collaboration between the medical writing department and representatives of the relevant development streams.

As part of the CTD, the proposed Summary of Product Characteristics (SmPC, EMA) or Prescribing Information (PI, USA) is prepared, which is also a collaborative effort of the 3 development streams and the international regulatory and marketing departments.

Finally, as part of the MA application file, the following documents should be submitted as well:

- a risk management plan (RMP, EMA) or risk evaluation and mitigation strategy (REMS, FDA);
- a paediatric investigation plan (PIP) or waiver or deferral for applications to EMA (FDA may request itself paediatric studies either pre- or post-approval).

The final preparation of the submission file may take from 3 to 6 months, and once submitted, MA can at best be granted about 12 months later. This can be shorter for fast-track procedures (drugs satisfying a high medical need, orphan drugs) or longer (if more time is needed to answer questions during clock stops). The project team should be stand-by at critical moments during the review process to answer questions, to prepare oral or written explanations, and to discuss the final versions of the SmPC, the RMP and the PIP.

6.3   Marketing authorisation

Obtaining a first marketing authorization (MA) is a capital milestone in the life cycle of a new drug and determines the switch from the pre-approval to the post-approval phase in late drug development. This section describes the different MA procedures available in Europe and the USA (both 'normal' and 'special' ones), the granting of a MA, as well as the conditions for exceptional use of unauthorised new drugs ('compassionate use' and 'medical need' programmes). It also introduces the concept of 'market access', i.e. the extra steps needed on top of obtaining a MA to get the new drug really available to patients.

6.3.1   Marketing authorisation procedures

6.3.1.1   Marketing authorisation of new drugs in the USA

The registration procedure for a medicine in the United States is initiated with the submission of a registration dossier and follows a discrete set of events described schematically in a flow chart as shown in Figure 6.19. For more details about the process and guidance, the reader is referred to the corresponding page of the website of the FDA [51].

The registration dossier, which is called a New Drug Application (NDA), is submitted to the Center for Drug Evaluation and Research (CDER, Chapter 3). The procedure starts with the validation of the submitted file. It is used to check whether the submission is complete and all the documents required for a critical assessment by FDA expert reviewers are included. If there are reasons for discontinuing the submission and the approval

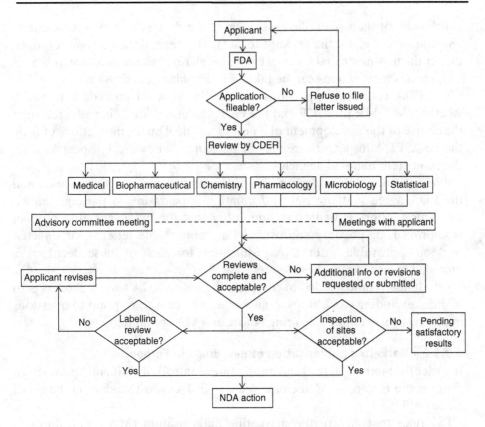

Figure 6.19 The NDA review process.

procedure, a "refuse to file" letter is sent to the sponsor with a request to submit the dossier with a complete set of data within 60 days of the submission.

When the dossier is 'fileable', the various modules are sent to the scientific review experts in the Center for Drug Evaluation and Research. For example, the clinical dossier containing the argumentation for the efficacy and safety of the medicinal product is circulated to the medical/clinical reviewers, who assess the efficacy and safety of the product. In most divisions, these reviewers carry out a full assessment of the safety data (clinical and nonclinical), the data on human pharmacology and animal toxicology, and the clinical data. This evaluation provides the basis of the final evaluation of the application. In addition, the biopharmaceutical, statistical, microbiological and chemical-pharmaceutical evaluations (CMC or Chemistry Manufacturing and Control section) are reviewed in parallel. As part of this evaluation process, meetings can be organised with the sponsor and advisory committees to allow the FDA to take into consideration the opinions of scientific experts outside the FDA. In the course of the evaluation process, the sponsor is able to defend the dossier to the FDA during specially organised meetings. Once the technical reviews are finalised, FDA experts prepare a report that includes the conclusions of their scientific evaluation of the dossier and may recommend amendments (e.g., for the package leaflet). The head of the division responsible for the new medicinal product evaluates all reviews and recommendations and decides what actions can be taken for the submitted dossier.

The FDA conducts inspections during the approval procedure to verify whether the GMP, the GCP and the GLP guidelines are being adhered to in the course of the development of a new medicine. During inspections outside the USA, FDA inspectors are/may be accompanied by local inspectors from the competent national agencies.

When the inspections do not lead to major remarks and the sponsor and the FDA agree that the right information appears in the package leaflet, an "action letter" is written stating either that the medicinal drug product is approved, or possibly approvable (an "approvable letter"), or rejected (a "non-approvable letter"). A justification for each of these decisions is provided together with these letters.

The standard time needed to complete the entire NDA review process is 10 months, excluding clock stops to allow the applicant to respond to questions in writing or to prepare a hearing before an FDA committee.

6.3.1.2 Marketing authorisation of new drugs in Europe

In order to standardise the registration (and control) of medicinal products in Europe, the European Medicines Agency (EMA) was founded on the 1st of January 1995.

The rules that govern the marketing authorisation (MA) procedures in Europe, apply in all member states of the European Economic Area (EEA), i.e. the current 28 member states of the European Union (EU) plus Iceland, Liechtenstein and Norway.

For some medicinal products (see further), the EMA coordinates the evaluation of MA applications via the European centralised procedure. For other products, there is the mutual recognition procedure and the decentralised procedure, wherein the EMA also plays a coordinating role in case of arbitration. In addition, separate national procedures still exist under the autonomy of the individual member states. All four procedures are briefly summarized, but more detailed information can be found on the websites of the EMA [52] and the European Commission [53].

European centralised procedure

All medicines for human use derived from biotechnology and other high-tech processes are to be approved via the centralised procedure coordinated by the EMA. The same applies to:

- advanced-therapy medicinal products (ATMPs);
- human medicines intended for the treatment of HIV/AIDS, cancer, diabetes, neurodegenerative diseases, auto-immune or other immune dysfunctions, and viral diseases;

–   as well as to all designated orphan medicines intended for the treatment of rare diseases.

For medicines that do not fall under any of the above-mentioned categories, companies can submit an application for a centralised marketing authorisation to the Agency, provided the medicine constitutes a significant therapeutic, scientific or technical innovation, or is in any other respect in the interest of patient health.

The European centralised procedure is schematically summarised in Figure 6.20.

Once an application is submitted to the European Medicines Agency, and deemed valid, it is transmitted to the Committee for Human Medicinal Products (CHMP) for a two-step scientific evaluation: the preliminary one within 120 days and the final assessment within another 90 days, leading to a CHMP

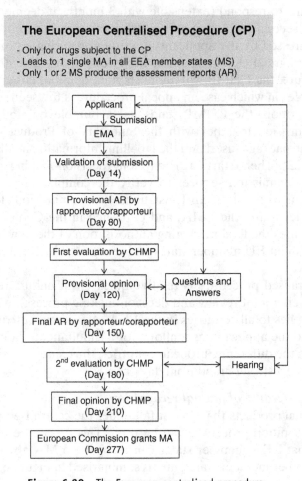

Figure 6.20 The European centralised procedure.

opinion within 210 days (excluding clock stops giving the applicant the opportunity to answer questions from the CHMP).

In order to streamline the evaluation process, a rapporteur and a co-rapporteur, i.e. two national regulatory authorities within the EEA, are designated by the CHMP to perform the scientific evaluation of the submitted dossier and prepare an Assessment Report for the CHMP so that officials of the other member states can comment and participate in the preliminary and final assessments. The rapporteur and co-rapporteur select the members of the assessment team from the list of experts, which is available on the website of the EMA (www.ema.eu.int/). The EMA informs the applicant for a marketing authorisation of the identity of the rapporteur and co-rapporteur. The EMA also sets up a Product Team that is charged with the administrative support of the procedure and the activities of the rapporteur and co-rapporteur.

At the end of the first evaluation period (120 days), the CHMP sends its preliminary conclusions and a list of outstanding issues to the applicant who has 3 months to respond (extensible with 3 months if deemed appropriate). During the second evaluation period (90 days), remaining outstanding issues can be addressed by the applicant in writing or during an oral explanation (again with agreed clock stops). At the latest on day 210 after the start of the procedure, the CHMP will adopt its final opinion, either favourable or unfavourable (in which case an appeal procedure is foreseen).

After adoption, the CHMP sends its favourable opinion to the European Commission together with the Summary of Product Characteristics (SmPC), the package insert and the labelling information in all EU languages (currently 22). Then, starts a 67-day long decision-making process by the European Commission services to verify the compliance of the marketing authorisation with European legislation. The Commission decision is sent to the applicant and the EMA, and published in the Community Register. This constitutes the final marketing authorisation of the new medicine, valid for 5 years in all EU member states and recognised by the 3 other members of the EEA.

The centralised procedure is relative quick (with unique requirements, a single dossier, a joint review and decision-making process), while the resulting MA applies to all countries in the EEA. A positive outcome is certainly beneficial to the applicant, as it allows for a simultaneous launch of the new medicine in the different European countries, thus reducing costs and potentially creating a strong brand from day one.

European procedure of mutual recognition
For medicinal products that do not fall under the centralised procedure, the mutual recognition procedure can be used. This procedure is based on the principle that EEA member states can recognise a MA already granted by any of the other member states, and is summarised in Figure 6.21.

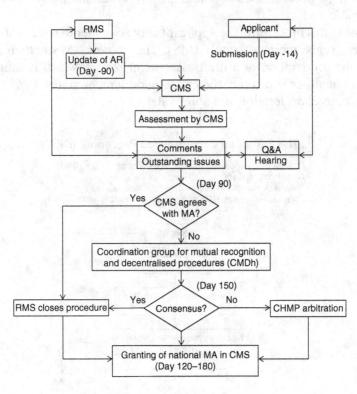

The European Mutual Recognition Procedure (MRP)

- Only for drugs not subject to the centralised procedure (CP)
- MA already obtained in one (reference) member state (RMS)
- Mutual recognition by concerned member states (CMS)

Figure 6.21 The European mutual recognition procedure.

The process is initiated when the holder of a marketing authorisation in one member state (the reference member state, RMS) files an application for a marketing authorisation in the other member states (the concerned member states, CMS). The concerned member states may then recognise the previously granted marketing authorisation in the reference member state and approve the application for a marketing authorisation in their territory.

Once an applicant who already holds a national MA in one country announces its intention to start a mutual recognition procedure, the RMS has 90 days to update its initial assessment report. The concerned member states then have 90 days to recognise the decision of the reference member state and in the case of agreement another 30 days to grant national MAs.

Since the concerned member states receive access to the application in a relatively late phase, they may have (very) different opinions and delay the procedure (see below).

European decentralised procedure

For medicinal products that fall outside the mandatory scope of the EMA via
the centralised procedure, and when no MA has been obtained yet, a drug
development organisation can also submit a marketing authorisation application using a decentralised procedure, which is schematically represented in
Figure 6.22.

Following this procedure, the applicant chooses a member state of the EEA
as the reference member state (RMS). The chosen RMS is then responsible for the preparation of a draft assessment report, which is submitted to
the other member states (i.e. the concerned member states, CMS) for their
simultaneous consideration and approval.

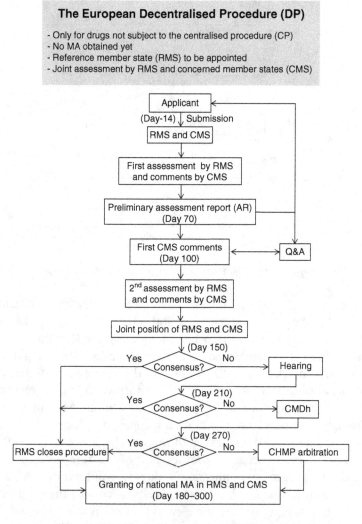

Figure 6.22   The European decentralised procedure.

In contrast to the procedure of mutual recognition, the concerned member states are allowed access to the application for registration of the medicinal product in an early phase, so that it is possible that any potential issues and concerns of the concerned member states can be dealt with quickly and efficiently, within a timeline of 210 days. This procedure is also considered more efficient than multiple national procedures, since a positive outcome will result in simultaneous approvals in several member states that can be chosen by the applicant.

In both the mutual recognition and the decentralised procedure, disagreement may arise between member states to recognise each other's decisions. In case such disagreements are based on grounds of 'potential serious risk to public health', the issues are escalated to the Coordination group for Mutual recognition and Decentralised procedures – human (CMDh) which operates under the umbrella of the Heads of Medicines Agencies (HMA) and has representatives of all EEA member states. The role of the CMDh is to try to find a consensus within 60 days, thus avoiding arbitration by the CHMP. If not, the matter is transferred to the CHMP for final arbitration.

Once agreement is reached the RMS closes the procedure and a MA is granted by all member states concerned within 30 days.

National procedures in Europe

Each member state in the EEA also has its own national procedure to authorise the marketing of a new medicinal product. The MA resulting from a national procedure is only valid in the member state where the registration dossier was submitted and approved. When a national marketing authorisation is granted, it may serve as the basis for the European mutual recognition procedure. If the application is rejected, the medicinal product can still be approved by other countries. However, separate applications are required for each member state, with usually different regulatory requirements and formats.

6.3.1.3 MA procedures in other countries

If a marketing authorisation is sought for in other countries outside the EEA or the USA such as Australia, Canada, Japan and the BRIC countries (Brazil, Russia, India and China), specific regulatory procedures have to be followed that are available on the websites of the respective health authorities.

6.3.1.4 Special MA procedures

Several countries and regions use special procedures to speed up development and authorisation of innovative drugs as compared to the standard process and procedures. They allow faster access of new drugs to patients with serious or rare conditions who are in desperate need of better treatments.

For example, the FDA has developed several approaches to improve access to important new drugs in the USA [54]. They are known as 'Fast Track', 'Accelerated Approval', 'Priority Review', and 'Breakthrough Therapy'. These procedural systems are used to speed up the approval of drugs when needed for particular therapeutic reasons.

Fast track   The FDA Fast Track Development procedure is intended to secure rapid approval of medicines for the treatment of severe life-threatening diseases and is requested by the sponsor. The fast track process is a process whereby:

- (more) frequent meetings are held between the sponsor and the FDA to discuss the development plan and to guarantee that all information that the FDA wishes to see at the time of submission will be available; and
- there is (more) frequent written correspondence on, for example, the design of a clinical trial to be conducted.

If relevant criteria are met, the fast track designation is also eligible for 'accelerated approval' and 'priority review'. Alternatively, a 'rolling review' can be agreed upon between FDA and the drug development organisation, whereby parts of the dossier that are already complete are submitted for review as soon as they become available.

Accelerated approval   This procedure allows new drugs for serious conditions filling an unmet medical need to be approved on the basis of clinical benefit demonstrated on softer surrogate or intermediate endpoints instead of the usual and more meaningful hard clinical endpoints. The FDA decides whether a proposed surrogate or intermediate endpoints is acceptable as substitute for real clinical benefit measures on the basis of the available scientific evidence.

The use of surrogate markers can substantially accelerate the development and approval process of a new drug, for instance when tumour regression can be used instead of overall survival in the assessment of clinical benefit in cancer patients. However, accelerated approval may not preclude that the FDA still requests a commitment from the applicant to demonstrate the drug's clinical benefit on hard clinical endpoints during post-approval clinical trials.

Priority review   Medicinal products for which a fast track status has been granted also receive from the FDA a 'priority review status'. This implies that the agency attempts to evaluate the product within 6 months of submission (instead of the standard 10 months). In fact, the FDA takes priority review into consideration for every NDA, especially when 'significant improvements' in existing therapy for serious conditions are foreseeable with the new drug. Alternatively, the applicant may also expressly request it.

Breakthrough therapy   This approach was recently added for drugs that may offer a substantial improvement over existing therapy in the treatment of serious conditions, on the basis of promising results on 'clinically significant endpoints' during early development. When requested by the drug development organisation, the FDA responds within 60 days. 'Breakthrough Therapy' status offers all the features of the Fast Track process and additional intensive senior advice from the FDA.

In Europe and other countries, similar procedures exist to bring important innovative drugs earlier to the patient. As an example, the CHMP has issued a guideline on Accelerated Assessment reserved for 'medicinal products of major interest from the viewpoint of health and in particular from the viewpoint of therapeutic innovation' [55]. If the request is properly substantiated, the CHMP opinion is given within 150 days (instead of the usual 210).

Another approach foreseen in the European drug legislation is the Conditional Marketing Authorisation [56], available to drugs for seriously debilitating or life-threatening diseases, for drugs used in emergency situations or orphan drugs. It can be requested by the applicant or proposed by the CHMP, and it is granted for 1 year (renewable) under certain conditions:

- the benefit-risk balance is considered positive based on less than comprehensive clinical data, but it is likely that the applicant will be able to provide additional clinical data within a reasonable time period (either from ongoing or new studies);
- the drug fulfills an unmet medical need; and
- the benefits to public health of the immediate availability outweigh the risk inherent in the fact that additional data are still required.

Further thinking along this line generated ideas about 'adaptive or progressive licensing' (also known as 'staggered or stepwise approval'), instead of the current 'all-or-nothing' marketing authorisation. In this approach the MA would not be granted at once for all patients, but would initially be restricted to a smaller number of patients (with an acceptable level of uncertainty about the benefit-risk balance) under the condition of further evidence accumulation in controlled circumstances (to further reduce this uncertainty). As more clinical evidence becomes available, the MA can be extended stepwise. This approach could become a standard for innovative drug approvals in the near future, as it combines timely access for patients with robust scientific evidence.

6.3.2 Granting of marketing authorisation

The granting of a MA for a new drug usually comes with a package of accompanying agreements between the applicant and the regulatory authorities on matters such as:

- the Prescribing Information (PI in USA) or Summary of Product Characteristics (SmPC in Europe), and the Package Insert (PI in USA) or

Patient Information Leaflet (PIL in Europe), to guide the prescriber and the patient in the correct use of the product;

– a Risk Management Plan (RMP in Europe) or a plan with Risk Evaluation and Mitigation Strategies (REMS in the USA), including a structured pharmacovigilance plan, to monitor continuously in real clinical practice the safety profile of the drug; and

– a Paediatric Investigation Plan (PIP in Europe), or similar requirement in the USA under the Pediatric Research Equity Act (PREA), to perform clinical trials in children.

If appropriate, and in the context of the discussion at the end of the previous section, the applicant also has to commit itself to perform additional studies within an agreed timeline in order to generate data that can fill an existing knowledge gap on the drug's efficacy, effectiveness or safety (Section 6.4).

Once the MA of a new drug is granted, it is generally announced in the news section of the concerned medicines agency's website together with the publication of a public assessment report (PAR), the SmPC or PI, the package insert (in as many languages as needed) and a press release. This information is usually quickly picked up by the news media and distributed worldwide, with potential consequences for the stock market value of the concerned MA holder company.

6.3.3   Compassionate use and medical need programmes

6.3.3.1   Compassionate use

In Europe, Article 6 of Directive 2001/83/EC [57] requires that medicinal products are authorised before they are marketed in the Community. Drug products that are not authorised in the European Community are only available to patients when they have entered an approved clinical trial.

However, the EMA allows treatment of patients who suffer from a disease for which no satisfactory authorised alternative therapy exists or who cannot enter a clinical trial, by means of an unauthorised drug product in what is called a 'compassionate use programme'. According to the concerned EMA guideline [58], a 'compassionate use programme is intended to facilitate the availability to patients of new treatment options under development'. In addition to such a compassionate use programme governed through European legislation, national compassionate use programmes make medicinal products available on a named patient basis or to cohorts of patients and are governed by individual Member States legislation.

The European view on compassionate use is strict. Article 83 of Regulation (EC) No 726/2004 [59], the legal framework for the EMA guideline, lists the criteria that should be fulfilled to make an unauthorised drug available through compassionate use:

– the drug product is to be made available to 'patients with a chronically or seriously debilitating disease, or a life-threatening disease, and who cannot be treated satisfactorily by authorised medicinal product' in the European Union;

– the compassionate use programme is intended for a 'group of patients';

– the medicinal product is either 'the subject of an application for a centralised marketing authorisation in accordance with Article 6 of Regulation (EC) No 726/2004 or is undergoing clinical trials' in the European Union or elsewhere.

In the USA, the use of drug products under a compassionate use programme is known as 'Expanded access' [60]. It allows the use of an investigational drug outside of a clinical trial in order to treat a patient with a serious or immediately life-threatening disease or condition who has no comparable or satisfactory alternative treatment options. FDA allows access to investigational drugs on a case-by-case basis either for an individual patient, or for intermediate-size groups of patients with similar treatment needs who otherwise do not qualify to participate in a clinical trial. Large groups of patients who do not have other treatment options available, are also eligible for expanded access only if more is known about the safety and potential effectiveness of a drug from ongoing or completed clinical trials.

Investigational drugs are expensive to manufacture. Some companies provide the drug for free to patients. Other companies charge patients costs associated with the manufacture of the drug. Most insurance companies will not pay for access to an investigational drug. In addition, there may be additional costs associated with administration and monitoring of the investigational drug by healthcare professionals.

6.3.3.2 Medical need

A similar set of rules exists for 'medical need programmes', i.e. the 'controlled off-label use' of a drug that already has a marketing authorisation in (at least) one indication, but is still in development in another indication, and where patients with the new indication are in need of treatment with this drug.

6.3.4 Market access

Obtaining a marketing authorisation is only the first (but legally necessary) step to allow a new medicine to be manufactured, distributed and sold on the market, prescribed by physicians and used by patients. In order for a new medicine to be successful on the pharmaceutical market other steps are mandatory (such as obtaining a fair price) or highly desirable (such as demonstrating extra value for money). Taken together these additional requirements are referred to as 'market access', i.e. the steps that allow a new medicine to be successful on the market. These steps are also known as 'the 4th hurdle', i.e. the demonstration of the 'value' of the new drug, on top of the first three requirements that have been taken into account at marketing authorisation (quality, efficacy and safety).

Successful market access can be achieved if and when the following criteria are met:

- a fair price for the drug is obtained;
- fair reimbursement conditions (based on sound cost-effectiveness studies) can be negotiated with the authorities;
- interesting marketing claims (on the basis of (extra) clinical data) can be substantiated;
- the new medicine has a 'good place' in clinical practice guidelines (again something that has to be earned by excellent clinical results).

Some of these issues can be addressed in studies performed in the post-approval phase of late development as described in Section 6.4. A more detailed description of market access is given in Section 8.2.

6.4   Post-approval development

6.4.1   Chemical and pharmaceutical development

When the drug has been approved by the regulatory authorities, the process of chemical/pharmaceutical development has not come to a halt. As a result of marketing experience, new opportunities arise that allow the development of products with an even better patient compliance profile such as the reduction of the pill burden or the development of dosage forms that are more patient friendly, for example, nasal sprays. The objective of chemical development is to continue the improvement of chemical processes that lead to a high-purity active ingredient as well as the increase of yield and the reduction of production cost. These development efforts take place on the background of full-scale manufacturing of the active ingredient and the drug product. If new synthesis procedures or improved manufacturing processes have become available they can only be implemented if approval for these changes is obtained from the regulatory authorities. These processes are called 'post-approval changes' and are described in specific regulatory guidance documents made available by the FDA and by the EMA, where they are described as post-approval changes and post-marketing variations, respectively. In addition, as a result of the globalisation, manufacturing site switches have become standard operations within major pharmaceutical corporations and these changes are also subjected to post-approval regulatory approval processes.

6.4.2 Nonclinical development

Once marketing authorisation has been received for the drug, the contributions of nonclinical development to post-marketing drug development reduces significantly when carcinogenicity studies have been finalised and the results reported before marketing authorisation. In cases of drugs that respond to an urgent unmet medical need (e.g. HIV, multidrug-resistant tuberculosis) marketing authorisation can be granted conditional on the finalisation of carcinogenicity studies in the post-marketing phase. When there is the intention to start a paediatric development plan and juvenile toxicology studies have already been started in the pre-approval phase of late development, such studies are continued and finalised after marketing authorisation to support the planning of clinical paediatric studies. Apart from the finalisation of the nonclinical studies already started before marketing authorisation, development support may also be required to address the relevance to humans of certain tumour types found in carcinogenicity studies by conducting targeted mechanistic toxicology studies (e.g. rat thyroid tumours, mouse pulmonary tumours, rat male mammary tumours). To understand new and unpredicted safety findings in the clinic, mechanistic toxicology and metabolism studies may be required to aid in defining a strategy to remove the problem (e.g. interaction with hepatocytic transport peptides in case of jaundice). Line extensions such as the introduction of new delivery technology (e.g. sustained release forms, fixed-dose combinations, nanonised formulation forms) or routes of administration (e.g. inhalation, intramuscular depot) require extensive pharmacokinetic evaluation prior to introduction in the clinic. To maintain the drug on the market a continuous follow-up is needed of the literature on the safety aspects of the drug and members of the same drug class and new testing is conducted to address concerns based on new science or outcomes from post-marketing investigator studies or pharmacovigilance surveillance programmes.

6.4.2.1 Pharmacokinetics

Toxicokinetics Toxicokinetic data from juvenile toxicology studies become available as soon as these studies are finalised and analysed for the support of paediatric studies. These data provide important information on the pharmacokinetic behaviour and metabolic pathways of the drug during the various phases of post-natal development. Comparison of the pharmacokinetic profile of the drug in juvenile animals with that of adult animals offers a knowledge-based adaptation of the therapeutic dose as a function of the age range of paediatric patients. Besides the *in vivo* data from juvenile toxicology studies also more mechanistic metabolism studies can be carried out such as the identification of the enzymes involved in the metabolism of the drug at various post-natal time points and in how much the drug influences the activity of these enzymes (e.g. inhibition or induction of cytochrome P450 isoforms). The differences identified between animals of different age range may contribute to the understanding of differences in sensitivity to the drug between juvenile and adult individuals. All these nonclinical data can also be used to estimate changes in pharmacokinetics in children using paediatric pharmacokinetic prediction computer models. When new routes of administration are explored, nonclinical pharma-cokinetic studies are required to assess the availability of the drug to the target site and to avoid toxicity. For the development of a sustained release intramuscular form of the drug, intramuscular pharmacokinetic studies are useful to help in the selection of excipients and formulation techniques to come to an optimal sustained release pattern that produces therapeutic systemic concentrations without causing local intolerance at the injection site. Another aspect of this type of treatment is that evidence should be delivered that the injection site is depleted completely over time without leaving any chemical residue. The development of drug forms for paediatric use such as syrups and small capsule, tablet or granule forms will also have to be evaluated nonclinically for their performance before being used in the clinic.

Drug-drug interactions   As the drug is used increasingly in medical practice, more data become available on the kind of other drugs that are combined with the drug in the intended patient population. When it concerns drugs that have not been investigated yet for drug-drug interactions during pre-approval development and that are known to be either an inhibitor or an inducer of one or more metabolising enzymes of the drug, an *in vitro* drug-drug interaction screen may be required to get an idea about the extent of interaction. In case of significant interaction, targeted clinical drug-drug interaction trials may be necessary to adjust the dose to the proposed combined treatment. Pharmacokinetic support to the development of fixed-dose combinations (e.g. drug combined with an inhibitor of an important metabolising enzyme such as CYP3A4 to increase systemic exposure) helps in finding the right ratio of both drugs to be combined in the right formulation to make sure that both drugs are systemically available at optimal concentrations.

6.4.2.2 Toxicology

Carcinogenicity   For drugs that are intended to be administered for long periods of time (more than 6 months) carcinogenicity studies have to be performed and most of the time the results obtained are reported in the sub-mission for marketing authorisation. Sometimes, marketing authorisation is granted while these studies are still ongoing. The outcome of carcinogenicity studies in rodents is in many cases difficult to interpret in terms of human relevance. In dialogue with the health authorities a research programme can be agreed upon to demonstrate that the tumours of concern are not relevant to man. If the sponsor fails to demonstrate that some of the tumours are not relevant to man they are reported on the label of the drug.

Juvenile toxicology   Juvenile toxicology studies that have been started before marketing authorisation within the framework of a paediatric development programme are continued in the post-marketing phase. The outcome of such a study in combination with the results of the entire reproductive toxicology programme may be sufficient to provide a sound basis for clinical paediatric studies. When effects are found such as retardation of development or sexual maturation, these have to be addressed first before starting studies in children. The findings of a first juvenile toxicology study may also indicate effects (e.g. neurobehavioural effects) that have to be addressed in a second more tailored juvenile toxicology study (e.g. by including more detailed neurohistopathology and more advanced behavioural tests).

Mechanistic toxicology   Mechanistic toxicology is applied when certain safety issues that are identified during nonclinical and clinical testing or medical practice need to be further addressed to enable knowledge-based decisions on how to resolve the problem and proceed with the development and marketing of the drug. Mechanistic toxicology fits in the concept of translational medicine where there is an intensive interaction between clinical practice and laboratory investigations. Mechanistic toxicology uses all available tools in biochemistry, molecular biology, cell biology and physiology to try to understand the underlying molecular mechanisms of toxicity and establish their relevance to man (in case it has been observed in nonclinical models) or their relevance to specific patient populations and their disease status. The increasing experience with novel techniques such as genomics, proteinomics and metabolomics certainly contributes to the effective elucidation of mechanisms of action in nonclinical species as well as in man. When delayed sexual maturation is observed in juvenile development toxicology studies, mechanistic studies are required to investigate possible endocrine disrupting effects of the drug (e.g. estrogenic, anti-estrogenic, androgenic, anti-androgenic). The testing battery for endocrine disruption of sexual hormones is very extensive and varies from *in vitro* (e.g. proliferation of breast cancer (MCF-7) cells, inhibition of aromatase, binding affinity to estrogenic and androgenic receptors, steroid biosynthesis, steroid metabolism and excretion) to a large variety of *in vivo* tests (e.g. uterotrophic assay, Hershberger assay, tailored extended reproductive toxicology tests). In many rodent carcinogenicity studies tumours are detected that are related to treatment. This does not necessarily mean that these tumours will also be produced in man. Many of the tumour types discovered in rodent species (mice and rats) and that are not based on a genotoxic mechanism of action are not relevant to man. To be able to dismiss these tumours for human cancer risk assessment evidence has to be provided for each or them that the generation of such tumours is not possible in man. Without that evidence the tumours are accepted by the regulatory authorities as relevant to man and are reported in the drug label. The differences that may exist between rodent species and man and make tumours species specific are the presence or not of metabolic enzymes that are essential in the pathways leading to the ultimate carcinogenic molecular species (e.g. reactive oxygen species (ROS), iminoquinones). Reactive oxygen species attack the cell membrane causing membrane rupture, ultimate cell death and regenerative cell proliferation leading to neoplasia. Iminoquinones bind to cysteine residues of essential structural proteins of the cell causing collapse of the cell structure and cell death leading to regenerative cell proliferation and neoplasia. Certain orphan nuclear receptors in hepatocytes (e.g. constitutive androstane receptor, CAR) trigger the induction of specific metabolising enzymes and cell proliferation in rodents but only produce enzyme induction in humans without cell proliferation. The cell proliferation step is here a prerequisite to the production of hepatocellular tumours. Apart from the qualitative difference in the capacity to form tumours there may be also quantitative differences between rodents and man. These may be based on differences in receptor populations on cell membranes or differences in the quantity and activity of certain metabolising enzymes in pathways that are present both in rodents and in man. It is much more difficult to have quantitative arguments in favour of the non-relevance of certain tumour types to man be accepted by regulatory authorities. Another example of the application of mechanistic toxicology is the discovery of QT prolongation in the clinic after chronic administration of an antiviral drug. QT prolongation was not identified in a complete battery of cardiovascular safety testing during nonclinical development including the cardiovascular safety assay in the conscious dog, nor was any effect seen in man during phase 1 testing in the clinic. The drug was clearly not interacting with the normal functioning of the potassium channels of the cardiomyocytes and still QT prolongation was observed. When this problem was presented to nonclinical mechanistic safety pharmacology to find out what was actually causing this effect, an explanation could be offered. The mechanism behind the QT prolongation was found to be a disturbance of the transport mechanism that traffics the freshly synthesised potassium channel peptide from the endoplasmatic reticulum to the cell membrane where it is embedded. Since this disturbance was only produced after longer-term treatment it was missed in single-dose and short-term cardiovascular safety experiments. The problem could be resolved by decreasing the dose without loss of therapeutic activity. To do this a tailored thorough QT prolongation study in the clinic was necessary.

6.4.3   Clinical development

Clinical drug development is certainly not finished once the drug gets its marketing authorisation as a medicine or medicinal product. There are many reasons why clinical drug development should continue once the medicine is available on the pharmaceutical market, but they finally end up in 2 main categories:

- to optimise the use of the new medicine in the approved indication in routine clinical practice; and
- to initiate new developments with the new medicine, either for new indications, new pharmaceutical formulations, or (new) combination therapies.

Post-authorisation studies within the approved indication are known as phase 4 studies, essentially 'therapeutic use' trials in the ICH guideline E8 [35] terminology, whereas new developments require a new clinical development plan, either restarting from the beginning (with new phase 1 trials) or at a somewhat later stage (phase 2a or b).

6.4.3.1   Phase 4 studies

Phase 4 clinical trials are defined as post-authorisation studies within the approved indication. Their main objective is to learn more about the optimal use of the new medicine in day-to-day clinical practice.

Commonly conducted phase 4 trials include studies in special populations (e.g. the elderly), on effectiveness (i.e. efficacy in routine clinical practice), on drug safety (pharmacovigilance), on pharmacoeconomics (cost effectiveness), but also studies of morbi-/mortality outcomes, more patient-centred outcomes (e.g. quality of life) and comparative effectiveness (when different treatment modalities are available).

The reasons for these studies as well as the initiators may be quite diverse:

- Some post-marketing studies are required by regulatory authorities as an integral part of the marketing authorisation. The MA for the new medicine is granted 'on condition' that the MA holder (MAH) commits himself to perform one or more post-authorisation studies to alleviate uncertainty. They are therefore also known as 'commitment studies' (in Section 6.2.3.3/Figure 6.18 an example is given for new anti-diabetic drugs). The same holds for safety studies agreed upon within the context of the EU risk management plan (RMP) or the US equivalent on risk evaluation and mitigation strategies (REMS), both on top of routine post-marketing safety surveillance.
- Other studies may be required or recommended to support decisions for health insurance or public health service coverage and/or reimbursement of the new medicine, or its uptake in clinical practice guidelines

or prescription formularies. They mainly include studies in relation to Evidence-Based Medicine (EBM), Comparative Effectiveness Research (CER), and Health Technology Assessment (HTA), i.e. studies that will allow clinicians, payers, and (health care) policy makers to identify the best treatment option with the best value for money, to the benefit of most patients.

– Many post-authorisation studies are initiated by interested investigators ('investigator-initiated trials' or IITs), rather than by the drug development organisation or marketing authorisation holder. This can be with or without the support of the MAH (e.g. manufacturing the drug and matched placebo, or giving financial support). Some of the CER is initiated by (international) investigator groups, such as the European Organisation for the Research and Treatment of Cancer (EORTC), that set up studies comparing or associating different treatment modalities already available on the market. Other CER is done by meta-analysis experts independent of MA holders, such as a Cochrane Collaboration Centre.

– Still other studies are performed by MAHs because they might confer to the new medicine an additional competitive advantage over already existing therapies, thus substantiating new marketing claims that can substantially expand its market share. Typical examples are morbi-/mortality studies, which, if successful although very expensive, may have an important impact on return of investment.

– Finally, the pharmaceutical industry may still initiate phase 4 'seeding' trials as part of the marketing strategy to launch a new product, to make it better known to future prescribers and ultimately to increase its sales. As the scientific value of these studies is mostly very limited, they are ethically not defendable.

6.4.3.2   Effectiveness versus efficacy

Randomised controlled trials are considered to generate the best form of evidence when assessing whether any new health care intervention, including a new drug in development, really works. However, results obtained in RCTs are not always generalisable to daily clinical practice, as the patients included in RCTs do not always reflect the population later treated in real life, and the applied clinical practice as requested in the trial may not entirely reflect real-life practice.

For any intervention, and for drugs in particular, the demonstration whether it is appropriate for routine clinical use implicates a positive answer to the following questions:

– can it work (in principle)?, demonstrated by its 'efficacy', i.e. it does more good than harm under ideal circumstances, as is the case in most pre-MA RCTs (in carefully selected patients, with no serious comorbidities, excluded concomitant medication, and good adherence to the trial protocol and study treatment);

- does it work in practice?, demonstrated by its 'effectiveness', i.e. it does more good than harm under real-life circumstances, as can be done in pragmatic RCTs (large studies in less selected and more diverse patient populations, with more comorbidities and associated medications, with less good adherence to treatment, and focused on more patient-centred outcomes such as quality of life), or in observational trials (e.g. cohort studies) in routine clinical practice;

- is it worth it?, demonstrated by its 'cost effectiveness' or 'value for money', i.e. the value of the health gain produced is worth the cost of it, as can be proved in specific health or pharmacoeconomic studies (looking at the health gains and at the reduction in healthcare costs induced by the benefits of the new treatment, versus the costs induced by deleterious side effects as well as the proper costs of the new treatment).

Phase 4 studies with medicines already on the market can still address aspects of its efficacy, either because the evidence available was only considered sufficient for MA on the condition of one or several additional commitment studies on efficacy, or either because the MAH wants to strengthen or widen the available evidence with post-authorisation studies (for instance, by studying morbi-/mortality outcomes instead of surrogate endpoints, or by trying to extend the licensed indication to a larger patient population). Other studies might focus on a better identification of treatment responders or treatment-resistant patients (predictable by a biomarker), or on the benefits of different dose regimens.

Otherwise, phase 4 trials are focused on demonstrating the drug's (comparative) effectiveness in everyday clinical practice. While some of these trials may be pragmatic RCTs, most of them are non-interventional or observational in nature, mainly cohort studies. In a pragmatic RCT, the selected study population resembles as closely as possible the one treated in clinical practice, patients are randomised in several groups (one receiving the new medicine and the others receiving alternative treatments), the practice as requested by the protocol is as close as possible to real-life practice, and the outcome variables are oriented on patient and caregiver benefits (functional status, quality of life, burden of disease). In a prospective cohort study, patients are treated in clinical practice as usual, some with the new medicine, others with another treatment from the same therapeutic class, or still others with another treatment from a different therapeutic class, are observed in parallel over a longer period of time, and results on effectiveness and safety are compared.

In many cases, new medicines do not perform as well on effectiveness in daily clinical practice as they do on efficacy during pre-MA clinical trials. This is called the efficacy–effectiveness gap. It is most often due to the greater biological heterogeneity of the clinical practice population versus the artificially created homogeneity of clinical study populations. Effectiveness data account a lot more for variability than efficacy data. This gap also skews some of the cost-effectiveness studies, especially when they use Markov models [61] based on efficacy data from clinical trials that do not well reflect routine clinical practice. That is precisely why payers and policy makers in the health care business insist as much as possible to have (comparative) effectiveness data available rather than just (comparative) efficacy data to decide whether a new drug deserves to be reimbursed by the social security system, and if so, under which conditions.

6.4.3.3   Comparative effectiveness research

Healthcare payers and policy makers, as well as clinicians and ultimately patients, are not only interested to know whether a new medicine is effective on its own right, but also want to know how it compares with the effectiveness of other available treatments. This is the subject of comparative effectiveness research (CER, more used in the USA) or relative effectiveness assessment (or REA, a term more used in the EU).

This becomes extremely important within a particular drug class with many (new and 'me too') representatives of first and later generations (e.g. angiotensin converting enzyme inhibitors and angiotensin receptor blockers, both acting on the renin-angiotensin-aldosterone system), but also within a particular therapeutic area with several older and new drug classes as treatment options (e.g. in type 2 diabetes mellitus and rheumatoid arthritis).

The paradigm of evidence-based decision making about treatment options, both at patient and population level, has become increasingly important in health care management. Many countries have introduced CER as the basis for decision making on reimbursement of new medicines, and in that sense it feeds into health technology assessment (HTA). Similarly, clinicians base their clinical practice guidelines on CER, which thus becomes also essential to evidence-based medicine (EBM).

As these various concepts are not always clearly defined, it is interesting to have a closer look at their definitions and the relationship between them. According to Luce *et al.* [62], the preferred definitions are as follows:

–   Comparative effectiveness research (CER) concerns essentially the comparative assessment of the effectiveness of interventions in routine clinical practice, and includes both evidence generation and synthesis. Its outputs are useful for clinical practice guideline development, evidence-based medicine (EBM), and health technology assessment (HTA).
–   Evidence-based medicine (EBM) combines evidence regarding the clinical effectiveness of interventions with patients' preferences in making

clinical decisions about their care. It is essentially a decision-making process, including some evidence synthesis, mainly used to assist individual patients' and/or physicians' decisions, but also useful on a broader scale for developing clinical practice guidelines, prescription formularies and pharmaceutical care.
– Health technology assessment (HTA) is a method of evidence synthesis that considers evidence regarding clinical effectiveness, safety and cost effectiveness. When broadly applied, it includes social, ethical and legal aspects of the use of health technologies (drugs, devices or procedures). Its major use is in informing reimbursement and coverage decisions about treatment options.

The relationships between these key evidence-based activities can be depicted as shown in Figure 6.23.

Several national and international initiatives support and promote these activities during drug development in order to generate data that are relevant downstream to multiple stakeholders such as regulators, HTA organisations, payers and patient groups. In the USA, the Patient-Centered Outcomes Research Institute (PCORI) is 'authorised by Congress to conduct research to provide information about the best available evidence to help patients and their health care providers make more informed decisions' [63]. The institute has a national priorities and research agenda to guide and fund comparative

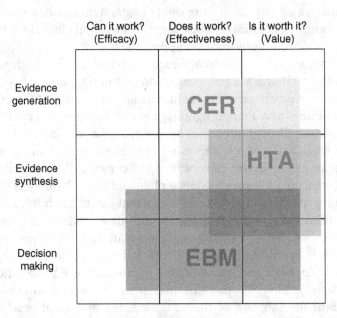

Figure 6.23 Relationship between key evidence-based activities(Source: Adapted from Luce *et al.* 2010 [62], figure 1, p. 260. Reproduced with permission of John Wiley & Sons).

effectiveness research (CER). In the EU, a European network for HTA was created (EUnetHTA), that developed a set of methodological guidelines for relative effectiveness assessment (REA) of pharmaceuticals, including guidance on clinical endpoints, composite endpoints, surrogate endpoints, safety, health-related quality of life, criteria for the choice of the most appropriate comparator(s), direct and indirect comparison, internal validity, and applicability of evidence in the context of REA [64].

6.4.3.4 Pharmacovigilance

The knowledge about the safety of a newly marketed medicine can only be regarded as provisional, because of the known limitations of pre-authorisation clinical trials to study drug safety. Therefore, it is extremely important that continued efforts are made to accumulate further evidence about the medicine's safety during its everyday use in clinical practice. These post-authorisation drug safety activities are an integral part of what is known as pharmacovigilance (PV).

Pharmacovigilance is essentially a risk management activity with the objective to identify, evaluate, investigate and minimise the risks associated with medicines in clinical use. It studies adverse drug reactions (ADR), i.e. unintended effects (side effects) that are noxious, with the intention to prevent them. In the past, the term pharmacovigilance was restricted to post-marketing surveillance (PMS), i.e. routine pharmacovigilance limited to collection of spontaneous ADR reporting, a rather passive activity. Today, it encompasses all aspects of drug safety assessment throughout the drug life cycle, including nonclinical studies, pre-authorisation clinical trials, as well as more proactive post-authorisation approaches.

Post-authorisation pharmacovigilance is part of the risk management plan (RMP in the EU) and the risk evaluation and mitigation strategy (REMS in the USA) agreed between drug regulators and marketing authorisation holders at the time a new marketing authorisation is granted. This RMP/REMS needs updating throughout the drug life cycle, i.e. when the existing MA is renewed, when a new MA is requested or whenever a new safety issue is identified. As an example, the European RMP consists of 3 sections: the safety specifications, the pharmacovigilance plan, and the risk minimisation plan.

The safety specifications describe important safety concerns, i.e. confirmed and potential risks, study limitations and areas with incomplete or missing information. The pharmacovigilance plan addresses how these safety concerns will be further evaluated and followed-up in practice, either by routine PV (passive and active PMS) or additional PV activities (specific safety studies). The risk minimisation plan contains additional measures to safeguard the safe use of the new medicine in clinical practice, such as limitations of use in the SmPC or drug label (e.g. dose reduction in renal insufficiency), educational initiatives for prescribers (e.g. a dear healthcare professional (DHCP) communication or dear doctor letter, or an information leaflet on drug-drug interactions), control of drug prescription (e.g. limited to medical specialists, or conditional to control of a safety variable such as white blood cell (WBC) count before clozapine re-prescription). The successful implementation of these measures has to be evaluated regularly and reinforced or adapted if needed.

Routine pharmacovigilance activities Routine post-authorisation pharmacovigilance is applicable to all new medicines. It mainly allows the detection of unexpected ADRs and is thus essentially hypothesis generating.

The cornerstone of post-marketing surveillance of drug safety is *spontaneous ADR reporting*, i.e. voluntary reporting of suspected unexpected ADRs of new medicines by healthcare professionals (physicians, pharmacists, nurses) or even patients and caregivers nowadays. Individual PV cases or individual case safety reports (ICSR) – identified by a patient code, a suspected ADR, a suspected drug, and a reporter – are collected on a paper or electronic 'yellow card' or FDA Form 3500. These forms are either sent to the MAH (who forwards them to the competent regulatory authorities within legal timelines) or directly to pharmacovigilance centres (set up by regulatory authorities on a national or international level), who store the information into databases (e.g. the EudraVigilance database at EMA, the FDA adverse event reporting system AERS, and the WHO Vigibase).

Spontaneous ADR reporting systems are extremely important in detecting 'signals' of previously unrecognised risks (especially rare, new or serious ADRs), allowing the generation of hypotheses that can later be tested in properly designed PV studies. Their advantages are that they are simple, quick and relatively cheap to run. The disadvantages are that they are far from being perfect, with problems such as false-negatives and false-positives, selective and underreporting (probably only 10% of all ADRs are voluntarily reported), and misinterpretation of the signals (causality is sometimes difficult to establish, especially when the background incidence of the event or 'noise' is high).

The availability of electronic healthcare records (HER) in large electronic databases, currently allows the identification and quantification of drug-specific or drug class-specific ADRs to be speeded up. Whereas spontaneous ADR reporting is a rather passive system to detect drug safety signals, the *data mining of large existing electronic databases* is a new, more proactive and more powerful approach for signal detection. Marketing authorisation holders as well as PV monitoring centres also actively and regularly *search the medical literature* for hitherto unrecognised ADRs of newly introduced medicines.

Additional pharmacovigilance activities   Routine pharmacovigilance may be complemented by additional monitoring activities such as:

- post-authorisation safety studies (PASS), mostly comparative observational pharmaco-epidemiological studies (case-control or cohort studies), which will be dealt with further;
- the use of registries, either disease- (e.g. orphan diseases) or drug-based (e.g. women who become pregnant while using a new drug), to study rare diseases or the effects of rare exposures;
- targeted clinical investigations (e.g. a specific PK–PD study in patients at risk), mechanistic nonclinical studies (e.g. is there a plausible underlying mechanism of action that could explain the unexpected safety issue?), or drug utilisation studies (see further).

Post-authorisation safety studies (PASS) are generally non-interventional or observational studies in real-life conditions using epidemiological methodologies. Whereas routine PV approaches (such as spontaneous ADR reporting) are only hypothesis generating, PASS allow statistical hypothesis testing.

They may be voluntarily initiated by the MAH, or required as mandatory commitment studies at the time of marketing authorisation. In PASS, essentially 2 types of design are frequently used, cohort studies and case-control studies.

In a prospective cohort study, a sample of users of the new drug (typically 10 000 patients), and eventually the same number of patients on a comparator drug, are followed over time to see which ADRs develop. The study population can either be selected by several investigators (in so-called field studies) or drawn from large electronic healthcare databases (e.g. the General Practice Research Database or GPRD in the UK). Cohort studies (Chapter 4) allow absolute as well as relative risks to be measured, but they are generally not sufficiently large to identify very rare ADRs.

Prescription-event monitoring (PEM) is a particular form of cohort study that is both useful to detect unexpected ADRs (hypothesis-generating) and to quantify more common drug safety signals (hypothesis testing). It was introduced in the UK by Bill Inman in the 1980s [65] as a proactive form of PMS during a brief period after the launch of new medicines (usually 1 year). General practitioners who prescribe the new medicine are asked to transfer *all events* recorded in the patient file on a 'Green Form' to the Drug Safety Research Unit (DSRU, an independent academic medical charity), responsible for the analysis of the data and the causality assessment. As the general practitioners do not have to worry whether the observed events are possibly drug related or not, PEM may identify ADRs that were not suspected of being drug induced.

In a case-control study (Chapter 4), a smaller number of patients presenting with the suspected ADR (the cases, usually 100 to 200) are selected and their former suspected drug use is compared with that of a somewhat higher number of similar controls (300 to 600) without the ADR of interest. A case-control study can only measure an odds ratio, an approximation of relative risk, but no absolute risk (as the number of cases has been pre-defined). Nevertheless, it is the only practical way to generate statistical evidence about rare ADRs.

Drug utilisation studies are an essential part of pharmaco-epidemiological studies with particular interest in the extent, nature and determinants of drug exposure. The data can be extracted from large electronic diagnosis-linked healthcare databases, such as the GPRD in the UK or databases of various health maintenance organisations (HMO) in the USA. They can be very informative about the use of (new) medicines in real life, as they allow study of the pattern of use (ideal for international drug consumption comparisons), the quality of use (adherence to prescription guidelines), determinants of use (drug, user, prescriber), as well as outcomes of use (health benefits, ADRs, economic consequences). In the context of pharmacovigilance, they are very useful to calculate rates of ADRs, to monitor the effects of regulatory risk minimisation measures, or to study off-label use (use outside the authorised prescription information in the SmPC or label).

Recent pharmacovigilance initiatives   The EU has from July 2012 updated its pharmacovigilance legislation, partly triggered by the benfluorex (Mediator°) case in France where a number of cardiac valvulopathies and deaths in overweight patients were allegedly associated with the use of the drug (both on- and off-label). The marketing authorisation holder, the French medicines agency, as well as the regional centres of pharmacovigilance were accused of not being sufficiently proactive in getting the drug off the market, while prescribers were held co-responsible for off-label use of the drug. The new EU legislation intends to manage safety risks of (new) medicines in a more proactive and more proportionate way, without increasing administrative burden, and with an explicit commitment to greater transparency and better communication. It is applicable to all medicines used in the EU, whether authorised via the central or national procedures.

The implementation of this new PV legislation is accompanied by a number of other initiatives that merit attention:

– the publication of Good Pharmacovigilance Practices, a set of several modules drawn up to facilitate the practice of pharmacovigilance in the EU;
– the creation of the Pharmacovigilance Risk Assessment Committee (PRAC) within the EMA, among other things responsible for the review and approval of Post-Authorisation Safety Studies (PASS);

–   the creation of a European Network of Centres for Pharmaco-
    epidemiology and Pharmacovigilance (ENCePP), issuing independent
    methodological standards and guidance for the proper planning and
    conduct of pharmaco-epidemiological and pharmacovigilance studies.

6.4.3.5   New developments

The first marketing authorisation of a new medicine is generally not meant to
be the only one conditioning the entire drug life cycle, but it allows first return
on investment and creates more room for further developments also known
as 'line extensions'. There may be many good reasons to continue to invest in
a new medicine that demonstrated a positive benefit-risk balance in its first
marketing authorisation. Drug developers and marketing authorisation holders are constantly looking for new opportunities that could either expand its
market potential (increase market share, open new markets) or extend its life
cycle (extend the patent-protected period, manage the patent cliff and generic
competition). When the new drug looks sufficiently promising, then some of
these new developments are even planned and started during the late development phase for the first MA.

The most common new developments for already available medicines
are briefly discussed below, and some of them are treated in more detail in
Chapter 7.

New indications   The simplest development of a new indication is by
extending the approved indication, e.g. from only severely affected patients
to moderate and mild patients, or from second-line to first-line treatment.
In general, this can be obtained with one well-designed and positive clinical
phase 3 trial. There are many examples of drugs that have been developed
in several indications during their life cycle. Most of them are closely linked
(such as anti-depressant drugs that are also indicated in anxiety disorders,
or some anti-cancer drugs that are indicated in several different cancers),
while others have indications that are far apart (e.g. minoxidil, a vasodilator
used as anti-hypertensive, that turned out to stimulate hair growth and
also became indicated in alopecia androgenica). The clinical development
programme in these new indications may be relatively simple or may require
a completely new development plan starting from a phase 2a proof-of-
concept trial.

In real-life clinical practice, new medicines are not always used within their
intended indication and according to the authorised prescription information
(SmPC or label). This is known as off-label use.

Off-label use can reveal unknown benefits of a new medicine, which can then
be explored in an additional development plan. More often, though, extensive
off-label use can be at the origin of serious safety issues with withdrawal of the
new drug from the market as a consequence.

New forms and formulations   These developments include new forms of the active pharmaceutical ingredient (API), such as a new ester, salt or other non-covalent derivative, with the intention to extend the patent life of the drug. In this case, the new development can be limited to bio-equivalence studies demonstrating that the new form is bio-equivalent to the already authorised one. Other developments in this category simply concern other versions of the finished product, such as a new strength or package size, which only need minimal pharmaceutical development.

A common one is the development of new formulations. The main reasons are to

- optimise drug efficacy and reduce ADRs, either by improving oral absorption, by circumventing a first-pass effect (via inhalation or trans-dermal), or by prolonging the therapeutic effect (sustained, extended or modified release tablets that slow or extend absorption, replacing initial immediate release tablets, allowing once daily administration and thus improving patient compliance);
- enhance patient convenience and compliance, such as the development of a suitable formulation for children, or the search for a non-injectable formulation of insulin (unsuccessful to date);
- to satisfy requirements for another indication, such as the development of minoxidil lotion for the topical treatment of hair loss (whereas for its first approved indication, hypertension, it was available as an oral tablet).

The development of new formulations requires intensive chemical phar-maceutical input and confirmation of therapeutic equivalence with the initially approved formulation by positive bio-equivalence studies in healthy volunteers.

(New) combination therapies   Many single diseases need to be treated by multiple drugs or even multiple treatment strategies (e.g. chemotherapy combined with radiotherapy and/or surgery for cancer treatment). The combi-nation of multiple drugs can be indicated to increase efficacy (e.g. several anti-hypertensive drugs with different mechanisms of action, L-dopa with a decar-boxylase inhibitor, amoxycilline with clavulanate), to decrease adverse events (e.g. anti-cholinergic agents diminish extra-pyramidal symptoms induced by anti-psychotics), or to prevent (multiple) drug resistance (e.g. multidrug chemotherapy in cancer, anti-HIV therapy, or anti-tuberculosis therapy).

In many of these instances, oral fixed-dose combinations (FDC) of mul-tiple drugs are developed, reducing the number of pills to be taken daily (thus enhancing compliance), and often allowing use of lower doses of the individual components. These FDCs are very popular for the treat-ment of hypertension (dual and triple therapy of different drug classes like ACE-inhibitors, beta-blockers, calcium antagonists and diuretics), ischaemic heart disease and stroke (the 'polypill' combining aspirin, a statin and 2 or 3 anti-hypertensives), or infectious diseases (HIV, tuberculosis). The clinical development plan of these drug combinations usually foresees one or two well-designed randomised clinical trials comparing the FDC with each drug given separately, and demonstrating superiority (an indication of possible synergism) or at least non-inferiority (see Chapter 7, Section 7.5).

Besides drug-drug combinations, several other combinations of treatment modalities are possible and merit a separate and specific development plan (sometimes from the start to get the first MA). These are particularly common in cancer treatment and fall into 3 categories:

- concomitant or concurrent systemic therapy, i.e. systemic medical treatment (chemo-, immuno- or hormonal therapy), is given at the same time as radiotherapy for instance;
- adjuvant systemic therapy, given after surgery for many types of cancer;
- neo-adjuvant systemic therapy, given before surgery.

Other examples of combined therapies are drug–device combinations such as drug-eluting coronary stents or dermal iontophoretic drug-delivery systems. Development of such combinations is more complex as it should be performed in agreement with both drug and device regulations.

Tailored/Personalised treatment   Historically, the development of tailored or personalised medicines started when some of these drugs were already on the market and the variability of response in clinical practice became more evident. By using a clinically validated predictive biomarker, a subset of patients can be identified that fare better on the drug. The biomarker can be linked to drug efficacy (e.g. BCR-BCL genotype tyrosine kinase positive patients with chronic myeloid leukaemia respond better to the kinase inhibitor imatinib), drug safety (e.g. the UDP-glucuronosyltransferase variant 1A1 identifies patients prone to serious ADRs when treated with the anti-cancer agent irinotecan), or drug resistance (e.g. the identification of HIV strains with specific mutations that confer resistance to (non-)nucleoside or nucleotide reverse transcriptase inhibitors and protease inhibitors). This 'retrospective' approach has led *a posteriori* to better patient stratification and the first tailored or personalised treatments based on biomarkers. Today, the identification of the subset of patients likely to be better responder is started 'prospectively' during the early development phase of new drugs. The predictive biomarker is then developed in parallel and proposed as 'companion diagnostic' at the time of marketing authorisation of the new medicine. Prescription (and reimbursement) of the drug may be conditional to positive testing of the patient to the companion diagnostic. Possible issues with this approach are for instance the consequences of false-negative results, i.e. the biomarker suggests that the drug will not be effective, whereas in reality it would have been effective. Another problem is that coverage decisions on biomarkers are done by decision makers other than for those on medicines, leading to a potential lack of coordination.

Evergreening In general, marketing authorisation holders will combine several of the above-mentioned development opportunities in order to increase revenues and to extend the post-authorisation phase of the drug life cycle for as long as possible. In particular, the so-called 'patent cliff' (the steep drop of revenue once the patent has expired) and the consequent generic competition should be pro-actively anticipated. In this battle, some pharmaceutical companies have been accused of 'evergreening', i.e. the attempt to use legal ways to extend the market exclusivity period of their drug so as to restrict or prevent generic competitors entering the market. Evergreening is an approach that is disapproved by the regulatory authorities and – in many cases – is indicative of a poor drug development pipeline.

6.4.4 Integration and decision making

In the post-authorisation phase of late drug development, integration and decision making – requiring the input of the 3 development streams – is particularly important at defined time points during the drug life cycle when authorities require updated integrated information on the (new) medicine.

Four of the these merit special attention: periodic benefit-risk evaluation reports (PBRER), risk management plans (RMP), marketing authorisations (MA) and health technology assessments (HTA).

Periodic Benefit-Risk Evaluation Reports (PBRER) Until the end of 2012, at defined time points after marketing authorisation, the MAH had to submit a report on the worldwide safety experience with the new medicine to the competent authorities, the Periodic Safety Update Reports (PSUR). As from January 2013, these reports have been replaced by the Periodic Benefit-Risk Evaluation Reports (PBRER), as detailed in Revision 2 of the ICH E2C guideline [66]. With the evolving insight that the risks of (new) medicines are most meaningful in the light of their clinical benefits, these reports now put more emphasis on the periodic evaluation of the benefit-risk balance of (new) drugs in the post-authorisation phase.

Their periodicity can vary between countries and regions, but is typically every 6 months during the first 2 years after MA, then yearly during the 2 next years, and thereafter every 3 years. The PBRER contains information on worldwide exposure and use of the (new) drug, new and cumulative safety data, an evaluation of the risks, new clinical benefit information, significant findings from clinical studies, and an integrated benefit-risk analysis for each approved indication. It concludes with recommendations for future actions, e.g. significant changes to the investigator brochure, the informed consent form for clinical study participants, the authorised SmPC or label, or the risk minimisation activities.

It is clear that this comprehensive evaluation of safety and benefit data by the MAH, as well as the critical analysis of the medicine's benefit-risk balance, requires intensive collaboration between the different development streams and the regulatory affairs department. After submission, PBRERs are reviewed by regulatory agencies worldwide. The analysis and recommendations by the MAH are either approved or amended for further implementation.

Risk management plans (RMP)   With the first marketing authorisation of a new medicine in Europe comes also an agreement on a risk management plan that has to be updated regularly during the whole drug life cycle.

Regular review of this RMP is essential when new safety signals are picked up, or when results of committed PASS become available, or when it turns out that the effectiveness of the implemented risk mitigation strategies is not as expected. Each time, the clinical development team together with the nonclinical safety team, the regulatory affairs department and marketing people will sit together to critically analyse the new information and to decide on additional measures. A new RMP is prepared as needed, with updated sections on safety specifications, the PV plan and risk mitigation strategies. It is submitted to regulatory agencies, reviewed by them and approved or amended for further implementation.

In the USA, an equivalent risk evaluation and mitigation strategy (REMS), requested by the FDA in the post-approval phase, may require similar periodic integrated risk management assessments.

Marketing authorisations (MA)   The initial marketing authorisation of a new medicine is also regularly updated during the whole drug life cycle. This can be for the 5-yearly renewals, addition of new indications, or the authorisation of new formulations. In the EU, marketing authorisation modifications or 'variations' can be related to administrative changes, quality changes, or safety, efficacy and PV changes. Each of these variations is classified as minor (type IA or IB) or major (type II), and according to the type of variation the conditions to be fulfilled, the documentation to be submitted and the regulatory procedure to follow is different. A similar classification exists for changes to an approved NDA in the USA, where 3 categories exist (minor, intermediate and major changes), each with specific regulatory procedures.

Depending on the nature and importance of the MA variation, different development teams will be involved in preparing the necessary documents.

In most cases, a new overall benefit-risk assessment will have to be done. The international strategy to apply for new marketing authorisations in different countries and world regions is decided together with representatives of worldwide regulatory affairs and marketing.

Health technology assessments (HTA) After the first marketing authorisation and each time a substantial variation has been approved (a new indication, a new formulation), health technology assessments will be performed in order to decide whether the costs of the new medicine will be (partly) covered by the health insurance or public health service system. As this is still a national matter, similar HTAs will be done in different countries by different authorities. In general, a *Core Value Dossier (CVD)* is drafted that can serve as template for customised submissions to various HTA authorities (NICE in the UK, IQWiG in Germany, CADTH in Canada, and the AMCP in the USA). A core value dossier is a summary of the clinical, economic and humanistic (quality of life) value of the new medicine and all the supporting evidence (Chapter 8). Drafting this dossier is a collaborative effort of many contributors, such as clinical epidemiologists (burden of disease), the clinical development team (clinical and humanistic outcome evidence), health economists (cost-effectiveness studies, budget impact analysis and economic modelling), and medical writers.

References

[1] CHMP Guideline Active Substance Master File Procedure, CPMP/QWP/227/02 Rev.2, 31 May 2013.
[2] CHMP Guideline Summary of Requirements for Active Substances in the Quality Part of the Dossier, CHMP/QWP/297/97 Rev.1, 2004.
[3] CHMP Guideline Chemistry of New Active Substances CHMP/QWP/130/96 Rev.1, December 2003.
[4] ICHQ11 *Development and Manufacture of Drug Substances*, May 2012.
[5] ICHQ8 (R2). *Pharmaceutical Development and Annex to Q8*, August 2009.
[6] ICH Q6A *Specifications: Test procedures and acceptance criteria for new drug substances and new drug products: chemical substances*, October 1999.
[7] ICH Q6A-*Specifications: Test procedures and acceptance criteria for new drug substances and new drug products: chemical substances – decision trees*, October 1999.
[8] ICHQ2 (R1). *Validation of analytical Procedures: Text and Methodology* October 1994/November 1996?
[9] ICH Q3A (R2). *Impurities in New Drug Substances*, October 2006.
[10] ICH Q3B (R2). *Impurities in New Drug Products*, June 2006.
[11] EMA-CHMP. *Guideline on the limits of genotoxic impurities.* EMEA/CHMP/QWP/251344/2006. London, 28 June 2006.
[12] ICH Q3C (R3). *Impurities: Guideline for Residual Solvents*, February 2011.
[13] ICH ICH Q1A (R2). *Stability Testing of New Drug Substances and Products*, February 2003.
[14] ICH Q1C *Stability Testing for New Dosage Forms*, November 1996.

[15] ICH Q1D *Bracketing and Matrixing Designs for Stability Testing of New Drug Substances and Products*, February 2002.

[16] ICH Q1B *Stability Testing: Photostability Testing of New Drug Substances and Products*, November 1996.

[17] ICH Q1E *Evaluation for Stability data*, February 2003.

[18] EMA/CHMP/BWP/534898/2008 *Guideline on the requirements for quality documentation concerning biological investigational medicinal products in clinical trials*, 18 February 2010.

[19] ICH M3 (R2). *Guidance on nonclinical safety studies for the conduct of human clinical trials and marketing authorization for pharmaceuticals*. 15 July, 2008.

[20] ICH S1A. *Guideline on the need for carcinogenicity studies of pharmaceuticals*. 29 November, 1995.

[21] ICH S1B. *Testing for carcinogenicity of pharmaceuticals*. 16 July, 1997.

[22] ICH S1C (R2). *Dose selection for carcinogenicity studies of pharmaceuticals*. 11 March, 2008.

[23] Klaassen CD, Hood AM. (2001) Effects of microsomal enzyme inducers on thyroid follicular cell proliferation and thyroid hormone metabolism. *Toxicologic Pathology* **29**(1), 34–40.

[24] Flamm WG, Lehman-McKeeman LD. (1991) The human relevance of the renal tumor inducing potential of d-limonene in the male rat: implications for risk assessment. *Regulatory Toxicology and Pharmacology*, **13**(1), 70–86.

[25] Ross J, Plummer SM, Rode A *et al.* (2010) Human constitutive androstane receptor (CAR) and pregnane X receptor (PXR) support the hypertrophic but not the hyperplastic response to the murine nongenotoxic hepatocarcinogens phenobarbital and chlordane in vivo. *Toxicological Sciences* **116**(2), 452–466.

[26] US FDA-CDER Guidance for Industry: *Non-clinical safety evaluation of pediatric drug products*, February, 2006.

[27] EMEA-CHMP. *Guideline on the need for non-clinical testing in juvenile animals of pharmaceuticals for pediatric indications*, EMEA/CHMP/SWP/169215/2005, London, 24 January, 2008.

[28] Cappon GD, Bailey GP, Buschmann J *et al.* (2009) Juvenile animal toxicity designs to support pediatric drug development. *Birth Defects Research* (Part B) **86**, 463–469.

[29] MEA-CHMP. *Guideline on the environmental risk assessment of medicinal products for human use*. EMEA/CHMP/SWP/4447/00 corr 1, 1st June 2006.

[30] DHHS-FDA-CDER-CBER. *Guidance for industry: Environmental assessment of human drug and biologics applications*, Rev 1, July 1998.

[31] ECHA. *Guidance on information requirements and chemical safety assessment. Chapter R.10: Characterisation of dose (concentration)-response for environment*, May 2008.

[32] *OECD Guidelines for the testing of Chemicals*, OECD publications, Paris, 2006 http://www.oecd.org/env/ehs/testing/oecdguidelinesforthetestingofchemicals.htm (accessed 30 September 2013).

[33] ISO guidelines http://www.iso.org/iso/home.html (accessed 30 September 2013).

[34] *OECD Principles on Good Laboratory Practice (as revised in 1997)*, ENV/MC/CHEM(98)17, OECD, Paris, 1998.

[35] ICH E8 guideline. *General considerations for clinical trials. International conference on harmonization*, 17th July 1997, Geneva.

[36] *CHMP assessment report on antidepressants (EMEA/CHMP/266019/2008)*. London, 30th May 2008.

[37] Sorenson C, Naci H, Cylus J *et al.* (2011) Evidence of comparative efficacy should have a formal role in European drug approvals. *British Medical Journal* **343**, d4849.

[38] EMA. Benefit-risk methodology. http://www.ema.europa.eu/ema/index.jsp?curl=pages/special_topics/document_listing/document_listing_000314.jsp&mid=WC0b01ac0580665b63 (accessed 18 September 2013).

[39] ICH Guideline S7B. (May 2005) The non-clinical evaluation of the potential for delayed ventricular repolarization (QT interval prolongation) by human pharmaceuticals, ICH, Geneva.

[40] ICH Guideline E14. (May 2005) Clinical evaluation of QT/QTc interval prolongation and proarrhythmic potential for non-antiarrhythmic drugs, Supplemented with Q&As (R2, March 2014). ICH, Geneva.

[41] Malhotra BK, Glue P, Sweeney K et al. (2007) Thorough QT study with recommended and supratherapeutic doses of tolterodine. *Clinical Pharmacology & Therapeutics* **81**, 377–385.

[42] Fulmer T. (2013) Rushing to abandon tQT. *BioCentury* **21**(30), 1–4.

[43] Cohen D. (2010) Rosiglitazone: what went wrong? *British Medical Journal* **341**, c4848.

[44] FDA Guidance for industry. (December 2008) Diabetes mellitus – Evaluating cardiovascular risk in new antidiabetic therapies to treat Type 2 diabetes, FDA, Silver Spring.

[45] EMA Guideline. (May 2012) Guideline on clinical investigation of medicinal products in the treatment or prevention of diabetes mellitus (CPMP/EWP/1080/00 Rev. 1), EMA, London.

[46] Hirshberg B, Raz I. (2011) Impact of the U.S. Food and Drug Administration cardiovascular assessment requirements on the development of novel antidiabetes drugs. *Diabetes Care* **34** (Supplement 2), S101–S106.

[47] Chawla AJ, Mytelka DS, McBride SD et al. (2014) Estimating the incremental net health benefit of requirements for cardiovascular risk evaluation for diabetes therapies. *Pharmacoepidemiology and drug safety* **DOI**: 10.1002/pds.3559.

[48] The UMBRA Initiative by the Centre for Innovation in Regulatory Science (CIRS): http://cirsci.org/UMBRA (accessed 18 September 2013).

[49] EMA webpage. The benefit-risk methodology project: http://www.ema.europa.eu/ema/index.jsp?curl=pages/special_topics/document_listing/document_listing_000314.jsp&mid=WC0b01ac0580223ed6 (accessed 18 September 2013).

[50] FDA webpage. Structured benefit-risk assessment: http://www.fda.gov/ForIndustry/UserFees/PrescriptionDrugUserFee/ucm326192.htm (accessed 18 September 2013).

[51] FDA webpage. New Drug Application (NDA): http://www.fda.gov/drugs/development approvalprocess/howdrugsaredevelopedandapproved/approvalapplications/newdrugapplicationnda/default.htm (accessed 18 September 2013).

[52] EMA webpage. Central authorisation of (human) medicines: http://www.ema.europa.eu/ema/index.jsp?curl=pages/about_us/general/general_content_000109.jsp&mid=WC0b01ac0580028a47 (accessed 18 September 2013).

[53] European Commission webpage. EU Legislation – Eudralex. The rules governing medicinal product in the European Union: http://ec.europa.eu/health/documents/eudralex/index_en.htm (accessed 18 September 2013).

[54] FDA webpage. Speeding access to important new therapies: http://www.fda.gov/ForConsumers/ByAudience/ForPatientAdvocates/SpeedingAccesstoImportantNew Therapies/ucm128291.htm (accessed 18 September 2013).

[55] EMA Guideline. (July 2006) Guideline on the procedure for accelerated assessment pursuant to Article 14(9) of Regulation (EC) No 726/2004. EMA, London.

[56] EMA Guideline. (December 2005) Guideline on the procedures for the granting of a marketing authorisation under exceptional circumstances, pursuant to Article 14(8) of Regulation (EC) No 726/2004. EMA, London.

[57] Directive 2001/83/EC of the European Parliament and of the Council of 6 November 2001 on the Community code relating to medical products for human use, as amended. *Official Journal of the European Communities* 28.11.2001, L 311/67–128.

[58] EMA Guideline. (July 2007) Guideline on compassionate use of medicinal products, pursuant to Article 83 of Regulation (EC) no 726/2004. EMA, London.

[59] Regulation (EC) No 726/2004 of the European Parliament and of the Council of 31 March 2004 laying down Community procedures for the authorisation and supervision of medicinal products for human and veterinary use and the establishing a European Medicines Agency. *Official Journal of the European Union* 30.4.2004, L 136/1–33.

[60] FDA webpage. Access to investigational drugs outside of a clinical trial (Expanded Access): http://www.fda.gov/ForConsumers/ByAudience/ForPatientAdvocates/AccesstoInvestigationalDrugs/ucm176098.htm (accessed 18 September 2013).

[61] Briggs A, Sculpher M. (1998) An introduction to Markov modelling for economic evaluation. Pharmacoeconomics **13**(4), 397–409.

[62] Luce BR, Drummond M, Jönsson B *et al.* (2010) EBM, HTA and CER: clearing the confusion. *The Milbank Quarterly* **88**(2), 256–276.

[63] Patient-centered Outcomes Research Institute, www.pcori.org (accessed 18 September 2013).

[64] European Network for Health Technology Assessment, www.eunethta.eu (accessed 18 September 2013).

[65] Shakir SAW. (2006) Bill Inman: drug safety physician and pharmaco-epidemiologist. *Drug Safety* **29**(3), 187–188.

[66] ICH Guideline E2C(R2). (November 2012) Periodic Benefit-Risk Evaluation Report (PBRER). ICH, Geneva.

7
Special Drug Developments

7.1 Introduction

Although every new drug development project is in fact unique, the previous chapters describe general principles of drug development that are valid for most of them. However, some projects allow or require special approaches for various reasons, such as specific characteristics of the targeted patient population or the drug (combination) under development. Some of these special drug developments are addressed in this chapter.

One of the most risky drug development projects that are carried out by drug development organisations is the development of orphan drugs. This is due to the fact that the drug development timelines and costs of orphan drugs are not much less than those of blockbuster drugs but with a potential market that is much smaller and in some cases may only constitute a few hundred patients. However, the medical need for these drugs is high and authorities have created an environment in which these drugs can be developed thanks to a range of regulatory incentives, such as extended market exclusivity.

Other projects that merit special attention are the development of new drugs for children (a largely neglected area in the past) and for the elderly (a vulnerable and rapidly growing patient population). Finally, the development of fixed-dose combinations and some other special projects are briefly discussed.

7.2 Development of orphan drugs

Orphan drugs are drugs that treat 'orphan' or 'rare' diseases. The approach to and principles of orphan drug development do not differ from the approach and principles of the development of non-orphan drugs. The requirements of quality, safety and efficacy that apply to non-orphan drugs, also apply

Global New Drug Development: An Introduction, First Edition.
Jan A. Rosier, Mark A. Martens and Josse R. Thomas.
© 2014 John Wiley & Sons, Ltd. Published 2014 by John Wiley & Sons, Ltd.

to orphan drugs. The major difference between the two development approaches is that there is regulatory opportunity for support – either scientific or financial – to allow orphan drugs to be developed and approved. There are still many orphan or rare diseases and conditions for which no effective and safe therapy is available. In February 2012, the Global Genes/ R.A.R.E. Project [1], a patient advocacy organisation that represents the rare-disease community, presented an overview of 7000 known rare diseases and disorders. It is assumed that about 95% of the medical conditions on that list do not have an approved drug treatment. Both in the EU and in the USA, legislation was passed in an attempt to encourage drug R&D organisations to develop drugs for orphan diseases.

In Europe, a drug is identified as an 'orphan drug' if it can be established that the following criteria are met [2]:

- the drug is intended for the diagnosis, prevention or treatment of a life-threatening or chronically debilitating condition affecting not more than 5 in 10 000 persons in the Community when the application is made; or
- the drug is intended for the diagnosis, prevention or treatment of a life-threatening or chronically debilitating condition and that without incentives it is unlikely that the marketing of the medicinal product in the Community would generate sufficient return to justify the necessary investment; and
- there exists no satisfactory method of diagnosis, prevention or treatment of the condition in question that has been authorised in the Community or, if such method exists, that the drug will be of significant benefit to those affected by that condition'.

EMA's Committee for Orphan Medicinal Products (COMP) was established in 2001 with the objective to examine and assess applications from companies or individuals wanting to develop drugs for rare diseases. Drug development organisations can apply for orphan drug designation of a new drug if they can justify that it meets the criteria of an orphan drug, and if they share with the authorities the approach that will be followed to develop the drug. The COMP will assess the application and may grant the proposed drug (treatment) the status of orphan drug or, alternatively, can advise the drug R&D organisation to conduct additional studies to clarify and support their arguments. For example, the COMP may request an additional pharmacokinetic or clinical study to elucidate the behaviour of the molecule in the patients concerned.

The COMP has also issued measures to encourage the development of orphan drugs. These measures are:

- Regulatory advice: The regulatory health authorities offer assistance in the development of protocols for clinical studies. The objective of this assistance is to increase the probability of success of having the drug approved during the marketing authorisation procedure.

- Market exclusivity: Over a period of 10 years orphan drugs benefit from market exclusivity in the EU. During this period, directly competitive products cannot enter the market.
- Fee reduction: Sponsors that develop orphan drugs will receive a reduction of the fee that is normally accompanied by marketing authorisation applications, inspections, variations and protocol assistance. In the case of SMEs (small and medium-sized enterprises) an additional fee reduction is possible.
- EU-funded research: orphan drug development sponsors may be eligible for EU funding such as the European Commission framework programme.

In the United States, the Orphan Drug Act [3] describes the conditions under which orphan drugs may be developed. Rare or orphan diseases are defined as any diseases or conditions which affect less than 200 000 persons, or more than 200 000 but then there is no 'reasonable expectation that the cost of developing and making available a drug for such disease or condition will be recovered from sales of such drug'. The sponsor of a development programme may request the FDA to designate a new drug as an orphan drug. In analogy with the EU-based COMP, the FDA Office of Orphan Products Development (OOPD) advances the evaluation and development of products that demonstrate promise for the diagnosis and/or treatment of rare diseases or conditions. It evaluates scientific and clinical data from sponsors to identify and designate products as promising for rare diseases and to further advance scientific development of such products. The OOPD also provides incentives for sponsors to develop products for rare diseases. Before the programme became effective, fewer than 10 orphan drugs entered the market between 1973 and 1983. Since 1983, when the Orphan Drug Act was passed, more than 400 drugs and biologic products for rare diseases became available [4]. If the FDA believes that the drug has therapeutic potential for a disease or a condition that is rare in the USA, the FDA provides written recommendations for the non clinical and clinical investigations that would be necessary for approval of such a drug for such disease or condition. If the FDA has approved an application for an orphan drug, it may not approve another application for such a drug for such disease or condition until seven years from the date of the approval. The FDA, however, withholds the right to approve another drug within the 7-year period if the supplier of the first orphan drug cannot assure the supply of the orphan drug to meet the demands of the patients suffering from the orphan disease or if the supplier of the first orphan drug has given the authorisation to approve another drug. As is the case in the EU, the FDA may make available grants to defray the costs of qualified clinical testing incurred in connection with the development

Table 7.1 Orphan drug development legislation in the USA and EU.

	USA	EU
Legal framework	Orphan Drug Act 1983	Regulation (CE) N°141/2000 (1999)
Authority involved	FDA OOPD: Office of Orphan Products Development	EMA COMP: Committee for Orphan Medicinal Products
Marketing exclusivity	7 years	10 years
Accelerated marketing authorisation procedure available?	yes	yes (via centralised procedure)

of drugs for rare diseases and conditions. Table 7.1 presents an overview of the orphan drug regulatory environment in the USA and in the EU.

7.3 Paediatric drug development

Most clinical development plans that were conducted during the previous decades only focused on adult volunteers and patients. However, there is an increasing need for children to have their own drug regimens developed and approved [5]. First, the simple dose reduction based on age, bodyweight or body surface does not appropriately address the needs of drug therapy in children. The biotransformation pathways present in children[1] do not necessarily operate at the same level as they do in adults. Especially in very young children there is scientific proof that biotransformation pathways have not reached the level of the maturity observed in adults. Secondly, in some diseases such as AIDS, particularly children have been infected in considerable numbers and there are no or limited appropriate child-specific therapies. Therefore, the clinical development of drugs for children has received an increased interest from the regulatory authorities. There are 4 important considerations that need to be addressed in the development of drugs for children:

- there exists an increasing need for child-specific drug dosage regimens whereby side effects need to be carefully explored;
- standard toxicology tests are performed with adult animals and the concept of juvenile toxicology to predict safety issues in children should be taken into consideration;
- there is a need for appropriate dosage forms for the treatment of children such as formulations that include taste masking technology and allow careful and accurate dosing and dilution, specific dosage systems, absence of toxic excipients (e.g. benzylalcohol that is toxic for preterm newborns); and

---

[1] Pre-term newborn infants; term newborn infants: 0–27 days; infants and toddlers: 1 to 23 months; children: 2–11 years; adolescents: 12–16 or 18 years.

– not the least important, there will be no safety compromise in the case of drug development projects for children.

The development of child-specific drug treatments can be classified into three major therapeutic areas: diseases that are exclusively paediatric, diseases that are serious and life-threatening and for which there is no cure neither for adults nor for children, and other non-life-threatening diseases for which there are no child-specific therapies.

In exclusively paediatric diseases such as some genetic and metabolic disorders, clinical studies should be conducted in the paediatric population except for the initial safety and tolerability studies that are to be conducted in healthy adult volunteers. For diseases that are not exclusively paediatric but are life threatening, the introduction of children in the clinical investigation should take place as early as possible in the drug development plan. In this case a 'Paediatric Investigation Plan' (PIP) has to be submitted to the EMA for approval by the Paediatric Committee (PDCO) [6]. For diseases that are not exclusively paediatric and are not life threatening, there is less urgency required to engage in a clinical trial with children but it should be initiated as early as phase 2 or phase 3 of clinical development or as a post-approval commitment to the authorities.

If no paediatric data are included in the original application, their absence should be justified in the Marketing Authorisation Application. In view of the central theme in the development of paediatric drugs that no safety compromise is to be made, the clinical development of non-paediatric or non-life-threatening diseases should be conducted in such a way that there are no risks for children and all data are first produced in adult patients or healthy volunteers. Essential in the development of new drugs for paediatric purposes is the question of the correct dose and dosage regimen. There are two approaches possible: either an appropriate dose is generated by means of a pharmacokinetic or PK-based dose selection or a paediatric clinical trial is conducted in order to identify an appropriate dosage regimen.

7.3.1 PK-based dose selection

The regulators' argumentation for using a PK-based dose selection for children is based on a number of conditions:

– the indication in the adult population is identical to the indication in the paediatric population;
– the underlying process and progression of the disease is identical in both populations;
– the expected result of the proposed therapy will be identical in both populations.

Only if these conditions are met should it be possible to develop an appropriate paediatric dosage form that leads to a pharmacokinetic profile that is suitable for children. In this case the dosage in the paediatric population will be driven by the potential of the formulation and its performance to generate similar PK profiles as in adults.

7.3.2   Clinical trial-based dose selection

If there is no relationship between the plasma concentrations of the drug and the efficacy, then a PK-based dose selection is not possible and the approach of developing a paediatric dose is based on a dose-response relationship observed in the paediatric population (which may be different from the dose-response relationship for adults). Therefore, paediatric clinical studies have to be conducted that are based on data from human pharmacology studies in adults, juvenile toxicology studies, a therapeutic exploratory study and a therapeutic confirmatory study in the paediatric population. When the drug development team decides to introduce a paediatric clinical trial in the development plan of a new drug, this will have to be communicated to the competent authorities and a paediatric investigation plan (PIP) prepared. The PIP is submitted to the authorities in order to obtain approval of the plan and to allow the study to be initiated and incorporated in the development project plan. PIPs should be submitted early in drug development and where appropriate before the marketing authorisation application.

In the United States, the Paediatric Research Equity Act (PREA) and the 'Best Pharmaceuticals for Children Act' (BPCA) authorises the FDA to require paediatric studies to be conducted and age-specific formulations to be developed and tested in the relevant paediatric group. Both Acts were amended in 2007 and authorise the FDA to require that data showing the safety and efficacy of a new drug would include the paediatric population. As a result, the FDA requires age-specific formulations and dosages to be included in the applications for marketing authorisations (NDA). Since July 2012, the PREA includes a new provision requiring future marketing authorisation holders of new drugs to introduce to FDA a Pediatric Study Plan before the start of phase 3 clinical trials.

The advice for paediatric developments offered by either the EMA paediatric committee or the FDA review division is free. There is a 6-month extension of the market exclusivity period as well in the EU as in the USA for products for which paediatric information is added. In Europe, if paediatric data are added to an application of an orphan drug, a 2-year market exclusivity period is added to the 10 years for orphan drugs. Table 7.2 offers a comparison between the paediatric drug development approaches in the EU and the USA.

7.4   Geriatric drug development

With the growing number of elderly people, the need for the development of drugs for geriatric patients has increased over the last decades [7, 8]. A general rule in clinical development is that the population that will be introduced in

Table 7.2   Paediatric drug development legislation in the EU and USA.

	EU	USA
Legal framework	Covered under regulation EC Nr 1901/2006 as amended, covering all aspects of paediatric drug development	Covered by two separate but complementary Acts: – the 'Pediatric Research Equity Act' that requires the conduct of paediatric studies; and – the 'Best Pharmaceuticals for Children Act' providing for additional marketing exclusivity
Paediatric development plan	A Paediatric Investigation Plan or 'PIP' is recommended for submission as early as possible, and **results** must be submitted at the time of the marketing authorisation application	A Pediatric Study Plan must be submitted with or before submission of the New Drug Application NDA
Authority involved	The PDCO or Paediatric Committee reviews the PIP, as well as the requests for waivers or deferrals, and adopts an opinion.	The Review Division of the FDA in which the drug is reviewed also reviews the Pediatric Study Plan. Waivers for paediatric studies must be approved by the FDA Pediatric Advisory Committee
Market exclusivity for new drugs	Additional marketing exclusivity of 6 months for products for which paediatric information is added to labelling. Two years of additional marketing exclusivity is provided for orphan drugs for paediatric patients (in addition to the 10 years exclusivity for orphan drugs)	Additional marketing exclusivity of 6 months for products for which paediatric studies are completed in accordance with a written Pediatric Study Request issued by the FDA (but only as an extension of another granted exclusivity)
Market exclusivity for off-patent drugs	Market exclusivity is 10 years for off-patent drugs developed for paediatric patients	No exclusivity available for developing paediatric drugs for off-patent medicines

the therapeutic confirmatory trials is representative of the market population. Following this principle every major clinical study should include a relevant subpopulation of geriatric patients. In addition, there is a high probability that elderly patients take multiple medications and the identification of drug-drug interactions for the drug under development becomes mandatory.

In order to develop appropriate dosages and dosage regimens for geriatric patients, two approaches are possible. One approach consists of conducting clinical studies in which geriatric patients constitute a significant number of subjects. For diseases that are not exclusively observed in geriatric populations, it is argued that a minimum of 100 geriatric patients should be enrolled in the clinical trial. When the clinical trial is finalised a database analysis (PK data and response parameters) may lead to differences between older and younger patients and to a change in the proposed dosage (regimen) between younger and older patients. For diseases that are exclusively geriatric such as Alzheimer's disease, the clinical trial enrolls almost exclusively geriatric patients.

When dosages or dosage regimens need to be modified in order to accommodate geriatric patients, three types of studies have to be addressed: formal PK studies conducted in the elderly, studies that focus on drug-drug interactions and PK-screening studies using phase 3 databases. Formal PK studies can be conducted in elderly patients or in healthy elderly volunteers whereby a pilot study can explore age-related differences in PK. If there are indications that such differences exist, there is reason to conduct PK studies designed to explore the age-related differences in PK parameters. Drug-drug interactions are particularly troublesome for elderly patients and hence the interference with digoxin, oral anticoagulants, cytochrome P450 inducers or inhibitors should be considered. Likewise, it is interesting to explore the individual PK profiles of participants during phase 3 clinical trials to study age-related differences in the pharmacokinetic behaviour of drugs. The knowledge acquired from such population kinetic data can provide guidance on how the dose can be adjusted for geriatric patients.

7.5   Development of fixed-dose drug combinations

Fixed-dose drug combinations (FDCs) are combinations of 2 or more drugs, with or without individual marketing authorisation (MA), in one single pharmaceutical form. They should only be developed if an advantage can be expected over the single drugs administered separately, either in therapeutic benefits, patient safety or patient compliance [9, 10].

FDCs are generally acceptable if they are based on valid therapeutic principles such as:

-   the efficacy of the drugs in combination is potentiated or supra-additive, without having cumulative toxicity, thus allowing the combination of lower doses of the individual drugs and still obtaining a better benefit-risk balance;
-   the overall efficacy remains intact while the overall safety profile has been improved, for instance in cases where one drug reduces the adverse effects of the other drug(s);
-   one drug in the combination improves the bioavailability of the other drug, and thus the exposure to that drug;

- the combined drugs have different mechanisms of action to treat the same disease, or different aspects of the same disease;
- the combination results in a simpler administration of therapy and hence a better patient compliance, because (far) less separate dose units need to be taken daily.

They may be indicated as:

- First-line treatment in patients previously receiving neither of the single substances.
- Second-line treatment in patients unsuccessfully treated with the mono-components.
- Substitution in patients adequately controlled with the same free combination of the individual drugs (at the same dose level) administered in separate formulations.

There are many rational fixed-dose drug combinations available, especially in the treatment of arterial hypertension, infectious diseases (e.g. HIV infection/AIDS, hepatitis, tuberculosis, malaria), diabetes, asthma and cancer. Some well-known examples are sulfamethoxazole/trimethoprim and amoxicillin/clavulanic acid as antibiotics, levodopa/carbidopa as anti-Parkinson drugs, ACE-inhibitor/diuretic or sartan/calcium channel blocker combinations as anti-hypertensives, metformin/sulfonylurea or gliptin/statin combinations as hypoglycaemic agents or hypoglycaemic/hypolipidaemic drugs in the treatment of diabetes type 2, and tenofovir/emtricitabine/efavirenz or lopinavir/ritonavir (the second low-dose protease-inhibitor as pharmacokinetic enhancer or booster of the first one) as anti-HIV drugs.

Fixed-dose drug combinations can be rather simple (i.e. a combination of two well-known or new active pharmaceutical ingredients) but can also be complex. For example, two components can be combined whereby one is delivered immediately to the systemic circulation while the other is made available by means of a delayed release or an extended release profile. The chemical and pharmaceutical development of these fixed-dose combinations is rather complex and requires specific drug-delivery expertise.

The regulatory requirements for the development of FDCs are different according to their regulatory status (components with or without MA), their current clinical use (free combination established or not), and their intended use (substitution, second line or first line). According to the most frequent situations, the clinical development plan can be summarised as follows:

- For a substitution indication, demonstration of clinical pharmacokinetic bio-equivalence between the FDC and the free combination of the single drugs (at the same dosage regimen) may suffice.
- If the FDC contains only authorised drugs that have not been used in combination before, then the human bio-equivalence study should be supplemented with a proper phase 2 dose-ranging clinical trial

demonstrating the superiority of the various FDCs studied versus placebo and the single components administered as monotherapy. In this case, one or two confirmatory phase 3 trials may be needed to generate the necessary therapeutic efficacy and clinical safety data, also in accordance with specific disease-related guidelines.

– If one of the constituents of the FDC is a new drug without prior MA, a full development plan is required as for any new drug.

As there are many scenarios conceivable, drug development organisations usually seek scientific advice from regulatory authorities on a case-by-case basis. This allows the adaptation of the development plan in a proactive way and increases the likelihood to be successful in the registration procedure.

7.6   Other special drug developments

Besides the development of orphan drugs, paediatric drugs, geriatric drugs and fixed-dose drug combinations there are other 'special' drug development programmes that can be identified. Examples are the development of anti-cancer drugs, drug-device combinations (e.g. drug-releasing stents), herbal medicinal products, radiopharmaceuticals, diagnostic agents and drug-diagnostic combinations (companion diagnostics). However, the discussion of each of these possible special drug development programmes is beyond the scope of this book.

References

[1] The global genes/RARE (Rare disease, Advocacy, Research, Education) project, http://www.globalgenes.org (accessed 26 September 2013).
[2] Regulation (EC) No. 141/2000 on orphan medicinal products, 16 December 1999.
[3] Orphan Drug Act. Relevant Excerpts (Public Law 97-414, as amended) – Last updated August 2013, http://www.fda.gov (accessed 26 September 2013).
[4] Haffner EM, Whitley J, Moses M. (2002) Two decades of orphan drug development. *Nature Reviews Drug Discovery* **1**, 821–825.
[5] ICH guideline E11. Clinical investigation of medicinal product in the pediatric population, July 2000.
[6] Communication from the EU Commission (2008/C243/01). Guideline on the format and content of applications for agreement or modification of a paediatric development plan and requests for waivers or deferrals and concerning the operation of the compliance check and on criteria for assessing significant studies, 24 September 2008.
[7] Stegemann S, Ecker F, Maio M *et al.* (2010) Geriatric drug therapy: neglecting the inevitable majority. *Ageing Research Reviews* **9**, 384–398.
[8] ICH Guideline E7. Studies in support of special populations: Geriatrics, June 1993.
[9] EMA. Guideline on clinical development of fixed combination of medicinal products, February 2009, under revision.
[10] FDA guidance for industry. Fixed dose combinations, co-packaged drug products, and single entity versions of previously approved antiretrovirals for the treatment of HIV, October 2006.

8
Drug Commercialisation

8.1 Introduction

The ultimate goal of drug discovery and development is to introduce the new drug in the market and generate return on investment. This final part of the drug life cycle is known as the commercialisation phase, the time to generate sales revenue, net income and profit.

This is a crucial part of the drug life cycle, as it hopefully allows the vast amount of money invested over many years in the development of the new medicine to be recovered. This money can be used to compensate for the costs of the many development failures, and to generate profit to invest in new innovative projects. As schematically depicted in Figure 8.1, the annual cash flow during the life cycle of a profitable drug shows some typical features:

- net income (represented by the area under the curve above zero) exceeds net investment (area under the curve below zero), but this does not take into account the cost of failures and the cost of capital for upfront investment;
- relatively modest costs of drug discovery and nonclinical development, compared to the sharp rise in costs associated with clinical development;
- important costs of launching the new medicine on the market, some paid upfront, together with the extra expenses to secure full market access, explain why the break-even point may only be reached several years after launch;
- gradual and steady increase in sales for years after launch, less the costs of manufacturing, marketing, promotion and continued R&D investments. The success of this phase is highly dependent on the intrinsic qualities of the new medicine, the marketing strategy deployed and the continued

Global New Drug Development: An Introduction, First Edition.
Jan A. Rosier, Mark A. Martens and Josse R. Thomas.
© 2014 John Wiley & Sons, Ltd. Published 2014 by John Wiley & Sons, Ltd.

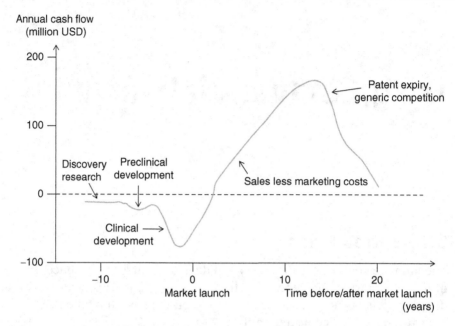

Figure 8.1 Annual cash flow during the drug life cycle. Source: Adapted from Rang 2006 [1], figure 22.4, p. 315. Reproduced with permission of Elsevier.

efforts in new developments (e.g. new indications, new formulations). It is also greatly facilitated by the fact that the drug is fully protected from generic competition during this period of market exclusivity before patent expiry,

–   sharp decline in revenue once the drug is off-patent and exposed to generic competition. This is known as the 'patent cliff' because sales can drop by 75 to 90% within one year.

It is clear that successful commercialisation of a new medicine requires thoughtful and proactive management of these cash flows during the whole drug life cycle. In order to maximise profitability, corporate management will want to:

–   reduce the costs of drug discovery and development;
–   reduce the time to market;
–   maximise sales before patent expiry; and
–   anticipate as much as possible the patent cliff to guarantee net income for as long as possible.

This chapter focuses on the following aspects of drug commercialisation:

–   market access, especially drug pricing and reimbursement, also known as the 4th hurdle;

- pharmaceutical marketing, with information on global marketing strategies and local marketing tactics as practiced by pharmaceutical companies;
- independent drug information, distributed by noncommercial organisations; and
- rational drug use, reviewing a number of measures to promote rational pharmacotherapy.

8.2 Market access

Obtaining a marketing authorisation (approval, licence, registration) for any new medicine is a necessary prerequisite but only a first step in its successful commercialisation. Marketing authorisation is granted on the basis of proof of 3 criteria: drug quality, efficacy and safety (the first 3 hurdles), resulting in therapeutic benefits that outweigh the potential risks. Full market access is only gained after taking a 4th hurdle based on proving the drug's value (for money). This includes demonstration of effectiveness and therapeutic benefit in routine clinical practice, as well as of cost effectiveness for society (payers, insurers), in comparison with alternative treatments. At this stage, costs arise as an additional criterion of choice for prescribing drugs.

Most countries have either a national health service (NHS) or a system of health insurance to cover costs of health care, that is either organised publicly (by a national social security system), or corporately (by companies for their employees), or privately (by private insurers). These healthcare insurers or payers cover or reimburse costs of health care, including prescription medicines, either totally or partly, depending on the local health care or pharmaceutical policy. Whereas the marketing authorisation of drugs is quite harmonised worldwide (partly thanks to ICH) not preventing that EMA and FDA to have divergent views on granting a MA on the basis of the same file and evidence price setting and coverage or reimbursement of drugs are still a national matter. This can lead to important differences in drug price and reimbursement policies between countries.

8.2.1 Drug pricing

The price of a new medicine is set by the marketing authorisation holder, normally a pharmaceutical company. The ex-factory price is determined by the costs of manufacturing and administration, but mainly by R&D and marketing costs. Currently, new drug prices are considered by many as (too) high. Pharmaceutical companies point out that high prices of branded prescription drugs are fuelled by high R&D costs, while critics argue that they are mainly driven by marketing, lobbying and administration costs. The total public price is further determined by the margins of drug wholesalers and retailers (pharmacies), as well as by taxes.

Drug prices, just as consumer goods, may vary from country to country, and this may be true at all levels of the constituents of the public price. As most prescription drugs are (partly) reimbursed by an insurance mechanism, it is not surprising that most countries have installed a national system of price regulation (with the USA as a notable exception). Well-known examples are:

- the Pharmaceutical Price Regulation Scheme (PPRS) in the UK, where the Department of Health, in a voluntary agreement with The Association of the British Pharmaceutical Industry, ensures that the National Health Service (NHS) 'gets access to good quality (branded prescription) medicines at a reasonable price' [2];
- the Patented Medicine Prices Review Board (PMPRB) in Canada, an independent body 'ensuring that the prices of patented medicines sold in Canada are not excessive' [3];
- different systems in use in several European countries, for example, aligning the price to prices in neighbouring countries, ceiling the price for reimbursement, payer-industry price-volume agreements, a premium price for drugs with 'considerable added therapeutic benefit' and a low reference price for drugs with 'no added benefit', payback and other rebate systems.

According to the complexity of the regulations and the resulting negotiations, the price setting for a new drug can take from several weeks to several months.

It is clear that a worldwide operating pharmaceutical company will have to manage carefully its global drug price policy in order to control possible parallel trade, a problem well known in the USA (where prices are higher than in Canada and Mexico) and the EU (mostly from Mediterranean or eastern to western European countries).

Once the branded new medicine loses its patent, generics enter the market with prices that are in the beginning at least one third lower than the original price, but that can drop further to just 25% as more generic competitors join in. This also requires proactive management of the originator company, for example, by anticipated development of its own (branded) generic version. One of the controversial issues in this field is that some companies pay generic drug makers to keep their generic version off the market for a specified number of years, with so-called 'pay for delay' settlements.

8.2.2   Drug reimbursement

As stated before, most countries have a public health service or a (social) health insurance system that covers or reimburses the costs of prescription medicines, either entirely (with no costs for the patient) or partly (with co-payment by the patient). In the USA this is limited to the Medicaid (for the poor) and Medicare (for senior citizens) programmes, but these are supplemented by corporate and private insurance systems.

In order to be eligible for coverage or reimbursement, new medicines have to prove their added value in terms of cost-benefit versus existing ones. This is where Health Technology Assessment (HTA) and pharmacoeconomic evaluation can help.

8.2.2.1 Health technology assessment (HTA)

The International Society for Pharmacoeconomics and Outcomes Research (ISPOR) defines HTA as 'A form of policy research that examines short- and long-term consequences of the application of health care technology. Properties assessed include evidence of safety, efficacy, patient-reported outcomes, real-world effectiveness, cost and cost effectiveness as well as social, legal, ethical and political impacts' [4]. It is a multidisciplinary umbrella term that bridges evidence analysis and decision making in 5 stages [5]: evidence analysis, outcomes analysis, cost analysis, cost-effectiveness analysis, and ethical/legal implications. In the context of drug reimbursement, it examines the medical, economic, social and ethical implications of the incremental value of a drug in health care, and helps insurers and payers decide whether the drug in question warrants coverage or reimbursement, and if yes, under which conditions.

HTA is increasingly being used by public payers and health care insurers across the world to make choices and set priorities on how to spend their money. Several countries have a long tradition of using HTA to inform their policy makers about integrated efficacy, safety and cost effectiveness of drugs (and other medical treatments). Well-known examples include: the Agency for Healthcare Research and Quality (AHRQ) in the USA, the Pharmaceutical Benefits Advisory Committee (PBAC) in Australia, the Canadian Agency for Drugs and Technologies in Health (CADTH), the National Institute for Health and Clinical Excellence (NICE) in the UK, and the Institute for Quality and Efficiency in Health Care (IQWiG) in Germany. Many of them require or recommend a cost-effectiveness analysis whenever they have to decide on coverage or reimbursement of a new drug.

8.2.2.2 Pharmacoeconomic evaluation

Pharmacoeconomics is a subspecialty of health economics. Its aim is to measure not only the benefits but also the costs of new medicines. Pharmacoeconomic studies provide a good basis for comparing the value for money of one drug versus another, and help to guide decisions about the optimal allocation of drug budgets.

There are several methods of pharmacoeconomic evaluation: cost analysis, cost-minimisation analysis (CMA), cost-effectiveness analysis (CEA), cost-utility analysis (CUA), and cost-benefit analysis (CBA). They will be briefly discussed below, but for more detailed information the reader is referred to a textbook on health economics [6].

Cost analysis
In cost analyses, health care cost related to drug treatment can be classified as direct (incurred by health care payers, such as the cost of hospitalisation or the cost of the drug itself, and relatively easy to measure), or indirect (incurred by society, such as loss of working days or loss of productivity, and more difficult to measure). Cost analysis should ideally focus on marginal costs rather than average costs, as they are closer to reality. For instance, reducing hospitalisation by 1 day versus the standard therapy, may be a substantial average cost saving, but the marginal cost saving may be limited (an empty hospital bed still has a fixed cost that remains unchanged). Opportunity costs should also be taken into account. It is the cost (as benefit lost) by not choosing the next best alternative. Spending money on the new drug should generate more benefit than spending it on the previous best therapy. That is why pharmacoeconomics is essentially interested in incremental analysis of costs and benefits in order to find out what the added value is of the new medicine over the old one.

Cost analyses are in principle always conducted to feed into CEAs, CUAs or CBAs (see below). Only in cost-minimisation studies are they useful as stand-alone analysis.

Cost-minimisation analysis (CMA)
This is the simplest method of comparative pharmacoeconomic analysis. It measures only costs and can only be used to compare 2 therapeutically equivalent drugs with different costs, such as a generic drug versus the original drug, or an oral versus an intravenous drug.

Cost-effectiveness analysis (CEA)
CEA quantifies both costs (in monetary units) and hard effectiveness outcomes, such as life-years saved, or hospital admissions avoided (in nonmonetary units). Then, the cost-effectiveness ratio (CER) can be calculated, for instance as the cost per life-year saved. Comparison between different drugs (or treatments) is mostly done on the basis of the incremental cost-effectiveness ratio (ICER), described by the equation $(C1 - C2)/(E1 - E2)$, where $C1$ and $E1$ are the costs and effectiveness of the new drug, while $C2$ and $E2$ the ones for the comparator drug.

Cost-utility analysis (CUA)
CUA adds the dimension of the quality of life, estimates the number of life-years lived in full health expressed as quality-adjusted life-years

(QALYs), and then compares the (incremental) cost-effectiveness ratio as (incremental) cost per QALY between different drugs (or treatments). A simple example will illustrate this concept:

–   with the new drug, the estimated survival is 2 years, the estimated quality of life (relative to perfectly healthy) is 0.6, and hence the number of QALYs 1.2 (2×0.6);
–   with the currently best available drug, the estimated survival is 1 year, the estimated quality of life 0.4, and the QALYs 0.4 (1×0.4).

The QALY gain from the new drug is $1.2 - 0.4 = 0.8$ QALYs. If the total cost of the new drug treatment is 20 000 EUR, then the cost per QALY gained is $20\,000/0.8 = 25\,000$ EUR.

Cost-benefit analysis (CBA)

Finally, CBA is considered to be the most absolute pharmacoeconomic approach, as it measures both costs and benefits in monetary units, allowing direct economic comparison of different drugs (or even treatments). There are several tools available to translate healthcare outcomes into monetary units, one of which is the 'willingness to pay' concept, i.e. the maximum amount a patient would be willing to pay, exchange or sacrifice in order to enjoy a certain benefit induced by the new drug (e.g. live 1 year longer).

Cost-effectiveness analysis (CEA), and its derivative cost-utility analysis (CUA), are currently the most widely used types of pharmacoeconomic evaluations. The two terms are often used interchangeably. Indeed, some authors prefer the term cost-effectiveness overall, whether outcomes are expressed as QALYs or other variables.

There are essentially 2 methods of performing these pharmacoeconomic evaluations, either:

–   directly during randomised clinical trials (preferentially pragmatic trials), capturing all necessary information about hard clinical outcomes, patient-preferred outcomes including quality of life, and permitting calculation of associated costs incurred or avoided; or
–   more indirectly applying modelling techniques that use existing data on clinical outcomes, quality of life, epidemiology and costs, to project the effects of the new drug on the target population. In particular, Markov models have become very popular for the pharmacoeconomic evaluation of drugs for chronic diseases [6].

Cost-effectiveness analyses are often visualised on a cost-effectiveness plane with 4 quadrants (Figure 8.2). Results plotted in the NW quadrant are less effective and more expensive (inferior and not recommended), those in the SE quadrant are more effective and less expensive (dominant

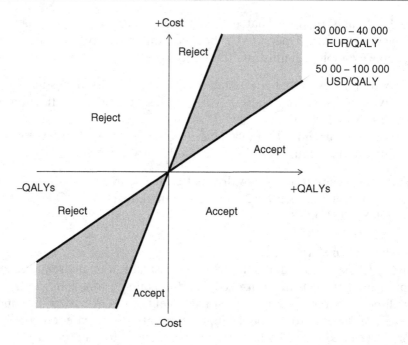

Figure 8.2   The cost-effectiveness plane. (QALYs: quality-adjusted life-years.) Source: Adapted from Andrikopoulos *et al.* [7], figure 1, p. 148. Reproduced with permission of Oxford University Press.

and recommended), those in the NE quadrant are more effective but more expensive, and those in the SW quadrant are less effective but also less expensive. Note that in the cost dimension, all health care costs are to be included, i.e. not only the cost of the treatment but also the potential savings in the health care sector, leading to a net cost of the new treatment versus the standard care. A straight line with slope K passes through the origin, with K being the maximum acceptable (incremental) cost-effectiveness ratio. Everything plotted below the line is considered cost effective. Most countries use (unofficial) thresholds for costs per QALY gained. In the UK, this is currently 30 000 GBP, in most European countries 30 000–40 000 EUR, and in the USA 50 000–100 000 USD. New drugs with a cost per QALY below these thresholds are more easily considered for coverage or reimbursement.

Even if a new medicine has demonstrated its added value versus existing therapies, pharmaceutical policy makers and payers are not always willing to fully cover or reimburse the new drug. In many countries, a budget impact analysis (BIA) is required in order to calculate the expected total costs for payers during the initial year(s) after market introduction, taking into account the expected number of treated patients and the price. In many cases, additional measures are taken to limit the impact of new and more expensive medicines on the escalating costs of drug budgets, such as:

- restricted coverage or reimbursement, limited for instance to the indication or patient subpopulation where cost effectiveness is demonstrated;
- conditional coverage or reimbursement, requiring prior authorisation from the payer, conditional on positive testing for a biomarker (e.g. HER2), or conditional on further evidence generation (of effectiveness or value), also known as 'coverage with evidence development' (CED);
- risk-sharing schemes, whereby pharma companies and payers agree to share the risks due to still existing uncertainties (e.g. about the real effectiveness of the new medicine, absence of meaningful long-term outcomes, the validity of the models used, and the budget impact).

Risk-sharing schemes can be:

- 'finance based', such as price-volume agreements (whereby the company gets a lower price once an agreed volume of sales is exceeded), or patient access schemes (with free drugs for an agreed period, or price- or dose-capping for an agreed period);
- 'performance or outcomes based', so-called 'no cure, no pay' schemes, introducing a lower price or delisting of coverage or reimbursement in patients without (the expected) response.

Some of these innovative policy measures may have a considerable negative impact on the commercial success of a new medicine. The risk-sharing deals, especially the finance-based ones, are considered by some in the pharmaceutical industry as poorly disguised price cuts, and they can have a domino effect from one region to another.

Overall, coverage or reimbursement negotiations can last for months and even years. It is considered to be a difficult and time-consuming step in the process of actual market access of new drugs.

8.2.3 Additional hurdles

Two other policy tools can further limit full market access of new medicines, namely clinical practice guidelines and drug prescription formularies.

Clinical practice guidelines primarily focus on improving the quality of care for patients, but they also advocate rational drug use for the treatment of a particular pathology. Being favourably cited in these guidelines or have a prominent place in the treatment strategy, can be very useful as a marketing tool and can give an important commercial boost to a new medicine.

Drug prescription formularies, either national or local, may further limit market access as they only contain a limited number of drugs for each indication. Once listed on a hospital formulary for instance, patients may get discharged from hospital with a maintenance prescription for long-term use of the new medicine.

Because of the potential impact of these additional hurdles on future revenue, it is not surprising that pharmaceutical companies spend substantial time with key opinion leaders involved in the development of guidelines and/or formularies to try and convince them with the necessary evidence that the new medicine already merits to be included in an updated version.

8.3   Pharmaceutical marketing

Pharmaceutical marketing can be defined as the process of promoting the sales of medicines. However, it implies more than just selling and advertising. In this section, it is limited to branded prescription medicines, and as it is practiced by pharmaceutical companies.

The topics that are addressed are some facts and figures about the worldwide pharmaceutical market, general marketing principles, an overview of typical pharmaceutical marketing activities, and some thoughts about drug promotion regulation.

For more detailed information the reader is referred to textbooks on pharmaceutical marketing [8] and drug life-cycle management [9].

8.3.1   The pharmaceutical market

The worldwide market of prescription medicines (pharmaceuticals, drugs), as part of the total health care market, evidently operates within the context of different economic systems (from a completely free-market economy, over regulated variants, to a totally centralised planned economy). In most countries, it is a typical example of a regulated market, i.e. with some intervention of governmental bodies (such as for market authorisation and market access). A further specific characteristic of this market and its marketing approach, is that pharmaceutical regulations in most countries (with the exception of the USA and New Zealand) do not allow direct communication between the pharmaceutical company and the consumer or patient. Most marketing activities for prescription drugs are thus focused on 'intermediate' targets, such as prescribers and third-party payers, operating in a so-called managed market.

Reliable information about the world market of prescription medicines, as well as the top selling products and top pharmaceutical players, is not readily available. Depending on the source, figures and rankings can vary widely. The information is gathered from what pharmaceutical companies make public, and it is not always easy to extract figures for (branded) prescription drugs only, as they are sometimes presented including revenues from generics,

Table 8.1 Global and regional spending on medicines from 2006 to 2016 [11].

Geographic area	Annual spending on medicines		
	2006	2011	2016
World	658	956	1200 (Bn USD)
United States	41	34	31 (%)
EU5	19	17	13
Pharmerging countries	14	20	30
Japan	10	12	10
Rest of the world	16	17	16

EU5: France, Germany, Italy, Spain, UK
Pharmerging countries: countries with >1 Bn USD spending growth over 2012–16, and Gross Domestic Product (GDP) per capita < 25 000 USD at purchasing power parity (PPP), i.e. Argentina, Brazil, China, Egypt, India, Indonesia, Mexico, Pakistan, Poland, Romania, Russia, South Africa, Thailand, Turkey, Ukraine, Venezuela and Vietnam

over-the-counter (OTC) drugs, or even nondrug health or personal care or other activities of some companies. On a global scale, IMS Health is the leading provider of this information to companies, payers and policymakers [10].

According to the IMS Institute for Healthcare Informatics in its July 2012 report 'The global use of medicines: outlook through 2016' [11], global spending on medicines (not only on prescription) was 956 billion USD in 2011, up from 658 billion in 2006, and estimated to reach 1.2 trillion by 2016, see Table 8.1.

Over this 10-year period, the major trends are:

- as summarised in Table 8.1, a decrease of the share of the developed markets (from 73% in 2006 to 57% in 2016), mainly due to continued cost containment measures, while the share of 'pharmerging' countries increases (from 14 to 30%), as their population and economic growth contributes to increased spending on medicines. IMS defines developed markets those in the USA, Japan, the top 5 EU countries (France, Germany, Italy, Spain, UK), Canada and South Korea. The pharmerging countries are defined as those with over 1 billion USD absolute spending growth over 2012–16, and that have a gross domestic product (GDP) per capita of less than 25 000 USD at purchasing power parity. They include 3 tiers: China (tier 1), Brazil, India, Russia (tier 2, both tiers also known as BRIC countries), and Argentina, Egypt, Indonesia, Mexico, Pakistan, Poland, Romania, South Africa, Thailand, Turkey, Ukraine, Venezuela, and Vietnam (tier 3),
- accelerated spending on generics (from 25 to 35% of total), but slow worldwide uptake of biopharmaceuticals (from 14 to 18%, as too expensive for many countries), and even slower replacement of original biopharmaceuticals by biosimilars,

Table 8.2   Top 15 prescription drug sales in the USA (Q2.2013) [12].

Rank	Generic name	Brand name	Main indication(s)	Company	Sales (Bn USD)
1	Aripiprazole	Abilify	Psychotic conditions	Otsuka	1.598
2	Esomeprazole	Nexium	Gastric ulcers	AstraZeneca	1.454
3	Adalimumab	Humira	Rheumatoid arthritis	AbbVie	1.342
4	Duloxetine	Cymbalta	Major depression	Eli Lilly	1.339
5	Rusovastatine	Crestor	Increased risk of CV complications	AstraZeneca	1.291
6	Fluticasone + salmeterol	Advair (Seretide)	Asthma, COPD	GlaxoSmithKline	1.241
7	Etanercept	Enbrel	Rheumatoid arthritis	Amgen	1.148
8	Infliximab	Remicade	Rheumatoid arthritis	Centocor (J&J)	0.996
9	Glatiramer	Copaxone	Multiple sclerosis	Teva	0.933
10	Pegfilgastrim	Neulasta	Neutropenia (cancer)	Amgen	0.861
11	Rituximab	Rituxan (Mabthera)	Cancer	Genentech (Roche)	0.826
12	Tiotropium	Spiriva	COPD	Boehringer Ingelheim	0.723
13	Efavirenz + emtricitabine + tenofovir	Atripla	HIV/AIDS	Gilead Sciences	0.714
14	Sitagliptine	Januvia	Diabetes mellitus	Merck & Co	0.693
15	Insulin glargine	Lantus	Diabetes mellitus	Sanofi-Aventis	0.682

Q2: second quarter of calendar year; CV complications: stroke, myocardial infarction; COPD: chronic obstructive pulmonary disease; HIV/AIDS: human immunodeficiency virus/acquired immunodeficiency syndrome

– increased spending on medicines for cancer, diabetes, asthma/COPD, and immunotherapy (top-selling therapeutic classes in 2016), with lipid-lowering and anti-ulcer drugs losing market share. Table 8.2 with the top 15 best-selling prescription drugs in the USA in 2013 [12] illustrates this trend.

Finally, Table 8.3 with the list of the top 15 pharmaceutical companies of 2013 [13] gives an idea of the most important players in this field (again not limited to revenue from prescription medicines).

8.3.2   General marketing principles

Marketing can be defined as the process of communicating the value of a product or service to customers. Classic models of marketing management, like the 4P model, are strictly producer oriented and centred around product, price, place (distribution) and promotion. More recent models are more

Table 8.3 Top 15 pharmaceutical companies of 2013 [13].

Rank	Company	Market capitalisation (Bn USD)
1	Johnson & Johnson	248.393
2	Pfizer	203.717
3	Novartis	173.4
4	Roche	166.477
5	Sanofi	148.381
6	Merck & Co	141.922
7	GlaxoSmithKline	112.511
8	Bayer	87.527
9	Bristol-Myers Squibb	67.657
10	AbbVie	64.584
11	Eli Lilly	64.687
12	AstraZeneca	62.475
13	Takeda	40.056
14	Astellas	23.888
15	Daiichi Sankyo	12.876

Ranking on 29 July 2013, based on market capitalisation, i.e. number of outstanding shares (on latest date published) times the share price (on that date)
Attn.: not conditioned solely by revenues of (prescription) medicines, but also by other activities of these companies

customer oriented, like the SIVA model, and focus more on solution (instead of product), information (instead of promotion), value (instead of price) and access (instead of place/distribution). In these models, customer relationship management (CRM) is of paramount importance. Current marketers tend to blend their marketing mix with elements of both (and still other) approaches.

Any marketing approach involves a number of consecutive steps:

- Analyse the strengths and weaknesses of the product/service (know yourself), and the opportunities and threats in the market (know your market and competitors), i.e. a classic SWOT analysis which is essentially forward looking. In this context, market research helps to understand market demand, while marketing research is broader and focuses on the product, its competitors and the customers.
- Define the marketing objective(s): how to increase sales by getting or keeping customers.
- Develop a marketing strategy: a long-term vision on *what* should be done to reach this goal, in complete alignment with overall business objectives.
- Document a marketing plan: concrete actions on *how* this should be done in practice.
- Implement the plan, review and improve it as needed. Whereas the international marketing strategy is defined on a corporate level, local implementation can be adapted according to local tactical and regulatory considerations.

One of the key elements of successful marketing is to create and maintain a sustainable competitive advantage (what makes your product different from competitors), and to be able to communicate this under the form of a unique selling proposition (USP). Equally important for success, is how to build a brand instead of just another product: a name, design, logo and slogan that catches attention and radiates confidence, so that customers are tempted to use that brand instead of another or are convinced to stay with it. The ultimate metric to measure success is market share, a key indicator of market competitiveness.

8.3.3   Pharmaceutical marketing activities

As a preamble, it is important to stress that any pharmaceutical marketing activity should be adapted to the different phases of the commercial life cycle of a new medicine (right part of Figure 8.1):

– Prelaunch period, the preparatory phase when the new drug is not yet on the market. This usually starts during drug development and might take several years, especially when awareness about a potential new market has to be developed (e.g. erectile dysfunction and Viagra°).
– Market launch period, an intense period of successive launches of the new drug on different markets around the globe.
– Ascending phase, a period of continuous annual growth in revenue leading to return of investment, stimulated by market exclusivity and the implementation of new developments (mainly new indications).
– Maturity phase, when maintenance of annual growth becomes more difficult and other new developments take over (such as new formulations and combinations).
– End-stage phase, when the patent expires and alternatives have to be sought, either by ways to extend the protection (evergreening), or by introducing a follow-on product, or by launching its own generic version (early-entry strategy), or by switching from prescription to over-the-counter status.

8.3.3.1   Market(ing) research

Marketing of a new medicine, like marketing in any sector, starts with gathering information about the market of the new medicine (e.g. for a new blood pressure lowering agent with a novel mechanism of action, it is the market of anti-hypertensive drugs). This activity is known as *market research*. It focuses both on:

– quantitative aspects, such as market size (e.g. total sales of anti-hypertensives, regional differences, sales per drug class, turnover as well as volume data, number of patients treated, number of prescribers,

figures of different market segments) and market dynamics (evolution versus previous month, quarter or year); as well as
-   qualitative aspects (why prescribers or patients chose one drug or drug class over another), such as prescriber or patient behaviour and motivation, their barriers and needs.

Quantitative data are somewhat easier to find, whereas reliable qualitative data are more difficult to get (from group discussions or interviews with prescribers or patients). Several providers such as Nielsen and IMS Health make these data available to pharmaceutical companies.

Market research analyses both the current situation and future trends. It also allows for market forecasts and the identification of opportunities and threats in the market.

Marketing research not only focuses on the drug's market, but also on the medicine itself and its competitors. It allows a full SWOT analysis, taking into account the strengths and weaknesses of the new product, as well as the opportunities and threats in the market. Figure 8.3 summarises some elements that can be important in such a SWOT analysis.

The ultimate goal of marketing research is to come up with answers to some of the following questions: 'how big, how old, how dynamic, how crowded is the market?', 'is there still room for differentiation?', 'are there still unmet needs?', 'what are the barriers?', 'has the new product at least one or more competitive advantages?', and 'are the new medicine's weaknesses manageable?'.

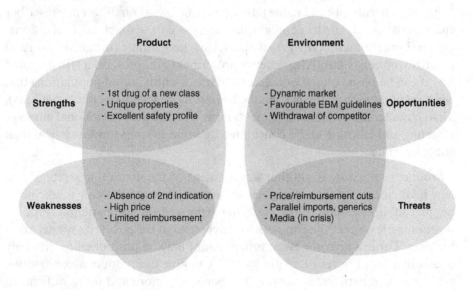

Figure 8.3   SWOT analysis in marketing research. EBM: evidence-based medicine.

Well-prepared, carefully conducted and critically analysed market and marketing research are essential building blocks for decision making about the marketing strategy to be implemented.

8.3.3.2 Marketing strategy

A marketing strategy for a new medicine is a long-term vision on what should be done to fill (or even create) market needs and reach marketing objectives, i.e. increase turnover and revenue. It should be in perfect alignment with the overall business and portfolio strategy and should be taken into consideration as early as possible during the development of a new medicine.

Three essential elements are discussed: market segmentation, product positioning, and customised targeting.

Market segmentation is based on the knowledge that not all customers are the same, but belong to several segments, clusters or niches who share similar needs and may require different marketing strategies. The market for a new prescription drug can be segmented grossly into prescribers, intermediate customers (hospitals and third-party payers) and patients, who may each need a different marketing approach. Within each of these segments, further segmentation can take place to find the most useful segments to target, the market space where the new medicine can win. However, not all pharmaceutical marketers are keen on market segmentation and niche focusing, as they consider that it might restrict the potential market share of the product (versus 'our product can benefit the whole market').

Market segmentation can be based on different or new market needs that can drive further product development (a new indication) and branding strategy (under another brand name). It can also be based on different prescriber characteristics that can be demographic (age or years of practice), professional (general practitioner (GP) versus specialist), geographic (urban versus rural practice), or behavioural (from heavy prescriber to no-prescriber). In the same way it can be based on patient characteristics identifying subpopulations that can benefit more from the new medicine (e.g. more severe or elderly patients). This character-based market segmentation can drive the promotional message targeting and tailoring and is considered by some as having more tactical than strategic value.

Product positioning is another key element of the marketing strategy of a new medicine. It refers to the decision where you want the new medicine to be 'placed' in the mind of the customers (prescribers and patients). Product positioning leverages the competitive advantage of the new drug versus existing ones. For example, a new anti-depressant may be positioned as 'the only one with a rapid onset of action', which can give the product a competitive edge over competitors. However, it is becoming more and more difficult to differentiate a new product from existing ones based on rational needs only such as superior efficacy and safety, or more convenience and added value. Emotional elements can also play a prominent role such as loyalty, or when prescribers think a certain marketing claim may make a real difference in the patients' quality of life, or when patients themselves feel better on the new medicine. Product positioning in pharmaceutical marketing is mainly driven by facts and figures, but added feelings can make up wonderful stories that can boost an ordinary product into a successful brand. The positioning of Viagra° and Cialis° in erectile dysfunction are examples of how this blend can help to make a marketing strategy successful.

Product positioning may need to be adapted to worldwide regional differences in regulation, medical practice, and coverage or reimbursement. Positioning can also change as the new medicine progresses through its profit cycle, which is often the case with multi-indication drugs in psychiatry and cancer, where the positioning may change with the arrival of a new indication. Another important strategic aspect is positioning of similar drugs within the product portfolio. Corporate management sees to it that internal competition within the same market is prevented by positioning similar drugs differently.

Not everyone can and needs to be reached by all promotional actions. *Targeting* is an approach whereby a subset of particular interest in a marketing segment is targeted with the idea that approaching this target will maximise promotional efficiency. *Customised targeting* is the application of different promotional strategies tailored to the needs of different market segments in order to reach maximal marketing efficiency. It allows the communication about the new medicine to be adapted to the needs of different audiences.

According to the innovation adoption model by Rogers [14], the acceptance of a new medicine by prescribers over time can be described as a bell-shaped curve. The curve starts off slowly with a first group of adopters called innovators, then followed by a bigger group of early adopters, and peaking with addition of the early majority. The curve comes down again when the late majority joins in, and finishes with a last group of people to accept the new product called laggards. Each of these profiles may need a different marketing strategy to reach the desired marketing effect.

Two additional marketing strategies merit attention, namely co-marketing and disease management.

Co-marketing is practiced when 2 pharmaceutical companies receive a separate marketing authorisation for the same medicine and co-market it under a different brand name in order to maximise market share. Most of the time it is preceded by co-development of the product. It is different from *co-promotion* where 2 companies co-promote the same medicine under a single brand. The innovator company is the marketing authorisation holder and the second (usually smaller) company joins in to maximise profit. Co-promotion is common practice to optimally cover the US market.

Disease management is aimed at improving quality and reducing cost of caring for patients with chronic diseases and carries some element of self-care (diabetes, COPD). For some pharmaceutical companies, it allows marketing of one or several products (anti-diabetic or anti-COPD drugs), to be bundled with a device (a glucometer and strips or a peak flow meter), and services (a lifestyle educational programme). The ultimate goal is to increase brand loyalty and to make better deals with payers than would be possible with the drug as stand-alone.

8.3.3.3   Marketing channels and tools
A multitude of different marketing channels and tools exist to convey promotional claims about a new medicine to different market segments and targets (prescribers, payers and patients). This is a short overview of the most important ones.

Prescribers
For prescription medicines for human use, prescribers remain the most important segment and target. According to the drug's indication, this may be general practitioners or medical specialists (and in some countries, nurse practitioners and pharmacists). The marketing toolbox for prescribers includes:

–   Detailing by sales representatives, pharmaceutical or medical reps, mostly during face-to-face meetings in the doctor's office. Although very expensive, this is still considered by pharma companies to be the most cost-efficient way to persuade prescribers. Big companies have more than ten thousand sales reps over the world. Sales reps generally use detail aids (visual aids, brochures and flyers) to support their promotional arguments, either in print or in digital format on a tablet computer. This material summarises the marketing claims with supportive data from clinical trials, underlining the drug's clinical benefits. As the time for a face-to-face meeting with a physician is limited (about 10 min), the promotional message has to be concise and persuasive.
–   Advertisements in medical journals. Publishers of international medical journals, especially multispecialty journals, depend heavily on advertisements for medicines. Pharmaceutical marketers consider it complementary to detailing and also a very cost-effective marketing tool. Although all medical journals have an advertising policy, generally stating that it is without influence on editorial content and decisions, some argue that this dependence on drug advertisements compromises their objectivity, and that they should not accept ads from companies with a commercial

interest in medicine (be it for drugs, devices, equipment or services). PLoS Medicine is one of the few exceptions that does not accept ads for drugs and devices.

- Continuous medical education (CME). The pharmaceutical industry is the largest sponsor of CME for physicians. By organising or sponsoring (by an educational grant) the organisation of medical congresses, conferences, symposia, seminars, workshops and meetings, they intend to have a say in the content management of the programme and the choice of speakers, panellist or moderators. In many countries, the regulation and codes of practices have drastically restricted the input from the pharmaceutical industry in CME (unconditional and unrestricted grants allowed only) in order to guarantee independence.

  The results of clinical trials with new medicines are often first revealed at big international medical congresses (at late breaking news sessions), commented by experts during a press conference, and published simultaneously in a top medical journal. The pharmaceutical industry also sponsors numerous 'satellite symposia' at these congresses, especially when a new medicine or a new indication is launched, or when new important clinical data become available. A more detailed version of the presentations is published simultaneously as a supplement to a respected medical journal, also sponsored by the pharma company. These journal supplements and reprints of clinical trial publications are later distributed to prescribing physicians (usually specialists) during detail calls or on other occasions.

  Finally, during medical congresses and similar meetings, many pharmaceutical companies sponsor a booth where drugs are promoted and (the latest) drug information is made available to congress attendants.
- Gifts, including invitations to restaurants, cultural or sporting events, but also payments and incentives for prescriptions. Again, this has largely been restricted to small gifts by regulations and codes of practice.
- Mailings (print and electronic) and telephone contacts (hotlines, call centres).
- Seeding, marketing or experience trials. These clinical trials are mostly set up during the launching phase of a new medicine. Their aim is to introduce the new medicine to selected physicians rather than to test scientific hypotheses. As the true objectives are sometimes hidden and payments may be disproportionate to the work required, they may exert undue influence and are considered by most as unethical.
- Sample distribution. This allows the prescriber to get a first experience with the new drug. In many countries, the number of samples that can be distributed is limited.
- Digital media and e-marketing tools. Because many busy prescribers find sales calls in their office rather intrusive, and because pharmaceutical

companies started to downsize their expensive sales forces, most pharma companies are gradually shifting their marketing efforts to digital tools to interact with prescribers. Examples are specific websites, web- or podcasts, webinars, online videos, live chats, apps that can be downloaded on tablets or smart phones, e-mail alerts, and many others. They provide information on (new) medicines, offer services, or run presentations by leading physicians speaking to peers. Today, digital marketing tools are still considered as supplemental to more traditional efforts, but in the future they are expected to replace them.

Key opinion leaders (KOL)

Key opinion leaders (KOLs) or thought leaders are experts in their therapeutic domain and can be very influential on prescribers. They are already contacted by pharmaceutical companies during the development of new drugs (as advisors and investigators), but they remain important consultants during the commercialisation phase of new medicines. The marketing channel by excellence to reach these KOLs is by personal contact. Depending upon the topic to be discussed, for example, the positioning of a new medicine or its uptake in clinical practice guidelines, they are contacted by an international or local (group) product or marketing manager, or occasionally, by the country or corporate top management. They may also be invited to medical congresses or meetings, either as a speaker, moderator or panellist.

Institutional HC providers, payers, insurers

Hospital pharmacies, managed care organisations and third-party payers may be approached directly by high-level marketing or sales people to inform them about new drugs or new developments, and to negotiate preferred agreements in order to get the drug on the hospital formulary or coverage plans.

Patients

In only two countries, New Zealand and the USA, is it permitted to promote prescription-only drugs directly to patients. In the USA, direct-to-consumer (DTC) advertising for medicines is big business. It uses popular channels such as TV, newspapers and magazines, radio and social media to inform patients about diseases and medicines to treat them. The concern of most countries is that patients influenced by DTC advertising may increase pressure on prescribers to prescribe drugs that are not strictly necessary.

An intermediate channel to reach patients is via patient organisations, i.e. non-profit organisations that defend and promote the interests of patients (and their families and carers) in general or groups of patients with a specific disease or medical condition. They exist at local, national, regional and international levels. Some pharmaceutical companies support these patient organisations through sponsorships and educational grants.

8.3.3.4   Marketing plan

The marketing plan summarises yearly or quarterly all the marketing activities described before, i.e. information about the (new) medicine, results of market research (sales, prescriptions, specific studies, trends), a SWOT analysis, the marketing objective(s), the marketing strategy (segmentation, positioning, targeting), and on top of that:

- the promotional plan, detailing how the marketing strategy should be implemented in practice, with emphasis on the promotional message(s) to be delivered and the promotional methodology to be used (the tactics);
- its follow-up and control (measure the implementation, analyse the situation and correct if needed);
- and last but not least as it may impact everything discussed above, the budget versus sales forecasts, minus cost of goods and marketing expenses, determining the drug's contribution to corporate profitability.

8.3.4   Drug promotion regulation

Legislation and regulation to control the promotion of prescription medicines is very different from country to country. In the USA, where direct-to-consumer (DTC) advertisement is allowed, several sections of the Federal Food, Drug and Cosmetic Act and the Code of Federal Regulations, as well as Guidances and Enforcement Actions describe the regulatory context wherein drug promotion should operate [15]. It is the mission of The Office of Prescription Drug Promotion (OPDP) within the FDA 'to protect the public health by assuring prescription drug information is truthful, balanced and accurately communicated. This is accomplished through a comprehensive surveillance, enforcement and education programme, and by fostering better communication of labelling and promotional information to both healthcare professionals and consumers'. Every promotional material has to be submitted to the FDA, but does not need prior approval, except in some enforcement circumstances and when it concerns TV ads.

Most other countries have minimal regulatory provisions, stating that prescription drug promotion should be in accordance with the approved labelling and that DTC advertising is prohibited, but encourage self-regulation by the players in the field. In this context, the WHO Ethical criteria for medicinal drug promotion from 1988 [16] have been the basis for a number of international and national pharmaceutical marketing Codes of Practices published by pharmaceutical company associations (IFPMA, EFPIA, ABPI) [17–19], that are regularly updated.

The enforcement of these regulations is not always easy. Several malpractices have been observed, such as off-label marketing, the use of exaggerated or false marketing claims, bribing of doctors, and fraud. They may be brought to the attention of enforcement bodies by prescribers (e.g. the Bad Ad programme of the OPDP helping healthcare professionals recognise misleading promotion and report it) or competitors filing complaints. Both systems, governmental or self-regulation, have led to legal actions and important settlement agreements [20].

8.4   Independent drug information

Most health care providers obtain their information about prescription medicines from pharmaceutical companies, and that information is often perceived as aggressive and distorted in favour of its own drugs. To counterbalance this dominant and biased source of drug information, several international and national non-profit organisations make reliable information available that is independent of pharmaceutical companies (some free of charge). Some examples are:

–   National drug formularies, such as the British National Formulary, updated twice a year and available both in paperback and electronic version [21]. It is much more than just a classic formulary (originally a recipe book for pharmacists to prepare remedies) or a list of drugs used in the National Health Service, as it has become a preferred independent reference guide for prescribers and dispensers of medicines in the UK (and elsewhere).
–   National drug bulletins, often edited by independent medicines information centres, such as Australian Prescriber, Der Arzneimittelbrief (Germany), Drug and Therapeutics Bulletin (UK), Prescrire (France), The Medical Letter (USA), and many more. Most of them are accessible from the website of the International Society of Drug Bulletins (ISDB) [22].
–   The Swedish institute for drug informatics (SIDI), founded at the Karolinska Institutet, promotes 'free access to evidence-based and objective information about medicines' [23]. It recently launched 2 initiatives: Drugle, a semantic search engine for drug information, and Drugline, a Q&A database from drug information centres in Scandinavia.
–   The independent drug information service (IDIS), a programme of the Alosa Foundation, initiated by Harvard Medical School in the US [24]. It is a form of 'academic detailing' by trained health professionals (pharmacists, nurses or others) to prescribers in their offices during a face-to-face visit, but noncommercial, evidence-based, and totally independent from the pharmaceutical industry. Academic detailing is also performed in Australia, Canada, the Netherlands, and the UK.

Independent information on comparative effectiveness, safety and costs of new medicines is considered a prerequisite for the rational use of medicines.

8.5 Rational use of medicines

According to WHO, rational use of medicines requires that 'patients receive medications appropriate to their clinical needs, in doses that meet their own individual requirements, for an adequate period of time, and at the lowest cost to them and their community' [25].

Irrational drug use may lead to overuse, underuse or misuse of medicines, all with potentially serious consequences for the patient and/or society, for example:

- overuse of antibiotics (resulting in microbial resistance) and polypharmacy (leading to drug interactions);
- underuse of drugs proposed in clinical practice guidelines based on solid evidence; and
- inappropriate self-medication, sometimes resulting in serious ADRs.

There are many contributing factors to irrational use of medicines and the most important ones seem to be lack of sufficient knowledge by prescribers, dispensers and patients; unethical promotion of medicines, and lack of a coherent drug policy.

Strategies to promote and improve rational use of medicines are multifaceted and are generally subdivided into 4 categories:

1. Educational:
   - Addressing healthcare professionals:
     - increase initial and continuous training in rational prescribing of medicines (based on the WHO Guide to good prescribing);
     - advocate further adoption of clinical practice or standard treatment guidelines, as well as principles of evidence-based medicine for drug treatment in individual patients;
     - promote wider availability of independent drug information;
     - give feedback to prescribers of own prescription profile compared to peers.
   - Targeting patients: educate patients to improve their adherence to drug treatment.
2. Managerial: promote the use of essential drug lists (based on the WHO model), and reinforce the use of preferred drugs listed in formularies such as the British National Formulary (BNF), local hospital formularies or the BNF for children.

3. Economic: stimulate generic substitution and avoid perverse financial incentives.
4. Regulatory: restrict choices (e.g. through control over marketing authorisation, price or reimbursement) and restrict pharmaceutical promotion of medicines.

The best results are obtained when the different interventions are implemented in concert. A well-functioning health care system with a coherent policy for the rational use of medicines is the perfect guarantee that the best medicine will be used, in due time, at the right dose, at the lowest cost, in patients who really need it.

References

[1] Rang HP. (2006) *Drug Discovery and Development*. Churchill Livingstone Elsevier, Edinburgh.
[2] The Association of the British Pharmaceutical Industry, Department of Health. (2008) The pharmaceutical price regulation scheme 2009. Available from: https://www.gov.uk [Accessed 14 September 2013].
[3] The Patented Medicine Prices Review Board (PMPRB). Available from: http://www.pmprb-cepmb.gc.ca [Accessed 14 September 2013].
[4] International Society of Pharmaco-economics and Outcomes Research (ISPOR). (2003) Health Care Cost, Quality, and Outcomes: ISPOR Book of Terms. Lawrenceville, NJ.
[5] Eddy D. (2009) Health technology assessment and evidence-based medicine: what are we talking about? *Value in Health* **12** (Suppl 2), S6–S7.
[6] Annemans L. (2008) *Health Economics for Non-economists*. Academia Press, Ghent.
[7] Andrikopoulos G, Tzeis S, Maniadakis N *et al.*(2009) Cost-effectiveness of atrial fibrillation catheter ablation. *Europace* **11**, 147–151.
[8] Rollins BL, Perri M. (2013) *Pharmaceutical marketing*. Jones & Bartlett Learning, Burlington, MA, USA.
[9] Ellery T, Hansen N. (2012) *Pharmaceutical lifecycle management: making the most of each and every brand*. John Wiley & Sons, Hoboken, NJ, USA.
[10] IMS Health. Available from: http://www.imshealth.com [Accessed 14 September 2013].
[11] IMS Institute for Healthcare Informatics. (2012) The global use of medicines: outlook through 2016. Available from: http://www.imshealth.com [Accessed 14 September 2013].
[12] Top 100 prescribed medicines by US National Sales in Q2 2013. Available from: http://www.drugs.com [Accessed 14 September 2013].
[13] Top 15 pharma companies of 2013. Available from: http://www.genengnews.com [Accessed 14 September 2013].
[14] Rogers EM. (2003) *Diffusion of Innovations* (5th edn). Free Press, New York.
[15] The Office of Prescription Drug Information (OPDP) Regulatory Information. Available from: http://www.fda.gov [Accessed 14 September 2013].
[16] World Health Organization (WHO). (1988) *Ethical criteria for medicinal drug promotion*. WHO, Geneva.
[17] International Federation of Pharmaceutical Manufacturers & Associations (IFPMA). (2012) *IFPMA code of practice*. IFPMA, Geneva.

[18] European Federation of Pharmaceutical Industries and Associations (EFPIA). (2011) EFPIA HCP Code. EFPIA code on the promotion of prescription-only medicines to, and interactions with, healthcare professionals. EFPIA, Brussels.

[19] The Association of the British Pharmaceutical Industry (ABPI). (2012) *Code of practice for the pharmaceutical industry* (Second 2012 edition). ABPI, London.

[20] Wikipedia. List of off-label promotion pharmaceutical settlements. Available from http://en.wikipedia.org [Accessed 14 September 2013].

[21] Royal Pharmaceutical Society of Great Britain, British Medical Association. (2013) British National Formulary. BMJ Group and Pharmaceutical Press, London.

[22] International Society of Drug Bulletins (ISDB). Available from: http://www.isdbweb.org [Accessed 14 September 2013].

[23] Swedish Institute for Drug Informatics (SIDI). Available from: http://www.sidi.org [Accessed 14 September 2013].

[24] The Independent Drug Information Service (IDIS). Available from: http://www.alosafoundation.org [Accessed 14 September 2013].

[25] World Health Organization (WHO). (2012) *The pursuit of responsible use of medicines: sharing and learning from country experiences.* WHO, Geneva.

Epilogue

As described in this book, the development of new drugs is very complex, costly and risky. Its success is highly dependent on an intense collaboration and interaction between many departments within the drug development organisation, external investigators and service providers, in constant dialogue with regulatory authorities, payers, academic experts, clinicians and patient organisations. Within the different phases of the drug life cycle, drug development is by far the most crucial part for the initial and continued success of a drug on the market.

As this book is intended as an introduction to drug development, it should not be considered as an exhaustive overview of all possible approaches that are currently used by drug development organisations to bring effective and safe drugs to the marketplace. To keep it simple, the traditional sequential phased strategy for the development of drugs was chosen as the backbone of this book, without referring too much to alternative approaches. Only the development of small molecule drugs for oral administration is described, since this is considered to be the best way to get a first impression of the complexity of the process of drug development, without having to explain the even more complex or more specific challenges of the development of biopharmaceuticals or vaccines or more sophisticated types of drug formulations.

This classic approach to the development of new drugs has been very successful in the past and was instrumental for the success of many blockbuster drugs (with an annual worldwide turnover of more than 1 billion USD). However, this paradigm has lost momentum, since its efficiency and return on investment are becoming problematic (drug R&D expenses have quadrupled over the last decade, without an apparent increase in the number of new chemical entities introduced into the market). More deviations from the classic

Global New Drug Development: An Introduction, First Edition.
Jan A. Rosier, Mark A. Martens and Josse R. Thomas.
© 2014 John Wiley & Sons, Ltd. Published 2014 by John Wiley & Sons, Ltd.

pattern of drug development are considered by drug development organisations in order to reduce clinical attrition rates, development cycle times and costs. New trends, paradigms, approaches and collaborations in drug discovery and development are emerging and the future will certainly bring more of them.

In the field of drug discovery, disruptive innovation is expected to be boosted through advancement of novel technology platforms, the wider implementation of bioinformatics and different omics approaches, the shift from drug discovery to *de novo* drug design, and the rise of open innovation.

In early drug development, initiatives from both industry and health authorities allow to further streamline the drug development process and increase its efficiency. The study of microdoses or subclinical doses in healthy volunteers in combination with the use of advanced technologies to quickly assess the pharmacokinetic behaviour of the drug candidate in man with a minimal safety database is one of these approaches. The growing use of biomarkers and genetic profiling will enable earlier safety and efficacy assessment of drug candidates and improve the selection of the appropriate patient population for clinical Proof-of-Concept studies. There is also more emphasis on lean development programmes where compounds are rapidly progressed from the pre-clinical phase to clinical Proof-of-Mechanism studies, and it is only when the relevance of the biological target has been clinically established in the case of a particular disease – largely by using novel clinical imaging and diagnostic techniques – that the lead compound is further characterised and developed pharmaceutically. This approach is a departure from the more classical approach where industry spends considerable effort in the pre-clinical phase without knowing the clinical relevance of a biological pathway of interest. Other trends such as the increased use of problem-driven approaches (rather than the traditional phase-based approach), quantitative modelling techniques (pharmacometrics) and adaptive clinical trial designs (seamless designs, enrichment strategies), enable further improvement of the success of early drug development.

The classic pattern of late drug development has also been challenged and is gradually evolving in new directions. Newer development strategies tend to be more proactive than reactive (to requirements of health authorities), especially in areas such as pharmacovigilance and risk management or pharmacoeconomics. New trends in drug marketing authorisation, e.g. the shift from all-or-nothing to stepwise (conditional) authorisations, allowing earlier access to new drugs for patients in need without jeopardising their safety, has an important impact on the way late (and especially peri- and post-approval) drug development is organised. New tools, such as big data analytics on large data sets of drug use in real life and new communication technologies (mobile devices and social media), allowing greater and more interactive participation of patients in clinical trials, will also contribute to revolutionise drug development strategies. Moreover, it is expected that patients through patient advocacy groups will become more involved and engaged in drug development and drug regulatory decision making.

Overall, drug development organisations will have to be more flexible and make smarter use of the different approaches available according to the specific needs of the actual drug in development.

Not only are the approaches to drug development changing, but also the way big pharma is organised to best perform drug development is challenged. The model of one big pharmaceutical company doing it all by itself is shifting towards new ways of collaboration with smaller-sized biotech, spin-off and start-up companies. Some companies have been successful in positioning themselves between discovery and the very costly late development. New molecules with a promising efficacy and safety profile are bought in and then developed up to the Proof-of-Concept level. The drug at that stage of development is then presented to larger pharmaceutical companies for late development and marketing. Pharmaceutical companies are currently setting up networks with small research organisations and academia and new partnerships and alliances are being created to boost the discovery of new and promising molecules. Big pharmaceutical companies that used to encompass all stages and activities of discovery and development are now shedding many activities and delegating them more and more to contract research organisations (e.g. toxicology testing, clinical development). In this way big and rigid industry silos are broken down and are replaced by a mosaic of smaller companies that work together in a network. In some therapeutic areas or rare diseases in high medical need for new treatments, consortiums of large and small companies, or public-private partnerships (PPPs) including academia are created to better tackle drug development.

The pharmaceutical industry has also been challenged on data transparency, in the sense that they are urged to be more proactive in their willingness to make results and even raw data of clinical trials publicly available. Especially in Europe, clinical trial data sharing is currently a hot topic involving different stakeholders (e.g. the Cochrane centres, the EMA and the European Federation of Pharmaceutical Industries and Associations or EFPIA) with divergent opinions on principles such as 'the right to know' versus protection of patient privacy and confidential commercial information. As the debate heats up, the question is no longer *whether* clinical trial data will be made public, but rather *how* this will be done in the near future.

On top of all these disruptive challenges intrinsic to drug development, shifts in external factors operating within the pharmaceutical market have also a huge impact on drug development and on the composition of the drug portfolio within pharmaceutical companies. To name just a few:

- the need for more specific anti-cancer drugs and the subsequent current development of hundreds of targeted drug therapies in oncology;

–   the success of biopharmaceuticals or biologicals (projected to represent soon more than half of the top 10 selling drugs);

–   the advent of combination products (e.g. drug-device, drug-companion diagnostic, antibody-drug conjugate) and new therapeutic strategies (e.g. nanomedical approaches to drug delivery, personalised medicines, therapeutic vaccines);

–   the increased competition from generic and biosimilar drugs (expected to reach more than half of prescription drug use); and

–   the rise in importance of 'pharmerging' countries (not only as a potential market, but as a consequence also holding the key for successful drug development).

In spite of these many significant challenges that will confront the pharmaceutical industry into the future, it remains the case that human diseases will continue to require treatment. To successfully meet these challenges, the industry will undoubtedly have to adapt itself both operationally and strategically, but its mission is still a noble one and as such it will continue to attract drug development scientists of the necessary calibre and commitment.

Index

Page numbers in *italics* refer to figures; those in **bold** refer to tables.

Global New Drug Development: An Introduction, First Edition.
Jan A. Rosier, Mark A. Martens and Josse R. Thomas.
© 2014 John Wiley & Sons, Ltd. Published 2014 by John Wiley & Sons, Ltd.

Printed in the United States
By Bookmasters